Securing Health

Lessons from Nation-Building Missions

Seth G. Jones • Lee H. Hilborne • C. Ross Anthony

Lois M. Davis • Federico Girosi • Cheryl Benard

Rachel M. Swanger • Anita Datar Garten • Anga Timilsina

Center for Domestic and
International Health Security

A RAND HEALTH PROGRAM

The research described in this report was carried out under the auspices of the RAND Center for Domestic and International Health Security, a program within RAND Health. Primary funding for the project was provided by a generous gift from David and Carol Richards.

Library of Congress Cataloging-in-Publication Data

Securing health : lessons from nation-building missions / Seth G. Jones ... [et al.].
    v. ; cm.
    "MG-321."
    Includes bibliographical references.
    Contents: Germany—Japan—Somalia—Haiti—Kosovo—Afghanistan—Iraq— Evaluating health reconstruction.
    ISBN 0-8330-3729-3 (pbk. : alk. paper)
    1. Medical assistance—Evaluation. 2. Medical assistance, American—Evaluation. 3. Health planning—international cooperation. 4. Public health—International cooperation. 5. Nation-building—Case studies. 6. War—Health aspects. 7. Post-war reconstruction—Health aspects. I. Jones, Seth G., 1972– . II. Rand Corporation
    [DNLM: 1. Health Planning. 2. Delivery of Health Care—organization & administration. 3. International Cooperation. 4. Public Health. 5. Social Planning. 6. War. WA 540.1 S446 2006].

RA390.A2S43 2006
362.1—dc22

                                                  2005032231

Cover photo: AP/Emilio Morenatti

Cover design by Eileen Delson La Russo

The RAND Corporation is a nonprofit research organization providing objective analysis and effective solutions that address the challenges facing the public and private sectors around the world. RAND's publications do not necessarily reflect the opinions of its research clients and sponsors.

RAND® is a registered trademark.

Published 2006 by the RAND Corporation
1776 Main Street, P.O. Box 2138, Santa Monica, CA 90407-2138
1200 South Hayes Street, Arlington, VA 22202-5050
201 North Craig Street, Suite 202, Pittsburgh, PA 15213-1516
RAND URL: http://www.rand.org/
To order RAND documents or to obtain additional information, contact
Distribution Services: Telephone: (310) 451-7002;
Fax: (310) 451-6915; Email: order@rand.org

Preface

This monograph presents the results of research conducted by the RAND Corporation on the health component of nation-building operations. The purpose of the research was to analyze the activities that countries, international institutions, and non-governmental organizations undertake in rebuilding public health and health care delivery systems after major conflict. In addition, this monograph outlines key principles for the success of such reconstruction efforts and identifies lessons for future nation-building operations. The findings are based on an examination of seven nation-building cases: two at the end of World War II (Germany and Japan); three in the 1990s (Somalia, Haiti, and Kosovo); and two after September 2001 (Afghanistan and Iraq).

The results of this study should interest policymakers, practitioners, and scholars concerned with the successes and shortcomings of past health efforts. Readers' comments are welcome and should be addressed to lead authors Seth Jones, Lee Hilborne, and Ross Anthony at the RAND Corporation. Primary funding for the project was provided by a generous gift from David and Carol Richards.

This study was conducted under the auspices of RAND Health's Center for Domestic and International Health Security. A profile of the Center, abstracts of its publications, and ordering information can be found at www.rand.org/health/healthsecurity/.

Contents

Figures

Tables

Summary

The number of nation-building missions has increased significantly since the Cold War ended.[1] From 1945 to 1989, roughly half a dozen cases of nation-building occurred, ranging from U.S. and European efforts to rebuild western Germany after World War II to the United Nations Operation in the Congo from 1960 to 1964.[2] Since the end of the Cold War, however, roughly 14 cases have occurred, equating to a 133 percent increase in one-third the time.[3]

We define *nation-building* as efforts carried out after major combat to underpin a transition to peace and democracy. Nation-building involves the deployment of military forces, as well as comprehensive efforts to rebuild the health, security, economic, political, and other sectors. The research we conducted focused on one aspect of nation-building—efforts to rebuild the public health and health care delivery systems after major combat. We looked at seven cases— Germany, Japan, Somalia, Haiti, Kosovo, Afghanistan, and Iraq. These are some of the most important cases since World War II in

---

[1] James D. Fearon and David D. Laitin, "Neotrusteeship and the Problem of Weak States," *International Security*, Vol. 28, No. 4, Spring 2004, pp. 5–43; James Dobbins et al., *America's Role in Nation-Building: From Germany to Iraq*, MG-1753-RC, Santa Monica, California: RAND Corporation, 2004; James Dobbins et al., *The UN's Role in Nation-Building: From the Congo to Iraq*, MG-304-RC, Santa Monica, California: RAND Corporation, 2005.

[2] Based on our definition of *nation-building*, Cold War cases include efforts to rebuild Germany, Japan, Korea, Vietnam, the Dominican Republic, and perhaps Lebanon.

[3] Examples include U.S., UN, and European efforts to rebuild Panama, Namibia, Mozambique, Haiti, Bosnia, Kosovo, Somalia, East Timor, Cambodia, El Salvador, Eastern Slavonia, Sierra Leone, Afghanistan, and Iraq.

which international institutions, non-governmental organizations (NGOs), and countries such as the United States have taken part in efforts to rebuild the health sector.

These missions also have important health components. To date, a significant amount of academic and policy-relevant work has been devoted to efforts to rebuild such areas as police and military forces. Little comprehensive work has examined efforts to rebuild public health and health care delivery systems, however. The work that has been done on health tends to focus on immediate humanitarian and relief efforts rather than long-term health reconstruction. The goal of our research was to fill this void.

The study has two core arguments. First, nation-building efforts cannot be successful unless adequate attention is paid to health. The area of health is strongly interrelated with other areas of nation-building in two ways (see Figure S.1): The health sector can have an independent impact on reconstruction and development, and other sectors can have an important impact on health. As Amartya Sen has argued, such areas as health, security, economic stabilization, and political development are deeply interrelated:

> Political freedoms (in the form of free speech and elections) help to promote economic security. Social opportunities (in the form of education and health facilities) facilitate economic participation. Economic facilities (in the form of opportunities for participation in trade and production) can help to generate personal abundance as well as public resources for social facilities.[4]

Second, successful health reconstruction depends on two factors: coordination and planning, and infrastructure and resources. The first factor includes the degree of coordination among the host government, NGOs, international organizations, and donor states, as well as the establishment of a plan for health. The second factor pertains to the existence of functioning hospitals, other infrastructure

---

[4] Amartya Sen, *Development as Freedom*, New York: Anchor Books, 2000, p. 11.

Figure S.1
Health and Nation-Building

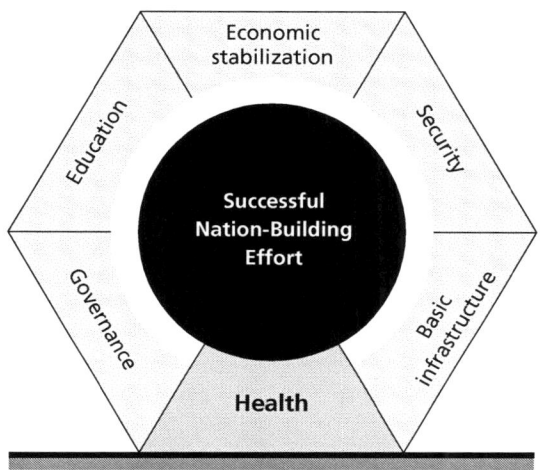

(such as water and power systems), and donor support. External actors have significant control over some of these factors and very little control over others, such as the condition that hospitals and clinics are in when reconstruction starts. The case studies show that policymakers often fail to adequately coordinate and plan health reconstruction and to provide sufficient infrastructure and resources.

Several cases we reviewed suggest that health can have an important effect—positive or negative—on security. In Japan, the introduction of powdered milk into schools created a reservoir of good will that contributed to a benign security environment. In Iraq, however, there is evidence that poor health conditions—especially poor sanitation conditions—contributed to anti-Americanism and support for the insurgency.

Measuring Success

The study asked two related questions: How successful have past efforts to rebuild public health and health care delivery systems during nation-building operations been? What are the most important lessons learned for future operations?

We define *success* as an improvement over time in several measures:

- Life expectancy rate
- Birth rate
- Death rate
- Infant mortality rate
- Infectious disease rate
- Malnutrition.

We also measured success in the context of broader nation-building efforts, since success or failure in rebuilding health can affect success in other areas of nation-building, such as security, economic stabilization, and infrastructure. We used quantitative and qualitative information from a variety of resources, such as the World Bank Development Indicators data set and statistics from the Pan-American Health Organization. We also conducted a simple factor analysis to compare data across cases.

Figure S.2 provides a conceptual framework for measuring the success of health interventions. It divides nation-building into five phases: pre-conflict, conflict, immediate post-conflict, reconstruction, and consolidation. All health efforts should aim to improve health conditions in relation to both the pre-conflict and the immediate post-conflict conditions. The endpoints in the figure (P1, P2, and P3) represent health outcomes *after* major reconstruction efforts have ended. (The reconstruction period has historically varied from less than three years to more than ten.) Endpoint P3 represents a decline in public health and health care delivery after reconstruction, which

Figure S.2
Phases of Nation-Building

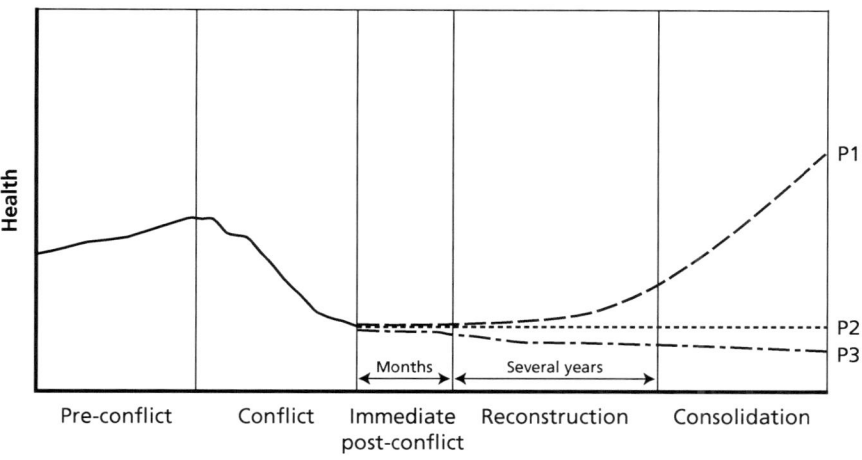

represents a failed health effort; P2 indicates little change from conflict health conditions; and P1 represents an improvement over both
pre-conflict and immediate post-conflict conditions, or, in other
words, a clear success.

Comparative Analysis

Figure S.3 plots the countries we examined in terms of the two
core factors of a successful health reconstruction effort: coordination
and planning, and infrastructure and resources. As can be seen, the
countries are clustered into three of the four quadrants. Japan and
Germany are the most successful cases; they had more of the elements
that contribute to a successful health reconstruction effort. Kosovo
and Iraq are mixed cases; they had high levels of some indicators and
low levels of others. And Haiti, Somalia, and Afghanistan had low
levels of all indicators and thus are the least successful.

Figure S.3
Distribution of Countries

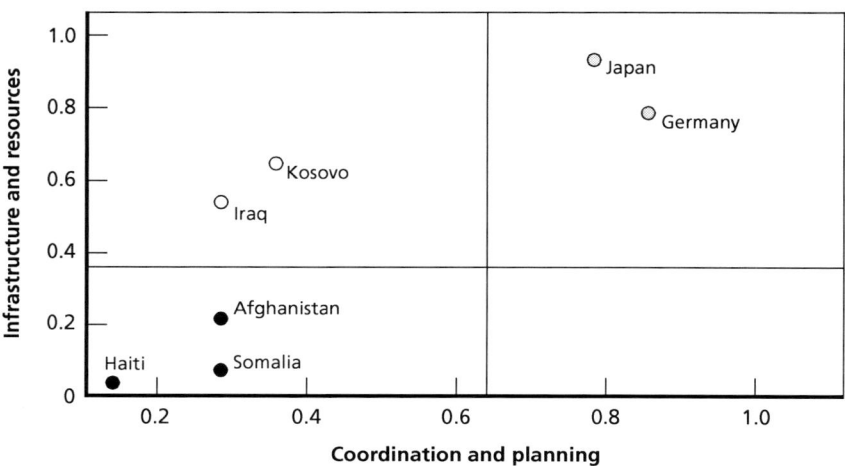

Note that none of the seven countries we examined is in the lower right quadrant, where countries would lie if their health reconstruction coordination and planning efforts were strong but their infrastructure and resources at the beginning of reconstruction were insufficient. Cases such as the United Nations effort in East Timor that began in 1999 might fall into this category.

Lessons Learned

The study also provided qualitative findings. Learning from and applying these lessons will improve the chances of success in rebuilding health. It will also increase the likelihood of improving water and sanitation conditions, infectious disease rates, mortality and morbidity rates, and food and nutrition conditions, and it will increase the likelihood that broader nation-building and development objectives will be achieved. The lessons fall into six categories: health as an independent variable, the impact of other sectors on health, coordination, sustainability and tipping point, exit strategies, and perform-ance metrics.

Health as an Independent Variable

Unless adequate attention is given to health, nation-building efforts cannot be successful. Indeed, health can have an important inde-pendent impact on nation-building and overall development. Several of the cases show that security is significantly impacted by the role health plays in helping to win "hearts and minds," an objective whose importance is illustrated by cases such as Iraq and Somalia. In both of these cases, the inability to win hearts and minds contributed to in-surgency, warlordism, and an unstable security environment. Coun-terinsurgency experts have long argued that winning hearts and minds is a key—if not *the* key—component in establishing peace. Health can play an important role in the effort by, for example, of-fering tangible health programs to the local population and meeting basic health needs, such as improving sanitation and nutrition condi-tions. Such programs should be designed to gain support for the host country, rather than for the United States or other outside actors; the local government should be the entity winning the hearts and minds of the population. In the early stages of nation-building operations, the absence of a local government may make it difficult to win hearts and minds. This was the case during the operations in Germany, So-malia, Kosovo, and Iraq. Over time, however, political authority in-variably shifts to local control. When it does, programs must be de-signed to gain support for the local government.

Health can have an important negative effect on security, as well. In Iraq, for example, there is some evidence that poor health conditions—especially poor sanitation conditions—contributed to anti-Americanism and support for the insurgency. Most early recon-struction efforts in the Iraqi health sector went into activities that were not immediately visible to Iraqis, such as establishing a surveil-lance system and creating a statistical database of hospitals and clinics.

Maximizing the effectiveness of health as an independent vari-able means paying close attention to the sequence of health steps. Nation-building programs will generally follow three broad, sequenced phases: immediate post-conflict, reconstruction, and consolidation. During the immediate post-conflict phase, at least three types of emergency health situations should take priority. Failure to address them well or quickly can complicate reconstruction in other areas and lead to animosity among the local population, whereas success can help win hearts and minds. First, the clinical consequences arising after the use of weapons of mass destruction must be quickly and adequately addressed. In Japan, this was not done; the treatment of survivors was left largely to the Japanese themselves. Allied doctors eventually brought in penicillin and plasma, but the slow and inadequate treatment of victims contributed to high casualty rates. Second, the outbreak—or potential outbreak—of communicable diseases needs to be met quickly to prevent spreading. Third, basic public health needs, such as food and sanitation, should be met as quickly as possible. Famine has been a particular concern. After Somali President Siad Barre was deposed in 1991, an estimated 300,000 people died of starvation over the next two years. The United Nations and United States provided immediate humanitarian assistance and saved an estimated additional 300,000 Somalis from famine.

Impact of Other Sectors on Health

Health conditions are deeply impacted by other key sectors, including security, basic infrastructure (such as power and transportation), education, governance, and economic stabilization. Amartya Sen argues that the linkages between these sectors are empirical and causal:

> [T]here is strong evidence that economic and political freedoms help to reinforce one another. . . . Similarly, social opportunities of education and health care, which may require public action, complement individual opportunities of economic and political participation and also help to foster our own initiatives in overcoming our respective deprivations.[5]

---

[5] Sen, *Development as Freedom*, p. xii.

The health sector is particularly sensitive to security in at least two ways: through direct effects, such as the inability of patients to visit doctors; and through indirect effects, such as the inability of health care facilities to function properly. A lack of security can impede progress in the reconstruction of water plants and hospitals, slow immunization campaigns, restrict delivery of needed supplies to health care facilities, and affect the labor force if healthcare providers are intimidated or threatened with kidnapping. Patients can also be deterred from seeking health care because of security concerns. Situations such as this (Iraq, for example), where there is a pervasive lack of security, cannot be fixed by ad hoc measures, such as providing security guards to hospitals and guarding water plants and pipes.

The success of the health sector is also tightly linked with progress in other sectors, such as basic infrastructure. In Iraq, for instance, hospitals and clinics operated at partial capacity and had to use power generators provided by international organizations. In general, a lack of clean water, sanitation, or power increases the likelihood of acute disease outbreaks or widespread epidemics, and makes it difficult to build a functioning health system. International organizations may spend time and resources refurbishing hospitals and clinics, training staff, and providing equipment. But unreliable power nullifies much of this effort. The success of the health care system is also linked to reconstruction of the financial, judicial, and education systems. For example, if financial systems are not working, it is difficult to acquire supplies and capital equipment, and equally challenging to develop health-financing mechanisms.

Coordination

The coordination of health efforts is a key challenge during reconstruction. Indeed, the World Bank argues that past nation-building efforts have suffered from "a lack of an overarching nationally-driven plan to which all donors agree, resulting in fragmentation, gaps or duplication in aid-financed programs."[6] Poor coordination can weaken fragile health systems by scattering assistance to an assortment of health projects and failing to sufficiently tackle key priorities.

In some ways, coordination and planning were easier in the post–World War II cases of Germany and Japan because there were fewer actors, which made it easier for government officials to coordinate policies and communicate among health personnel. The number of actors involved in health reconstruction has exponentially increased since the end of the Cold War. The greater the number of actors, the more difficult the coordination.[7] Two steps can help improve mission coordination: encouraging and rationalizing a lead-state or lead-organization system for health, and learning from and replicating successful on-the-ground organizational innovations.

First, the need to overcome coordination and collaboration problems makes it important to establish institutional arrangements that increase efficiency in rebuilding health. There are a variety of options: donor coordination units within a host state's Ministry of Health, a lead national actor, lead regional or local actors, regular collective Ministry of Health consultations with donors, and sector-wide approaches. A lead actor approach is usually the most effective coordinating strategy for planning and funding, especially when the host government is barely functional. In the health sector, experience suggests that the lead actor(s) should be an international organization rather than a state. It can be difficult to agree on a lead actor, since donor states, international institutions, and NGOs generally have different priorities, interests, and strategies. But a lead actor is critical to ensure efficiency and effectiveness. This can include coordinating and overseeing the undertaking of joint assessments, preparing shared

---

[6] United Nations Development Programme and World Bank, *An Operational Note on Transitional Results Matrices: Using Results-Based Frameworks in Fragile States*, New York: United Nations Development Group and World Bank, January 2005, p. 2. Also see *Health Policy Formulation in Complex Political Emergencies and Post-Conflict Countries: A Literature Review*, London: London School of Hygiene and Tropical Medicine, November 2002.

[7] Mancur Olson, *The Logic of Collective Action: Public Goods and the Theory of Groups*, Cambridge, Massachusetts: Harvard University Press, 1971, p. 2.

strategies, coordinating political engagement, establishing joint offices, and introducing simplified arrangements, such as common reporting and financial requirements. In theory, the lead actor can be a donor state, international organization, or NGO. In practice, however, only states and international organizations have the resources and legitimacy necessary to be lead actors. Two elements crucial to the task of establishing a lead actor are buy-in from the host government and support from key donors, international organizations, and NGOs.

Second, there is a strong need to consolidate lessons learned and best practices in coordinating activities. NGOs and other organizations have worked out effective ad hoc organizational arrangements at national and local levels to improve coordination. One important aspect should be to coordinate with international institutions or NGOs that were involved in health and health-related efforts before and during the conflict. Their experience provides an invaluable understanding of the health care system, the health status of the population, and the major health challenges within a country. Since reliable statistical information on health conditions is often unavailable during the initial post-conflict phase, prior knowledge is crucial. Bilateral donors, international institutions, and NGOs should utilize actors with in-country experience to assist in coordination and planning.

Sustainability and Tipping Point

Health sector reform must encourage long-term sustainability. Indeed, the ultimate objective of health reconstruction should be to reach a "tipping point": the point at which the local government begins to assume substantial responsibility for managing the health sector. This point will be different in every nation-building case, and will likely take longer to reach in less-developed states. It took Germany approximately two and a half years to reach the tipping point; however, U.S. advisors continued to observe, inspect, advise, and report on health activities. Haiti never reached the tipping point. The United States largely withdrew after three years, and the Haitian government never developed the capacity to implement health programs and to administratively operate them.

The training of indigenous personnel is critical to sustainability. Without it, the programs neither reflect favorably on the host government nor remain effective once outside forces and personnel have departed. Another critical aspect is assessment of the national and private health institutions' capacity to engage in needs assessment and implementation. Capacity has important implications for recovery and planning. From an operational perspective, it makes sense to distinguish between two types of post-conflict situations: strong national capacities and weak national capacities. These distinctions should not be regarded as absolute, but as two ends of a continuum. Most countries are located between these extremes.

In countries with strong national health capacities, such as Germany after World War II, health progress may be more rapid. Since national contributions and ownership are likely to be high, planning can be oriented beyond the short-term (0 to 18 months) to include the medium-term (18 to 36 months) recovery and development needs. In countries with weak health capacities, national and private health institutions usually lack the capacity to make substantial contributions to the needs assessment and implementation. In Somalia, warlords did not support relief efforts and attacked, looted, or extorted payments from relief convoys. In Afghanistan, tribes and local strongmen, rather than the central government, have historically controlled most of the country, making it difficult to create a self-sufficient and sustainable health system. The variation in initial nation-building conditions places a premium on correct determination of governance institution effectiveness and the nature of the conflict. Much like Afghanistan, states with a weak national capacity can face a series of challenges after major conflict:

- Severely deteriorating health conditions, especially if civilians and civilian structures were targets of violence
- Institutional collapse
- Social cleavages between groups manipulated by the parties to the conflict
- Lack of accountability mechanisms because there is no legitimate government.

The curves of decline and recovery are likely to be different for these cases, especially when there has been a long-term degradation of health. Challenges are deeper, and progress should be expected to be slower before reaching a tipping point. The health infrastructure, administrative capacity, and physical infrastructure may have ceased to exist—or may never have existed at all. Such situations require a reconstruction effort strongly shaped by the goal of development. In Afghanistan, the international community geared up for a standard post-conflict reconstruction effort instead of acknowledging that what it largely faced was a development challenge.

If development is the goal, an important question arises: Will health recovery plans perpetuate a tradition of national dependence on the external design, delivery, and financing of health care that will jeopardize sustainability? Unfortunately, the main health challenges in countries with weak national capacities are not amenable to quick fixes. The population must become stronger and healthier through improved nutrition and access to clean water and sanitation. A new generation of health care professionals has to be recruited, trained, and motivated to work in rural areas. Some long-standing habits and attitudes, particularly related to marriage, family, and the status of women, must change. And the country needs years of stability and security for these changes to occur and take hold.

Exit Strategies

Short-term medical care is valuable, but to change a state's health care system requires time and sustained effort. In Haiti and Somalia, for example, outside powers wanted to withdraw as fast as possible. The search for a fixed exit strategy is illusory, if this means a certain date in the near future when full control of health care facilities can be handed back to local authorities. Exit requires a functioning health care system that has at least reached the tipping point.

Duration is a critical variable and cuts across all aspects of reconstruction. Based on the cases we examined, no effort to rebuild health after major combat has been successful in less than five years. The cases of postwar Germany and Japan *underestimate* the time needed to rebuild health because both countries were fairly developed in 1945. Nation-building efforts in developing countries, such as Somalia and Afghanistan in this study, would have to continue for much longer than five years to be successful. With little health infrastructure to begin with, such countries require the time needed to achieve local buy-in, build hospitals and clinics, conduct immunization programs, train health personnel, and improve sanitation and nutrition conditions.

An interesting point about duration is that while staying for a long time does not always guarantee success, leaving early usually assures failure. U.S.-led efforts to rebuild Somalia and Haiti were short-lived. The bulk of health assistance lasted for only three years, and continuing political instability in Haiti led the international community to withhold all aid by 2000. The cost of early departures is clear: It is difficult to ensure success in rebuilding health. This brings us to the last lesson.

Performance Metrics

Health programs have often fallen into the trap of emphasizing outputs, rather than outcomes, as a measure of success. Success should not be measured by the number of hospitals constructed or the percentage of doctors and nurses trained. These are important, but they tell us little about the overall state of health. Health assistance can be broken into three categories: inputs, outputs, and outcomes.

Inputs are the amount of resources used in reconstructing health, such as the amount of financial assistance and international personnel deployed. *Outputs* are the first-order results of the assistance program—for example, trained doctors and nurses, and functional hospitals. (Many people call these outputs *proximate* or *intermediate* outcomes.) *Outcomes* are conditions that directly affect the public. They are not *what* governments and international institutions do; rather, they are the consequences of what they do. Nation-building missions may want to create a performance matrix that lists key health goals, inputs, outputs, and outcomes over time. This effort should include gathering information on baseline conditions and, perhaps, relevant non-health indicators. Most importantly, the matrix should track metrics over the course of reconstruction to monitor whether they are improving or getting worse.

Without the ability to measure performance, policymakers lack an objective method for judging success and failure in ongoing crises, which makes midcourse corrections more difficult. Key measures of health outcomes include life expectancy, birth rate, death rate, infant mortality rate, infectious disease rate, and malnutrition. Since these outcome measures may not always be readily available, more-tactical and short-term measures (e.g., vaccination rates, percentage of births with skilled attendance, access to timely basic health care, and adequacy of health care supply) may also be appropriate to give policymakers some indication of performance. Building such assessments into current and future assistance programs and encouraging host nations to undertake such assessments will make foreign actors better placed to optimize assistance programs.

Performance indicators should also vary somewhat for different countries. Some more-developed states may face a window of opportunity for rapid structural reform. For some less-developed states, however, rapid structural reform may be destabilizing, so immediate priorities should instead focus on rebuilding familiar administrative and service delivery functions. The timelines of performance measures should be adapted to a country's particular circumstances.

Moving Forward

What are the policy implications of rebuilding health for international institutions, NGOs, and donor states? Many recent cases, such as Afghanistan and Iraq, have reinforced well-worn lessons. Of the many lessons about health and nation-building that the international community learned during the 1990s, few have been applied in Afghanistan or Iraq.

Applying these lessons will not ipso facto guarantee success. But, on the basis of our findings, we believe it will vastly improve the chances of success, as measured by improvements in sanitation conditions, infectious disease rates, mortality and morbidity rates, and nutrition conditions. Our findings also support the use of these metrics as criteria by which to judge success. Given the likelihood of future nation-building missions, it may be worthwhile for interdisciplinary experts to define the possible dimensions of "success." While each nation-building mission will, of course, differ somewhat in overall objectives and data availability, it is nonetheless critical to develop a framework for monitoring and measuring inputs and outputs.

Acknowledgments

Several people at RAND made important contributions during the course of the project. Bradley Stein and Jerry Sollinger offered valuable input and insights. Tom Sullivan offered constructive suggestions and provided useful data for the Iraq chapter. In addition, Ambassador James Dobbins and Robert Wilensky provided frank and insightful reviews, which greatly improved the final manuscript. Nathan Chandler, Jennie Breon, and Karen Stewart helped assemble the final report and provided invaluable research and administrative support.

We are also grateful for the comments from participants at the Academy Health "Health in Foreign Policy Forum" conference in Washington, the "Health as a Bridge for Peace" conference at the United Nations Headquarters in New York, and the Global Public Health Conference in Lexington, Kentucky. We wish to thank the following individuals: Abdul Razzaq Raghbat and Said Mujtaba for facilitating visits to clinics and hospitals in Kabul and Kandahar, Afghanistan; Kaivon Saleh, Health Advisor with the Afghan Reconstruction Group, for providing useful insights into on-the-ground difficulties of health sector reconstruction; Georg Jakob Illi, of the German Medical Service, for providing information derived from 30 years of medical work in Afghanistan; Dr. Ellyn Cavanagh, of Rabia Balkhi Hospital, for offering us important data related to women's and children's health; and Soraya Sadeed, Mohammad Yousuf Jabarkhail, Aziz Shamal, and Dr. K.R. Quarga, of Help the Afghan Children, for arranging focus group discussions in their clinics.

Finally, we thank David and Carol Richards. Work on this study would not have been possible without their generous support.

Acronyms

ABCC	Atomic Bomb Casualty Commission
ADB	Asian Development Bank
AIHA	American International Health Alliance
CARE	Cooperative for American Remittances to Europe
CDC	Centers for Disease Control and Prevention
CPA	Coalition Provisional Authority
DFID	Department for International Development
DHSW	Department of Health and Social Welfare
DOTS	direct observation therapy strategy
DTP	diphtheria, tetanus, and pertussis
EC	European Commission
EERP	Emergency Economic Recovery Program
EU	European Union
FMC	family medicine center
FRY	Former Republic of Yugoslavia
GAO	Government Accountability Office (formerly General Accounting Office)
GARIOA	Government and Relief in Occupied Areas
GDP	gross domestic product
HDI	Human Development Index
ICRC	International Committee of the Red Cross

IDB	Inter-American Development Bank
IDP	internally displaced person
IMC	International Medical Corps
IMCI	integrated management of childhood illnesses
IO	international organization
IPH	Institutes of Public Health
IPSE	Internal Public Security Force
JMA	Japan Medical Association
JTF	Joint Task Force
KFOR	Kosovo Force
KLA	Kosovo Liberation Army
LARA	Licensed Agencies for Relief in Asia
MHSW	Ministry of Public Health and Social Welfare
MICIVIH	Mission Civile Internationale en Haïti (International Civilian Mission in Haiti)
MNF	multinational force
MTS	Mother Theresa Society
NCCI	NGO Coordination Committee for Iraq
NGO	non-governmental organization
OAS	Organization of American States
OFDA	Office of Foreign Disaster Assistance
OMGUS	Office of the Military Government, United States
OSCE	Organization for Security and Co-operation in Europe
PAHO	Pan-American Health Organization
PCO	Project and Contracting Office
PHW	Public Health and Welfare
PTSD	post-traumatic stress disorder
SACB	Somali Aid Coordination Body
SCAP	Supreme Commander of the Allied Powers

SNA	Somali National Alliance
SRSG	United Nations Secretary-General's Special Representative
STI	sexually transmitted infection (formerly STD, sexually transmitted disease)
SWNCC	State, War, and Navy Coordinating Committee
UN	United Nations
UNAMA	United Nations Assistance Mission in Afghanistan
UNHCR	United Nations High Commissioner for Refugees
UNICEF	United Nations Children's Fund
UNITAF	Unified Task Force
UNMIK	United Nations Mission in Kosovo
UNOSOM	United Nations Operation in Somalia
UNRRA	United Nations Relief and Rehabilitation Administration
USAID	United States Agency for International Development
WFP	World Food Programme
WHO	World Health Organization

CHAPTER ONE

Introduction

Since World War II, the United States and its allies have invested significant resources in rebuilding health in the aftermath of interstate wars and civil unrest. Most articles and books on health efforts tend to be case studies that evaluate single operations, such as Vietnam, Bosnia, Kosovo, Haiti, and East Timor.[1] This is also true in the broader social science literature on nation-building. There are several good historical accounts of U.S. and European reconstruction efforts after World War II in Germany and Japan, as well as of more recent efforts carried out after major conflicts. Over the past decade, scholars and policymakers have devoted particular attention to U.S. and European nation-building operations in such areas as the Balkans and Somalia and, most recently, Afghanistan and Iraq.[2] Several United

---

[1] See, for example, Robert J. Wilensky, *Military Medicine to Win Hearts and Minds: Aid to Civilians in the Vietnam War*, Lubbock, Texas: Texas Tech University Press, 2004; World Health Organization, *Case Study of the WHO/DfID Peace Through Health Programme in Bosnia and Herzegovina*, Sarajevo: WHO, 1998; World Health Organization, *WHO Disaster Preparedness and Response Operation in Kosovo: Evaluation of Kosovo Programme, 19992000*, Pristina: WHO, 2002; Francine Tardif, *Building a Bridge for Peace or Servicing Complex Political Emergencies? A Study of the Case of the Health Humanitarian Programs in Haiti*, Port-au-Prince: World Health Organization, 1998; National Academies Press, *Initial Steps in Rebuilding the Health Sector in East Timor*, Washington, D.C.: National Academies Press, 2003.

[2] See, for example, Marc Trachtenberg, *A Constructed Peace: The Making of the European Settlement, 1945–1963*, Princeton, New Jersey: Princeton University Press, 1999; John W. Dower, *Embracing Defeat: Japan in the Wake of World War II*, New York: W.W. Norton & Company, 1999; Walter Clarke and Jeffrey Herbst (eds.), *Learning from Somalia*, Boulder, Colorado: Westview Press, 1997; Ivo H. Daalder and Michael E. O'Hanlon, *Winning Ugly: NATO's War to Save Kosovo*, Washington, D.C.: The Brookings Institution, 2001; John D.

Nations (UN) operations, such as those in El Salvador, Cambodia, and East Timor, have also been examined.

The body of literature on specific areas of nation-building is growing. For instance, significant work has been done on post-conflict policing and justice sector reform, as well as on administrative practices and governance during nation-building operations.[3] But the work on health has been limited. Much of what has been done on health and nation-building focuses on immediate humanitarian and relief efforts rather than long-term reconstruction. Perhaps even more important, however, is that few health studies have attempted to examine a comprehensive set of cases, compare the quantitative and qualitative results, and outline best practices and lessons learned. Indeed, the scope, historical breadth, and comparative approach developed in this study are what make it valuable for both policymakers and academics.

While health is critical to nation-building, it is but one of several key areas. These areas and the roles they play are as follows:

- Security: Provides peacekeeping; law enforcement; a justice sector; and demilitarization, demobilization, and reintegration of ex-combatants.
- Health: Rebuilds the public health and health care delivery systems.
- Governance: Gives the local administration the resources and advice needed to provide basic public services and to begin longer-term capacity building.
- Economic stabilization: Establishes a stable currency and provides a regulatory framework in which local and international commerce can resume.

Montgomery and Dennis A. Rondinelli (eds.), *Beyond Reconstruction in Afghanistan: Lessons from Development Experience*, New York: Palgrave Macmillan, 2004.

[3] James D. Fearon and David D. Laitin, "Neotrusteeship and the Problem of Weak States," *International Security*, Vol. 28, No. 4, Spring 2004, p. 5; Simon Chesterman, *You, The People: The United Nations Transitional Administration, and State-Building,* New York: Oxford University Press, 2004, p. 5; Francis Fukuyama, *State-Building: Governance and World Order in the 21st Century,* Ithaca, New York: Cornell University Press, 2004.

- Democratization: Builds political parties, a free press, a civil society, and a legal and constitutional framework for elections.
- Infrastructure: Provides agricultural assistance and infrastructure
  improvements such as electricity, transportation, and water.

Figure 1.1 provides a conceptual framework for measuring the
success of health interventions. It divides nation-building into five
phases: pre-conflict, conflict, immediate post-conflict (which consists
of immediate humanitarian and relief efforts), reconstruction, and
consolidation. The objective of all health efforts should be to improve
health conditions with respect to their pre-conflict level. The three
endpoints in the figure represent possible health outcomes *after* major
reconstruction efforts have ended. The lowest endpoint, P3, depicts a
decline in public health and health care delivery, which represents a
failure. P2 indicates little change from pre-conflict health levels. P1
depicts an improvement in health conditions from both pre-conflict
and immediate post-conflict levels, which represents a success.

Figure 1.1
Phases of Nation-Building

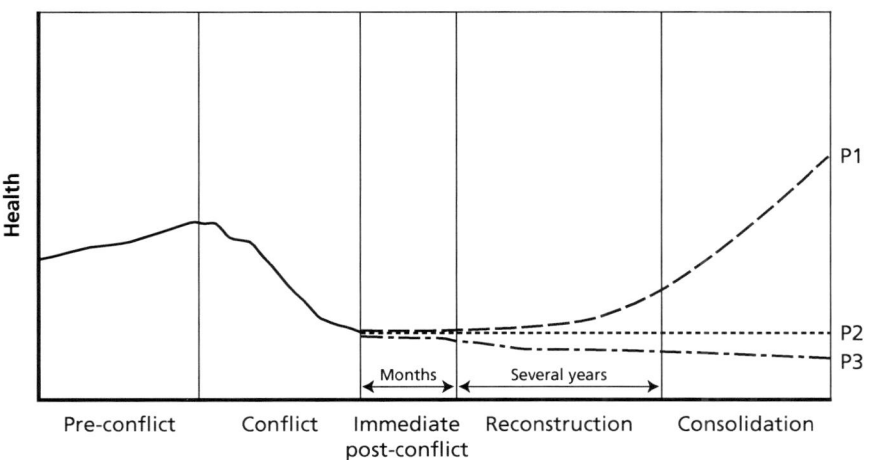

Definitions

For this study, we define the term *nation-building* as efforts carried out after major combat to underpin a transition to peace and democracy. Nation-building involves the deployment of military forces and includes comprehensive efforts to rebuild the health, security, economic, political, and other sectors. In some cases, nation-building occurs in a benign security environment with little or no resistance. In others (such as Somalia, Afghanistan, and Iraq), the violence and insurgent activity are significant. In addition, we define *success* in the health sector as an improvement over time in several outcome measures: sanitation conditions, infectious disease rates, mortality and morbidity rates, and nutrition conditions.

Other terms have been used for the activities just described: state-building, peace-building, occupation, stability operations, peace enforcement, peacekeeping, stabilization, and reconstruction. For example, some have argued that *state-building* is the most appropriate term, since *nation-building* implies the creation of a common nationality.[4] A nation, as British academic Ernest Gellner argues, includes a group of people who share the same culture, language, territory, and history.[5] The UN tends to use the term *peace-building*, which it defines as "comprehensive efforts to identify and support structures which will tend to consolidate peace and advance a sense of confidence and well-being among people."[6] U.S. policymakers frequently used the term *occupation* to refer to the U.S. and coalition efforts in Iraq after the 2003 war. This term was eventually adopted in official

---

[4] Fearon and Laitin, "Neotrusteeship," p. 5; Chesterman, *You, The People*, p. 5; Fukuyama, *State-Building*.

[5] Ernest Gellner, *Nations and Nationalism*, Ithaca, NY: Columbia University Press, 1983, p. 7. On nationalism, also see Benedict Anderson, *Imagined Communities: Reflections on the Origin and Spread of Nationalism*, New York: Verso, 1991; Ronald Grigor Suny, *The Revenge of the Past: Nationalism, Revolution, and the Collapse of the Soviet Union*, Stanford, California: Stanford University Press, 1993.

[6] United Nations, Supplement to *An Agenda for Peace: Preventive Diplomacy, Peacemaking, and Peacekeeping*, New York: United Nations, 1992, para. 55.

United Nations Security Council documents that dealt with Iraq,[7] but there has been a recent shift to the terms *reconstruction* and *stabilization*. Two good examples of this shift are the U.S. government's decision to establish an Office of the Coordinator for Reconstruction and Stabilization in the U.S. Department of State, and the British government's creation of a Post-Conflict Reconstruction Unit.

We use *nation-building* for two reasons. First, it is the most commonly used term to describe these activities. By using the word *nation*, however, we do not mean to imply that the cases we examine each have one culture, language, territory, and history, as Gellner and others have argued that a nation must. Countries such as Afghanistan and Iraq clearly are not nations in this sense. Rather, we use *nation* as a synonym for *country*, following a Merriam Webster definition for *nation*: a "community of people composed of one or more nationalities and possessing a more or less defined territory and government."[8] Second, nation-building encompasses the full range of health, political, economic, security, and humanitarian activities that we seek to analyze. We believe the term *nation-building* and our definition of it capture as well as any the nature of the issue addressed.

Methodology

This study used two methodologies. The first was a qualitative case study of seven cases: Germany, Japan, Somalia, Haiti, Kosovo, Afghanistan, and Iraq.[9] We chose these cases because they are some of the most important instances since World War II in which U.S. and

---

[7] UN Security Council Resolution 1546, for example, formally recognizes the shift from U.S. "occupation" to "the assumption of full responsibility and authority by a fully sovereign and independent Interim Government of Iraq" (United Nations Security Council Resolution 1546, on Iraq, June 8, 2004).

[8] *Webster's Third New International Dictionary of the English Language Unabridged*, Springfield, MA: G&C Merriam and Company, 1963, p. 1505.

[9] Alexander L. George, "Case Studies and Theory Development: The Method of Structured, Focused Comparison," in Paul Gordon Lauren (ed.), *Diplomacy: New Approaches in History, Theory, and Policy*, New York: Free Press, 1979, pp. 43–68.

other military forces have been used to rebuild health, security, economic, political, and other sectors after major combat. We also chose them because they vary widely in terms of input variables (such as degree of coordination and level of donor support) and success. For each case, we examined variation over time in several quantitative indicators, such as life expectancy, birth, death, infant mortality, and infectious disease rates. Subsequent research could focus on other cases that fall under our definition of nation-building—for example, efforts to rebuild Panama, Congo, Namibia, Mozambique, Bosnia, East Timor, Cambodia, El Salvador, Eastern Slavonia, Sierra Leone, Lebanon, Korea, and, perhaps, Vietnam.

The second methodology we used was a simple factor analysis of public health and health care delivery variables to support our qualitative analysis. The specifics of this analysis are in Appendices A and B.

Monograph Outline

Chapters Two through Eight present our case studies of the U.S. and allied operations for our seven countries: Germany, Japan, Somalia, Haiti, Kosovo, Afghanistan, and Iraq. Because our goal was to draw out "best practice" policies for nation-building operations, we adopted a common approach for our case studies. In each chapter, we first provide pertinent historical context and briefly describe the subject country's health history. Second, we describe the scope of the problem—What were the major public health and health care delivery challenges at the beginning of the operation?—with a particular interest in such areas as communicable diseases, water and sanitation, nutrition, health facilities and providers, consumables and equipment, and mental health. Third, we describe the roles of the major actors: the United States, other major donors, UN agencies (such as World Health Organization [WHO]), World Bank, the private sector, and non-governmental organizations (NGOs). We then examine how each operation developed over time: Did important health indicators get better, worse, or stay the same? Were humanitarian and relief needs met? Fourth, we compile the most important lessons learned that may be useful for current and future nation-building operations.

Chapter Nine has three major sections. The first uses factor analysis to assess the outcome of health efforts in the seven cases, with particular attention paid to finding those variables that contribute to success in rebuilding public health and health care delivery systems. In the second section, we compile and analyze the major lessons learned across the cases. These range from the importance of security as a precondition for health reconstruction, to the provision of programs that provide tangible improvements in the health of the population. The third, and final, section offers policy implications for current and future nation-building operations.

CHAPTER TWO

Germany

In the early morning hours of May 7, 1945, German General Alfred Jodl unconditionally surrendered all German forces to the allies in Reims, Germany. He was met by delegations from the United States and Great Britain, as well as representatives from France and the Soviet Union. Germany's surrender signaled the end of World War II in Europe, allowing the allies to begin the process of postwar rebuilding.

This chapter argues that health reconstruction efforts in the U.S. sector of Germany were largely successful. U.S. and German health authorities improved nutrition and sanitation conditions, helped decrease infectious and other types of diseases, and rebuilt Germany's health care delivery system. The Office of Military Government, United States (OMGUS) was established in October 1945 to oversee the rebuilding of the U.S. sector. Reconstruction of Germany's health system was carried out under the Public Health Branch of OMGUS's Civil Administration Division.

Reconstruction of the public health and health care delivery system in Germany differed from that in most of the post–Cold War cases (e.g., Haiti, Bosnia, and Iraq) for at least two reasons. First, World War II was significantly more destructive than these later conflicts. A total of 61 countries were involved in World War II, 110 million people were mobilized for military service, 55 million soldiers and civilians were killed, and participating countries spent over $1 trillion on the war. The United States alone spent approximately $306 billion on the war between 1941 and 1945—roughly three times its gross national product in 1940.[1] The breadth and intensity of World War II ensured that the process of reconstruction would be difficult and wrenching. Much of Europe was a wasteland, and German cities such as Berlin, Dresden, and Hamburg were reduced to rubble. Second, Germany was a highly developed country. Germany possessed an educated population, substantial economic resources, and an efficient government structure. These assets greatly facilitated reconstruction.

Historical Context

Germany's health system has been overseen by a strong state since at least the era of Otto von Bismarck, the German chancellor beginning in 1871. Bismarck, according to historian Theodore Hamerow, "believed that government had a right to regulate the interaction of classes and interests for the advancement of the general welfare."[2] One of his most significant health objectives was to establish the first national health insurance program. In 1883, Bismarck helped pass the Sickness Insurance Act, which required all workers earning a certain income or below to be insured by a sickness fund. The law also mandated employer-employee contributions, or premiums, and guaranteed that all members of a sickness fund would receive physicians' services, medication, eyeglasses, and hospital treatment.[3]

Bismarck was thus able to coordinate health programs already in existence under the banner of the state and help make Germany's

---

[1] These figures do not include China. Alan S. Milward, *War, Economy, and Society, 1939–1945*, Berkeley, California: University of California Press, 1979, Ch. 3; John J. Mearsheimer, *The Tragedy of Great Power Politics*, New York: W.W. Norton, 2001, p. 61; Melvyn P. Leffler, *A Preponderance of Power: National Security, the Truman Administration, and the Cold War*, Stanford, California: Stanford University Press, 1992, pp. 1–3.

[2] T. S. Hamerow (ed.), *The Age of Bismarck*, New York: Harper and Row, 1973, p. 233.

[3] Jan Blanpain, Luc Delesie, and Herman Nys, *National Health Insurance and Health Resources: The European Experience*, Cambridge, Massachusetts: Harvard University Press, 1978.

public health and health care delivery systems among the best in Europe. Membership in Germany's health insurance system gradually increased over the years. Roughly 23 percent of the population was insured by 1914, 28 percent by 1933, and nearly 50 percent by World War II.[4] The pervasive role of the state in German health affairs marked an important difference from later reconstruction efforts in such countries as Somalia and Afghanistan, which lacked strong, competent central governments.

Germany also enjoyed a health care delivery system that had a core of strong and competent physicians. Physicians played little role in the initial formulation of national health strategies under Bismarck. They were not recognized under law as a profession and did not have the extensive legal privileges of a profession.[5] But this changed between the beginning of the 20th century and World War II. In 1900, a group of physicians founded the Hartmann Bund, an organization dedicated to protesting the growing control of the sickness funds over the practice of medicine.[6] The Emergency Regulation of 1931 gave physician associations the legal authority to negotiate fee schedules with the sickness funds and to monitor physicians' practices. This authority led to the transformation of physician organizations into powerful political entities.[7]

---

[4] Laurene A. Graig, *Health of Nations: An International Perspective on U.S. Health Care Reform*, 3rd ed., Washington, D.C.: Congressional Quarterly, 1999; K.D. Henke, "The Federal Republic of Germany," in Richard Scheffler and L.F. Rossiter (eds.), *Advances in Health Economics and Health Services Research*, Greenwich, Connecticut: JAI Press, 1990, pp. 145–168.

[5] Donald W. Light, "Values and Structure in the German Health Care Systems," *Milbank Quarterly*, Vol. 63, No. 4, 1985, p. 620. Also see Donald W. Light and Alexander Schuller (eds.), *Political Values and Health Care: The German Experience,* Cambridge, Massachusetts: MIT Press, 1986.

[6] Deborah Stone, "Professionalism and Accountability: Controlling Health Services in the United States and West Germany," *Journal of Health Politics, Policy and Law*, Vol. 2, No. 1, Spring 1977, pp. 32–47.

[7] Bradford Kirkman-Liff, "Physician Payment and Cost-Containment Strategies in West Germany: Suggestions for Medicare Reform," *Journal of Health Politics, Policy and Law*, 1990, pp. 69–99; Graig, *Health of Nations*, p. 59.

When Adolf Hitler and the National Socialist party gained power in 1934, one of Hitler's most significant changes to the health system was to establish a Director of Public Health, in the Ministry of Interior, who was responsible for all health programs throughout Germany. Several other federal departments shared health responsibilities, such as the Ministries of Education, Labor, Propaganda, and Commerce and Food. German scientists and physicians were on the cutting edge of advanced technology; they developed or greatly improved the use of electronic computing devices, electron microscopes, atomic fusion, and data-processing technologies. While the German public health and health care delivery systems were among the best in Europe, German physicians were complicit in Nazi crimes against humanity. For many physicians, the seductive power of National Socialism lay in its promise to cleanse German society of its "corrupting elements." This included substances such as metallic lead and addictive tobacco, but also people: communists, Jews, homosexuals, and the mentally ill.

Health Challenges

By the end of World War II, Germany faced a number of health challenges, including acute malnutrition, significant damage to the sanitation system, high infectious disease rates, and the destruction of hospitals and equipment. As the United States Strategic Bombing Survey's study entitled *The Effect of Bombing on Health and Medical Care in Germany* noted:

> The events in the air succeeded in greatly lowering the standard of health throughout Germany by destroying facilities for the maintenance of environmental sanitation, by creating the most acute conditions of overcrowding which have been encountered in the western world, by denying civilians hospital care and ade-

quate drugs, and by changing three meals a day from an individual habit to an object of individual ingenuity.[8]

The allied strategic bombing campaign was particularly destructive to the public health and health care delivery systems. Allied military and civilian policymakers adopted a variety of strategies to defeat Germany. They ranged from precision attacks on key economic bottlenecks to cripple the German economy, to the use of incendiary bombs against cities and towns to break the population's morale.[9] For example, British Royal Air Force planners argued that in order to shatter German morale, "[W]e must achieve two things: first, we must make [German towns] physically uninhabitable and, secondly, we must make the people conscious of constant personal danger."[10] Allied bombers attacked 61 major cities and 31 towns and razed 128 square miles—or 50 percent—of their urban area. Over 7 million people were rendered homeless.[11] The consequences were devastating. Hunger reigned. Farmlands were despoiled, cattle slaughtered, and herds dispersed throughout Germany. Transportation facilities were wrecked. Demolished bridges and sunken vessels clogged the Danube and Rhine rivers, railroad roadbeds were destroyed, ports were severely damaged, and coastal shipping sunk.

Public Health

The bombing campaign and allied ground advance across western Germany caused numerous public health challenges. One of the most

---

[8] United States Strategic Bombing Survey, *The Effect of Bombing on Health and Medical Care in Germany*, Washington, D.C.: War Department, October 30, 1945, p. 1.

[9] Robert A. Pape, *Bombing to Win: Air Power and Coercion in War*, Ithaca, New York: Cornell University Press, 1996, pp. 254–313. On incendiary bombs, see United States Strategic Bombing Survey, *Physical Damage Division Report (ETO)*, Physical Damage Division, Washington, D.C.: War Department, April 1947.

[10] Air Staff, "The Value of Incendiary Weapons in Attack on Area Targets," September 29, 1941, in Towns Panel of the British Bombing Survey Unit, *Effects of Strategic Air Attacks on German Towns,* London: HMSO, 1947, p. 50.

[11] Larry J. Bidinian, *The Combined Allied Bombing Offensive Against the German Civilian, 1942–1945*, Lawrence, Kansas: Coronado Press, 1976, pp. 29, 35.

acute was malnutrition. Bombing decreased the production capacity of the oat and barley mills in Germany's key regions by 20 percent and the production capacity of the sugar industry by 38 percent.[12] By the beginning of 1945, damage to the food supply system caused significant problems for the Ministry of Food and the Public Welfare Agency, which was charged with feeding the population of areas under military attack. A decrease in the amount of daily calories and protein among the population led to a reduction in body weight and deficiencies in calcium and vitamins A, B_1, and C.[13] Inmates of German concentration camps also suffered from severe malnutrition and starvation.

The bombing of German cities devastated the country's sanitation system. Allied planes severely damaged Germany's water supply system, including water mains, wells, water towers, feed lines, and pumping stations.[14] On January 29, 1944, for example, 814 planes from the United States Eighth Air Force dropped 2,014 tons of bombs on Frankfurt, causing over 2,000 breaks in water mains and feed lines.[15] Fires, the loss of electricity, and the decreasing availability of chlorine further damaged the water system, as did allied targeting of water treatment facilities. Bombing and general war conditions also interfered with garbage collection and disposal. The shortage of manpower, declining availability of gasoline, and devastation of buildings and streets made it difficult to pick up garbage, which cluttered German cities. The public water supply and the sanitary conditions at congregation points for displaced persons, such as caves

---

[12] United States Strategic Bombing Survey, *The Effect of Bombing on Health and Medical Care in Germany*, p. 266.

[13] United States Strategic Bombing Survey, *The Effect of Bombing on Health and Medical Care in Germany*, p. 290.

[14] United States Strategic Bombing Survey, *Physical Damage Division Report (ETO)*, p. 76.

[15] United States Strategic Bombing Survey, *The Effect of Bombing on Health and Medical Care in Germany*, p. 236. On the targeting of Germany's sanitation system, also see United States Strategic Bombing Survey, Physical Damage Division Report (ETO), pp. 76–80.

and tunnels, also presented major challenges. Allied medical staff and physicians from the United Nations Relief and Rehabilitation Administration attended to the health of displaced persons, liberated prisoners of war, and the surviving inmates of concentration camps.[16]

The war increased the incidence of some diseases in Germany. During the allies' ground offensive in early 1945, allied public health personnel encountered serious problems with typhus fever and other infectious diseases. They disinfected with DDT powder all displaced persons and others likely to have been exposed to diseases at such locations as the *cordon sanitaire* at the Rhine River crossing and refugee centers.[17] As Figure 2.1 illustrates, a notable rise occurred in scarlet

Figure 2.1
Disease Rates, Germany, 1938–1944

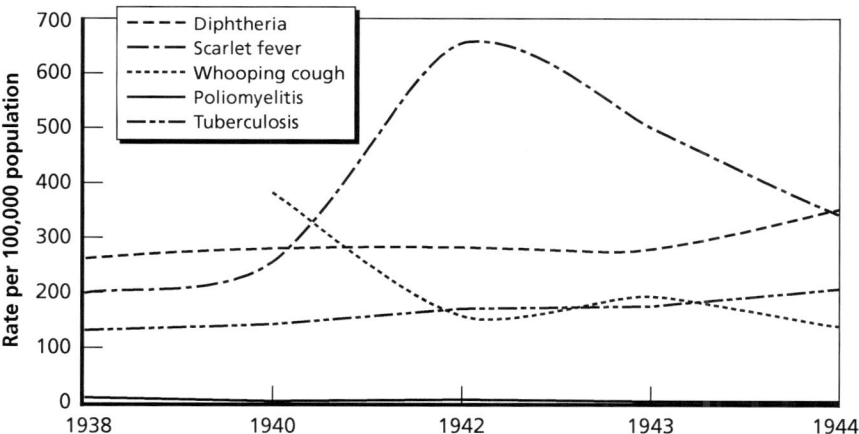

SOURCE: United States Strategic Bombing Survey, *The Effect of Bombing on Health and Medical Care in Germany*, pp. 30–105.

RAND *MG321-2.1*

---

[16] Joseph R. Starr, *Denazification, Occupation, and Control of Germany, March–July 1945*, Salisbury, North Carolina: Documentary Publications, 1977, p. 67.

[17] Starr, *Denazification, Occupation, and Control of Germany*, p. 66.

fever, diphtheria, and tuberculosis. Typhus fever also dramatically increased from a rate of 0 per 100,000 people in 1938 to 5.51 in 1944.[18] A number of factors may have contributed to this rise: a decline in sanitation conditions, the physical destruction of hospitals and health clinics, the poor nutritional state of the people, overcrowded and unsanitary conditions at air raid and emergency shelters, the influx of foreigners into Germany before and during the war, and the disruption of heating facilities. These factors also contributed to an increase in illnesses exacerbated by psychological stress, such as ulcers and coronary heart disease.

Mortality rates increased and the birth rate decreased during the war, as noted in Figures 2.2 and 2.3. The infant mortality rate rose from 59 per thousand people in 1938 to 97 per thousand in 1944. The annual mortality rates for a number of diseases (e.g., diphtheria, scarlet fever, and tuberculosis) also increased. The birth rate for Germany, which steadily rose until 1939, fell consistently during the war years. In a sample of 13 German cities, birth rates declined from 17 per thousand people in 1938 to 11 per thousand in 1944.[19] Much like the disease rates, the rise in mortality rates and the decline in the birth rate were most likely a result of both the cumulative hardships of wartime—including infrastructure destruction, poor sanitary conditions, and malnutrition—and direct attacks from the allied ground and air campaigns. In sum, German public health was in poor shape after World War II. The German population suffered from acute malnutrition, a damaged sanitation system, a rise in infectious diseases, and increasing mortality and morbidity rates.

---

[18] United States Strategic Bombing Survey, *The Effect of Bombing on Health and Medical Care in Germany*, p. 31. On concerns about typhus, also see Oliver J. Frederiksen, *The American Military Occupation of Germany, 1945–1953*, Darmstadt, Germany: Historical Division, Headquarters, United States Army, Europe, 1953, p. 109; Starr, *Denazification, Occupation, and Control of Germany*, p. 66.

[19] United States Strategic Bombing Survey, *The Effect of Bombing on Health and Medical Care in Germany*, pp. 120–121, 125.

Figure 2.2
Infant Mortality and Birth Rate, Germany, 1938–1944

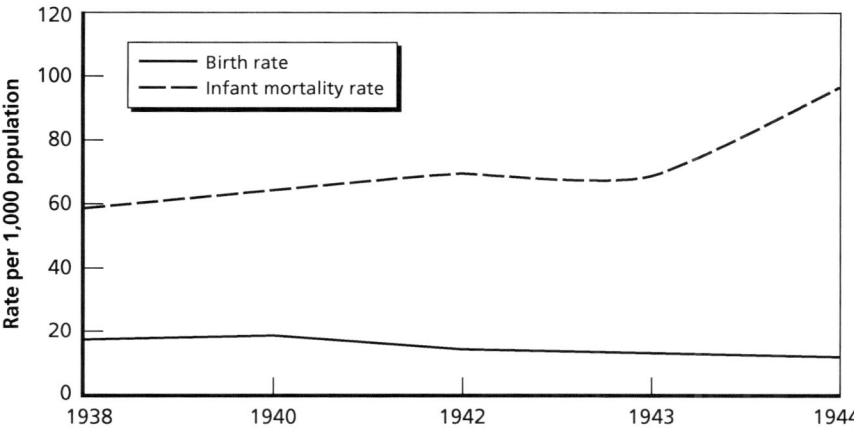

SOURCE: United States Strategic Bombing Survey, *The Effect of Bombing on Health and Medical Care in Germany*, pp. 117–158.

RAND *MG321-2.2*

Figure 2.3
Mortality Rate for Several Diseases, Germany, 1938–1944

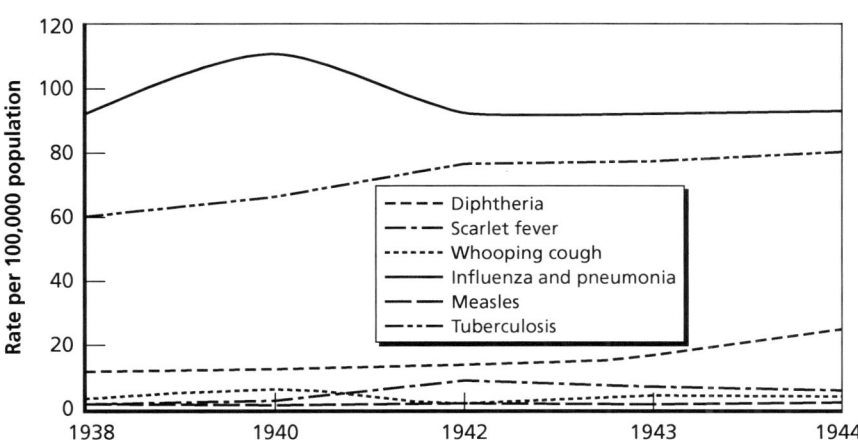

SOURCE: United States Strategic Bombing Survey, *The Effect of Bombing on Health and Medical Care in Germany*, pp. 30–105.

RAND *MG321-2.3*

Health Care Delivery

One of the most dramatic developments of World War II was the allied destruction of hospitals and medical facilities. As the United States Strategic Bombing Survey unabashedly noted:

> In total war, hospitals are not spared as experience in Germany and Great Britain has shown. Many large hospitals have been completely obliterated. . . . Indeed, the opinion has been expressed that in total war the red cross on the brilliant white background is no longer a shield of safety on the roof of a hospital but a pinpoint for orienting pilots over a blackened city on a moonlit night.[20]

Bombing by high-explosive and incendiary bombs significantly damaged western Germany's hospitals and hospital facilities. Table 2.1 illustrates the damage to hospitals in Essen, Germany. The damage was greatest in cities with a military-industrial infrastructure

Table 2.1
Damage to Hospitals in Essen, Germany

Hospital	Total Damage	Occupants Killed
Staedtisches Krankenhaus	Heavy	10
Krupp (Lazarett Strasse)	Heavy	Unknown (est. 85)
Krupp-Altenhof	Moderate	None
Lambertus-Recklinghausen	None	None
Huyssenstift	Slight	None
Elizabeth Krankenhaus	Moderate	1
Franz-Sales Haus	Heavy	30
Knappschaft-Stehle	Slight	None
Laurentius Hospital	Slight	None
Evangelisches-Stehle	Slight	None
Josephs-Kupferdreh	Slight	None

SOURCE: United States Strategic Bombing Survey, *The Effect of Bombing on Health and Medical Care in Germany*, p. 215.

---

[20] United States Strategic Bombing Survey, *The Effect of Bombing on Health and Medical Care in Germany*, p. 182.

because of their high-value targets. Data for the pre-war bed capacity of hospitals suggest that the number of total beds was between 350,000 and 700,000 in Germany. This number translated into a range of between 4.6 and 9 beds per thousand inhabitants.[21] The aerial bombing campaign had a particularly devastating effect on the bed capacity, though there are no reliable estimates for total capacity at the end of the war. The U.S. Strategic Bombing Survey suggests that as much as 45 percent of the beds in Germany's general hospitals were destroyed by allied bombing. For example, in Kassel and Hamburg, the bed capacity in 1945 was one-half of what it was in 1939; in Cologne, it was one-fifth; and in Frankfurt, one-half. Other cities, such as Dortmund, experienced little change.[22] Hospitals responded to the infrastructure damage and decrease in bed capacity by establishing auxiliary and emergency hospitals (usually outside of towns and cities), shortening patient stays, and, in rare cases, rebuilding hospitals during the war.

Hospital equipment and consumables were in short supply. Allied bombing destroyed significant quantities of specialized instruments, such as cystoscopes, surgical instruments, x-ray equipment, and other laboratory material. Allied strikes against German pharmaceutical facilities and railroads significantly decreased the number and availability of sulfonamides, insulin, and glandular extracts.[23] Karl Brandt, the General Commissar of German Health, informed Hitler in April 1945 that 20 percent of all essential medical supplies throughout Germany were destroyed, 40 percent of those in stock were partially damaged and would last two months, and the remain-

---

[21] United States Strategic Bombing Survey, *The Effect of Bombing on Health and Medical Care in Germany*, p. 184.

[22] United States Strategic Bombing Survey, *The Effect of Bombing on Health and Medical Care in Germany*, pp. 186, 220.

[23] United States Strategic Bombing Survey, *The Effect of Bombing on Health and Medical Care in Germany*, p. 294.

der would meet German health needs for four additional months if transportation could be restored.[24]

The war had little effect on some areas of health care delivery. There was no overall shortage of medical and nursing personnel. However, civilian hospitals sometimes experienced shortages when physicians and nurses were taken into the German armed services. Despite the extensive damage to many hospitals in Germany, there were few casualties among patients and among doctors, nurses, and other personnel. As one French Army report concluded: "Although villages in the Palatinate were often found devoid of medical help, nearly all communities east of the Rhine have at least an embryo organization, usually comprising a doctor, nurses, and midwives."[25]

Like public health, much of the health care delivery system was severely damaged by the allied ground offensive and strategic bombing campaign. German hospitals suffered significant infrastructure damage, and hospital equipment and consumables were in short supply.

Health Approach and Assessment

After the war, the United States, Soviet Union, Britain, and, eventually, France established military governments in their respective sectors. The U.S. sector included a large swath of territory comprising Greater Hesse, Baden-Württemberg, and Bavaria, as well as separate enclaves in Berlin and Bremen. This section outlines key participants and donors, examines U.S.-led efforts to rebuild Germany's public health and health care delivery systems, and provides an overall assessment.

---

[24] United States Strategic Bombing Survey, *The Effect of Bombing on Health and Medical Care in Germany*, p. 339.

[25] Quoted in Starr, *Denazification*, Occupation, and Control of Germany, p. 67. Also see United States Strategic Bombing Survey, *The Effect of Bombing on Health and Medical Care in Germany*, p. 215.

Key Participants and Donors

The U.S. sector was organized under the command of OMGUS. Acting "in the interest of the United Nations," U.S. officials argued that they had the authority to occupy and control Germany, "including all powers possessed by the German Government, the High Command and any state, municipal, or local government or authority."[26] This included the authority to operate and control the German public health and health care delivery systems, which were carried out under the Public Health Branch of OMGUS's Civil Administration Division. The United States gradually shifted responsibilities to German authorities over the course of reconstruction. By January 1948, German Laender health authorities took over full responsibility for health services. But OMGUS retained responsibilities in narcotics control and the venereal disease control program for the duration of the occupation, and it continued to observe, inspect, advise, and report on health activities.[27]

OMGUS also coordinated the efforts of numerous NGOs, which appointed a liaison to the U.S. Military Government. Much like U.S. efforts in Japan after World War II, a few international and local NGOs participated in health reconstruction. Major NGOs included CARE (Cooperative for American Remittances to Europe), Council of Relief Agencies Licensed for Operation in Germany, International Committee of the Red Cross, United Nations Relief and Rehabilitation Administration, Innere Mission, Caritas Verband, and a number of smaller, German NGOs.[28]

---

[26] United States Department of State, *Occupation of Germany: Police and Progress, 1945–1946*, Washington, D.C.: U.S. Government Printing Office, 1947, pp. 8, 79–80.

[27] Office of Military Government for Germany, United States, Report of the Military Governor, *Public Health and Medical Affairs*, No. 31, Washington, D.C.: OMGUS, January 1948, p. 29. On the handover of power to German health officials, also see Office of Military Government for Germany, United States, *Public Health and Medical Affairs*, No. 10, May 20, 1946, p. 1, and No. 31, October–December 1947, p. 1.

[28] Lucius D. Clay, "From General Lucius Clay Personal for Echols," May 18, 1946, CC 5314, in Jean E. Smith (ed.), *The Papers of General Lucius D. Clay: Germany 1945–1947* (2 vols.), Bloomington, Indiana: Indiana University Press, 1974, pp. 206–208.

Public Health

The nutritional health of Germans gradually improved over the course of reconstruction, as Figure 2.4 indicates. However, the results were not encouraging in the immediate postwar period. The German population experienced a notable decline in average body weight and an increase in malnutrition after the war because of a lack of food. The ration level for Germans dipped to as low as 1,200 calories per day, impeding the population's productivity.[29] The average weight of German males decreased to 133 pounds in 1946, and then steadily increased to 141 pounds by late 1949. The average weight of females experienced a similar fall and rise, decreasing to 119 pounds in 1946 and then increasing to 128 pounds by 1949.[30]

Figure 2.4
Average Body Weight of Adults, Germany, 1946–1949

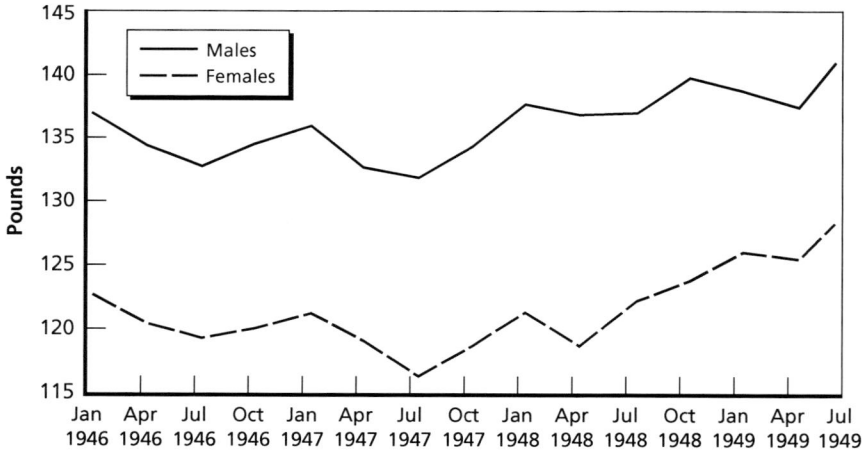

SOURCE: Office of Military Government for Germany, *Statistical Annex*, No. 49, July 1949, p. 52.

RAND *MG321-2.4*

---

[29] Office of Military Government for Germany, *Public Welfare*, No. 9, April 20, 1946, p. 2; and Clay, "From General Lucius Clay personal for Echols," p. 208.

[30] Office of Military Government for Germany, *Statistical Annex*, No. 49, July 1949, p. 52.

The U.S. Military Government organized three programs to evaluate the nutritional health of the German population. The first was a "street-weighing program." The *Kreisarzt*, or German district medical officer, weighed random population samples each month in cities within the U.S. zone with populations of 10,000 or greater. The second was a "school-weighing program" in which schools within the U.S. zone recorded the average weights and heights of children. The third program involved the deployment of nutrition survey teams to those cities with a population of greater than 25,000. The teams compiled information on weight, height, and diet, and took blood samples for laboratory analysis.[31] Health officials in the U.S. Military Government collected the information from all three programs, assessed the nutritional health of the German population, and supervised efforts to ameliorate malnutrition.

The most significant postwar sanitation tasks included alleviating severe water shortages, improving access to safe water supplies, inspecting refugees and refugee stations, and controlling the number of rats and other pests. Shortages of water pumps, materials, and labor slowed improvements to the water system. A lack of transportation, fuel, and tires interfered with garbage and refuse collection.[32]

Local German authorities organized most reconstruction and chlorination of the water supply, though Military Government officials assisted in a number of small towns in the U.S. sector. Financial assistance from the European Recovery Program, the U.S. program to help rebuild European nations after World War II, was critical in helping city governments clear their rubble and improve sanitation conditions.[33] U.S. and German health authorities established 68 refugee centers throughout Germany to process refugees, disinfect them

---

[31] Office of Military Government for Germany, *Public Health and Medical Affairs*, No. 18, November 1–December 31, 1946, pp. 4–6.

[32] Office of Military Government for Germany, *Public Health and Medical Affairs*, No. 12, July 20, 1946, pp. 45, and No. 28, August–September 1947, p. 11.

[33] Jeffry M. Diefendorf, "America and the Rebuilding of Urban Germany," in Jeffry M. Diefendorf, Axel Frohn, and Hermann-Josef Rupieper, *American Policy and the Reconstruction of West Germany, 1945–1955*, New York: Cambridge University Press, 1993, p. 350.

with DDT powder, and inspect them for infectious diseases.[34] The United States initially established a program of rodent and pest control under the supervision of the German Land Health Officer in Greater Hesse and then expanded the program to the rest of the U.S. sector.[35] A civilian mosquito control program, inaugurated in Berlin in June 1946, utilized power spray units mounted on trucks and barges.[36]

Many of the vaccination programs that existed before World War II disappeared during the war, making it critical that new programs be set up after the war. The U.S. Military Government targeted refugees, displaced persons, and children, in addition to the general population. Health officials spent significant resources vaccinating people at zonal border control stations, where high rates of infectious diseases were diagnosed.[37] As Figure 2.5 illustrates, U.S. and German health authorities vaccinated the general population for smallpox, diphtheria, typhoid fever, and scarlet fever over the course of reconstruction. By early 1946, the Military Government handed over operation of the vaccination program to German federal and Laender health authorities.

Disease rates generally declined over the course of reconstruction, and usually to below pre-war levels. As Figure 2.6 highlights, these included diphtheria, dysentery, and whooping cough. By 1949, disease rates were declining for almost all infectious diseases except scarlet fever. In several cases, such as tuberculosis and typhoid fever,

---

[34] Frederiksen, *The American Military Occupation of Germany*, p. 109; Office of Military Government for Germany, *Public Health and Medical Affairs*, No. 14, September 20, 1946, p. 3, and No. 10, May 20, 1946, p. 1.

[35] Office of Military Government for Germany, *Public Health and Medical Affairs*, No. 10, May 20, 1946, p. 5.

[36] Office of Military Government for Germany, *Public Health and Medical Affairs*, No. 14, September 20, 1946, p. 3.

[37] Office of Military Government for Germany, *Public Health and Medical Affairs*, No. 14, September 20, 1946, p. 3; No. 18, November 1–December 31, 1946, p. 3; No. 10, May 20, 1946, p. 4.

Figure 2.5
Cumulative Vaccination Rates, Germany, 1946–1948

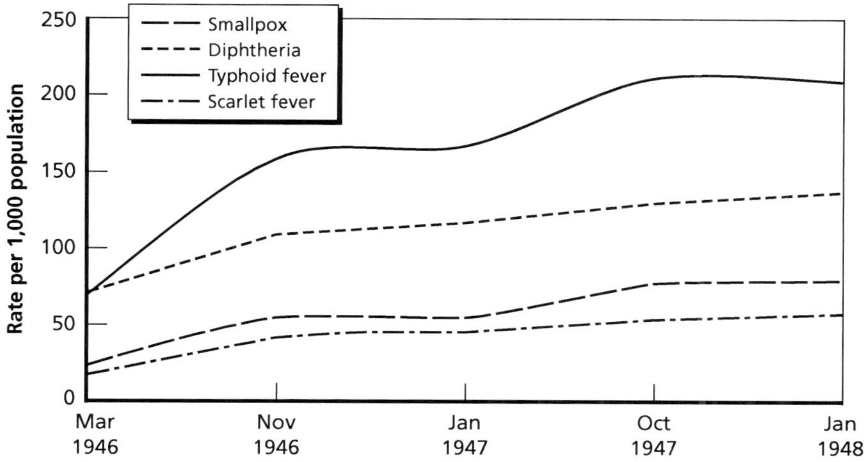

SOURCE: Office of Military Government for Germany, *Statistical Annex,* various, 1946–1948.

RAND *MG321-2.5*

disease rates increased during reconstruction and then fell by the end of the decade. Tuberculosis was a significant problem because of the shortage of hospital facilities for treating active cases. While the Military Government encouraged the German civil authorities to expand hospital beds for isolation and treatment of tuberculosis patients, there was little improvement during the occupation.[38] Typhoid fever was also a problem. In 1946, for example, an epidemic of typhoid fever, caused by the contamination of a central water supply, occurred in Bavaria, leading to 380 cases and 35 deaths. U.S. and German authorities coordinated the response and used a number of control measures, including quarantine, hyperchlorination of the water

---

[38] Office of Military Government for Germany, *Public Health and Medical Affairs,* No. 28, August–September 1947, p. 3, and No. 31, October–December 1947, pp. 3–5.

Figure 2.6
Disease Rates, Germany, 1938–1949

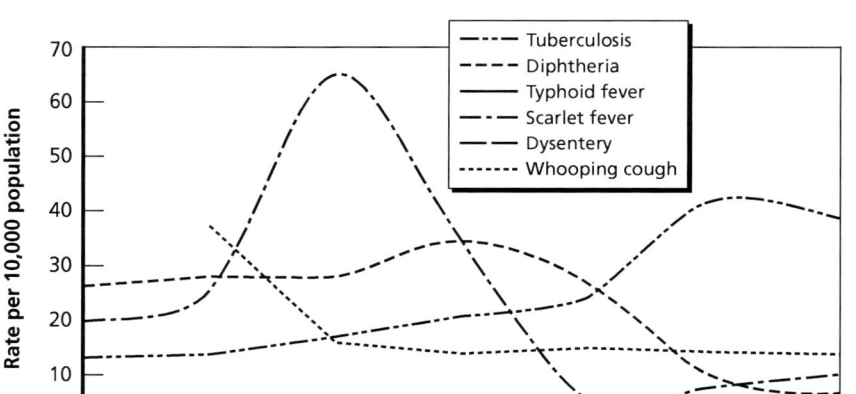

SOURCE: Office of Military Government for Germany, *Statistical Annex*, No. 49,
July 1949, p. 41.

RAND *MG321-2.6*

supply, immunization of the population, closing of schools, and prohibition of gatherings.[39]

Venereal diseases, such as syphilis and gonorrhea, significantly
increased in 1946 and 1947 and then dropped.[40] U.S. health officials
made a special effort to control the spread of venereal diseases among
the German population to safeguard the health of U.S. troops. In
August 1946, for example, they established a Venereal Disease Control Board to monitor the spread of venereal diseases. In addition,
U.S. European Command adopted a policy relieving the commander
of any U.S. military unit having a venereal disease rate that exceeded

---

[39] Office of Military Government for Germany, *Public Health and Medical Affairs*, No. 18,
November 1–December 31, 1946, p. 3.

[40] Office of Military Government for Germany, *Statistical Annex*, No. 49, July 1949, pp. 41,
49.

the average for U.S. European Command for three consecutive months.[41]

Figure 2.7 shows that the infant mortality rate rose significantly at the end of the war and then dropped to pre-war levels. Birth rate and mortality rate both remained largely unchanged.[42] Death rates for a number of major diseases also declined after the war, as Figure 2.8 illustrates. These included tuberculosis, diphtheria, poliomyelitis, scarlet fever, and whooping cough. The decline in mortality rates was likely caused by U.S. and German efforts to improve nutrition and sanitation conditions, as well as to vaccinate refugees, displaced persons, and the general population.

Figure 2.7
Mortality and Birth Rates, Germany, 1938–1949

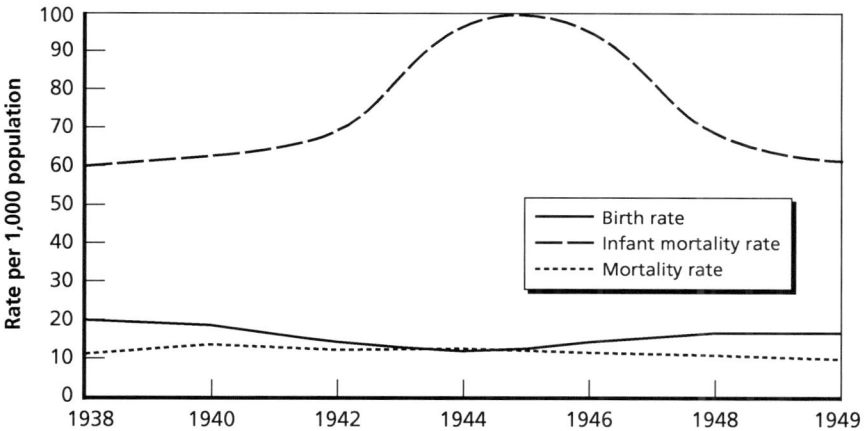

SOURCE: Office of Military Government for Germany, *Statistical Annex*, No. 49, March 1949, pp. 41–43.

RAND *MG321-2.7*

---

[41] Frederiksen, *The American Military Occupation of Germany*, p. 109.

[42] Office of Military Government for Germany, *Statistical Annex*, No. 48, June 1949, pp. 34–35.

Figure 2.8
Mortality Rate for Several Diseases, Germany, 1938–1949

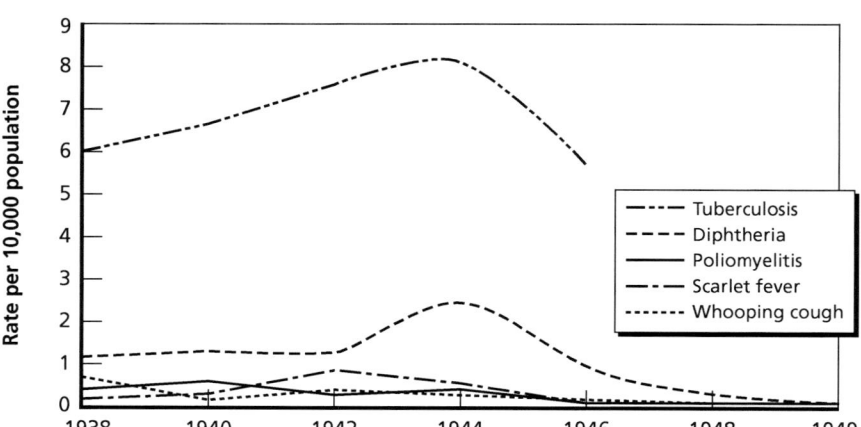

SOURCE: Office of Military Government for Germany, *Statistical Annex*, No. 49, July 1949, p. 41.

American efforts to ensure public safety were largely successful, thus facilitating the reconstruction of Germany's public health and health care delivery systems. U.S. forces in the U.S. sector suffered no casualties, despite initial concerns about German "werewolves," the irregular German units organized by Heinrich Himmler in 1944 to attack allied military forces and target Germans who cooperated with allied troops. These units disbanded shortly after the war ended.[43]

Soviet and Western military forces remained in Germany and adopted occupation duties after they defeated the *Wehrmacht*. In May 1945, the United States had 61 divisions and a total of 1.6 million soldiers in Germany. They manned border crossings, maintained checkpoints, and conducted patrols throughout the U.S. sector. Rapid demobilization quickly reduced the forces' levels, especially after the Japanese surrender in August. U.S. planners developed an Occupation Troop Basis goal of 404,500 for the following year,

---

[43] Perry Biddiscombe, Werwolf! *The History of the National Socialist Guerrilla Movement, 1944–1946*, Toronto: University of Toronto Press, 1998.

which was later reduced to 370,000. To meet both the Occupation Troop Basis goal and the security gap, the United States deployed a temporary constabulary force until a professional German police force could be trained and deployed.[44] The constabulary force was formally established in July 1946 and played an effective role in ensuring public safety.

In short, U.S. and German efforts to rebuild public health were largely successful. The nutritional health of Germans improved, sanitation conditions recovered, and mortality rates decreased to below pre-war levels in many instances. For some conditions, however, such as the incidence of tuberculosis and typhoid fever, the German population was worse off in 1949 than it had been before the war.

Health Care Delivery

Results in health care delivery were similarly positive. As Table 2.2 notes, bed capacity decreased in 1946 and then increased by 1947. The initial drop was probably caused by shortages in building materials and labor, which delayed the construction of new hospitals and the reconstruction of damaged and destroyed ones. As one OMGUS report concluded: "There is little prospect of any significant increase

Table 2.2
Civilian Hospital Beds, Germany

Beds	1945	1946	1947	1948
Number available	150,469	150,522	183,862	186,458
Number per 1,000 persons	9.9	9.3	10.1	10.0
Percent occupied	87.3	90	88.3	87.3

SOURCE: Office of Military Government, United States, *Statistical Annex*, No. 38, March 1948.

---

[44] On the U.S. constabulary force, see Earl F. Ziemke, *The U.S. Army in the Occupation of Germany, 1944–1946*, Washington, D.C.: U.S. Government Printing Office, 1990, pp. 339–341; Roy Licklider, "The American Way of State Building: Germany, Japan, Somalia, and Panama," *Small Wars and Insurgencies*, Vol. 10, No. 3, Winter 1999; Robert M. Perito, *Where Is the Lone Ranger When We Need Him? America's Search for a Postconflict Stability Force*, Washington D.C.: United States Institute of Peace, 2004, pp. 60–68.

in hospital capacity from major repairs of unused buildings or new construction, as materials and labor for such projects are not available," as well as that the increase in hospital beds was "barely keeping pace with the increase in population."[45] The assignment of some civilian hospital facilities for use by displaced persons also decreased the number of beds. Such policies as those contained in Joint Chiefs of Staff directive 1067 (JCS 1067) prohibited U.S. officials from rebuilding some infrastructure, such as destroyed or damaged houses, that would improve the German standard of living.[46] But assisting in the reconstruction of hospitals and hospital infrastructure fell under the JCS 1067 escape clause allowing measures to prevent "disease and unrest."[47]

The shortage of hospital buildings, beds, and other equipment in the initial postwar period hampered some programs, such as treatment of tuberculosis.[48] According to one OMGUS report, "The provision of additional hospital bed capacity for general hospitalization and for isolation and treatment of tuberculosis continues to be the most critical problem now facing German health authorities."[49] NGOs played an important role in increasing the number, quality, and bed capacity of health care facilities. Organizations such as Innere Mission, International Refugee Organization, and United Nations Relief and Rehabilitation Administration frequently built or refurbished hospitals. The U.S. military evacuated some hospitals for civilian use in 1945 and 1946, but many needed significant renova-

---

[45] Office of Military Government for Germany, *Public and Medical Affairs*, No. 28, August–September 1947, p. 15.

[46] Diefendorf, "America and the Rebuilding of Urban Germany," pp. 331–351.

[47] JCS 1067, "Directive to Commander in Chief of United States Forces of Occupation Regarding the Military Government of Germany" in *Occupation of Germany: Policy and Progress, 1945–1946*, Washington, D.C.: Department of State, Government Printing Office, August 1947, p. 155.

[48] Office of Military Government for Germany, *Public Health and Medical Affairs*, No. 10, May 20, 1946, p. 5; No. 14, September 20, 1946, p. 2; No. 18, November 1–December 31, 1946, p. 2.

[49] Office of Military Government for Germany, *Public Health and Medical Affairs*, No. 14, September 20, 1946, p. 4.

tions. For example, the U.S. Army handed over a hospital in Lesum to German authorities. It consisted of empty buildings that were partially stripped of necessary utilities, and Laender public health authorities believed that it would require nearly a year to renovate and equip. Innere Mission refurbished the hospital.[50] It also constructed makeshift hospitals for refugees and displaced persons and handed them over to German health authorities for general use when the number of refugees and internally displaced persons began to decline.[51]

The number of German physicians and other medical personnel was generally adequate during reconstruction (see Figure 2.9). However, since America's denazification process extended to doctors and other medical personnel, there was concern in the initial post-conflict period that there would be too few medical personnel. The March 1946 Law for Liberation from National Socialism and Militarism required every resident of the U.S. sector over 18 years old to submit a *Meldebogen*, a questionnaire that asked respondents to list their membership in National Socialist and military organizations.[52] Those with chargeable associations had to appear before local tribunals and could face fines, be sent to prison, or have their medical licenses revoked.[53] By May 1947, the Military Government and German authorities designated as "unacceptable" 4,055 physicians, 1,474 nurses, 1,965 dentists, and 1,793 other medical personnel because of their affiliation with the Nazi party or German military. Many had their licenses revoked, though half were retained and given temporary revocable

---

[50] Office of Military Government for Germany, *Public Health and Medical Affairs*, No. 31, October–December 1947, p. 14, and No. 28, August–September 1947, pp. 9–10.

[51] Office of Military Government for Germany, *Public Health and Medical Affairs*, No. 12, July 20, 1946, p. 6, and No. 9, April 20, 1946, p. 5.

[52] Ziemke, *The U.S. Army in the Occupation of Germany*, pp. 430–431.

[53] Office of Military Government for Germany, *Public Health and Medical Affairs*, No. 12, July 20, 1946, p. 1; No. 9, April 20, 1946, pp. 1–2; No. 10, May 20, 1946, pp. 1–2.

Figure 2.9
Number of Civilian Medical Personnel, Germany

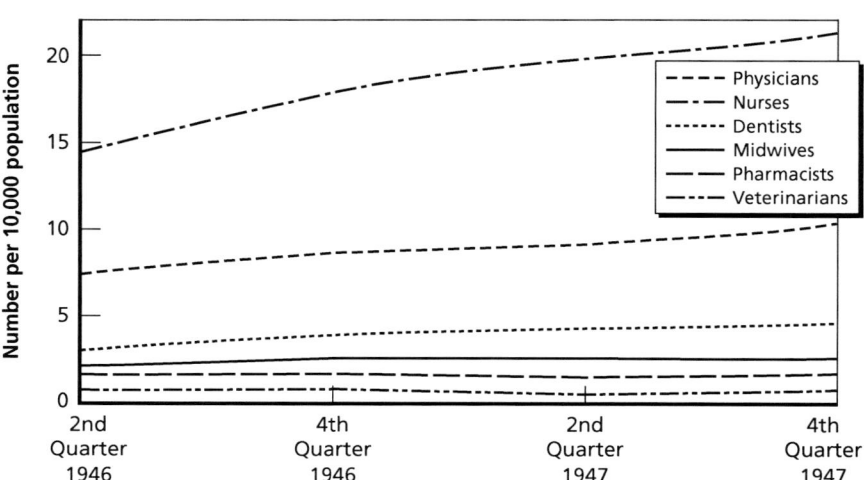

SOURCE: Office of Military Government for Germany, *Statistical Annex*, various, 1946–1948.

RAND *MG321-2.9*

licenses because of the need for health providers.[54] While the denazi-fication process did not adversely affect staffing levels for most medical personnel, it did cause some temporary personnel shortages among German Laender health authorities.[55]

Health authorities in the U.S. sector faced a temporary shortage of nurses from 1945 to 1947 because the prevalence of venereal disease, tuberculosis, and other conditions grew and thus increased the health care delivery load.[56] Nurse's aides supplemented the nursing staffs in most hospitals. By April 1946, the Military Government

---

[54] Office of Military Government for Germany, *Public Health and Medical Affairs*, No. 10, May 20, 1946, pp. 1, 8.

[55] Office of Military Government for Germany, *Public Health and Medical Affairs*, No. 28, August–September 1947, p. 1. Also see Office of Military Government for Germany, *Public Health and Medical Affairs*, No. 9, April 20, 1946, pp. 1–2, and No. 10, May 20, 1946, p. 1.

[56] Office of Military Government for Germany, *Public Health and Medical Affairs*, No. 31, October–December 1947, p. 14.

helped open 83 nursing schools in the U.S. sector, including ten in the U.S. sector of Berlin.[57] The Swiss Red Cross trained several hundred German nurses from the U.S. sector through a six-month postgraduate course. In some cases, local leaders shortened the two-year course requirement for general nurse training by six months to alleviate the shortage.[58]

Disease outbreaks occasionally caused U.S. and German health officials to seek outside help. In response to a 1947 poliomyelitis epidemic in Berlin, for example, German health officials requested the assistance of epidemiologists from the United States. The U.S. physicians flew to Berlin, where they advised German authorities on steps to improve control and treatment of the disease and offered instructions to German doctors and nurses on the latest developments in treatment. They also offered instructions on how to use respirators, which had not previously been used by German hospitals. The U.S. physicians visited Berlin hospitals and patients' homes, and they inspected environmental conditions surrounding the places of outbreak.[59]

There were increasing shortages of some essential medical supplies, such as soap, insulin, penicillin, and codeine. Between 1945 and 1947, a lack of domestic production in the U.S. sector, the depletion of current stocks, and an inability to import sufficient quantities of consumables created a problem. In addition, the distribution of consumables was hampered by a lack of vehicles for cargo transportation and shortages of motor fuel. In Baden-Württemberg, for example, 50 percent of ambulances were still inoperative in late 1946 because of a shortage of either tires or gasoline.[60]

---

[57] Office of Military Government for Germany, *Public Health and Medical Affairs*, No. 9, April 20, 1946, p. 4.

[58] Office of Military Government for Germany, *Public Health and Medical Affairs*, No. 31, October–December 1947, p. 14.

[59] Office of Military Government for Germany, *Public Health and Medical Affairs*, No. 28, August–September 1947, pp. 9–10.

[60] Office of Military Government for Germany, *Public Health and Medical Affairs*, No. 10, May 20, 1946, p. 2, and No. 14, September 20, 1946, pp. 1–2.

Acquiring supplies from captured *Wehrmacht* stockpiles made up some of the shortfall in medical supplies.[61] But when these stocks were depleted, their import became critical. The United States exported to Germany large quantities of insulin and penicillin, which were used for treating such venereal diseases as gonorrhea and syphilis. Joint U.S. and British funds were also used to import some consumables. When consumables could not be imported, alternatives for them were found. For example, U.S. and German health officials used sulfonamides in the absence of penicillin, though this often led to longer hospital stays and overcrowded hospitals.[62]

Shortages were particularly acute in the U.S. sector of Berlin, which required a constant supply of sanitary napkins, neosalvarsan,[63] dental x-ray films, disinfectants, and other medical supplies.[64] By late 1947, however, German production of most medical supplies— including insulin and penicillin—was sufficient, so imports were phased out.[65] One negative development was a rise in the number of illegal narcotics, which came from ex-*Wehrmacht* stocks that fell into the hands of traffickers prior to the war's end.[66] The Military Government helped set up a Narcotics Subcommittee of the Laenderrat Health Committee to keep zonal records of production and consumption; it also submitted periodic reports on narcotics traffic and regulated distribution.

---

[61] Office of Military Government for Germany, *Public Health and Medical Affairs*, No. 12, July 20, 1946, p. 2, and No. 28, August–September 1947, p. 16.

[62] Office of Military Government for Germany, *Public Health and Medical Affairs*, No. 18, November 1–December 31, 1946, p. 2.

[63] An arsenic-containing drug used historically for treating syphilis; it is now replaced by penicillin.

[64] Office of Military Government for Germany, *Public Health and Medical Affairs*, No. 28, August–September 1947, p. 16, and No. 14, September 20, 1946, p. 5.

[65] Office of Military Government for Germany, *Public Health and Medical Affairs*, No. 28, August–September 1947, p. 1, and No. 31, October–December 1947, p. 15.

[66] Office of Military Government for Germany, *Public Health and Medical Affairs*, No. 12, July 20, 1946, p. 5.

Overall Assessment

U.S. efforts to rebuild Germany's health system were largely successful. During World War II, the allied strategic bombing campaign and ground war destroyed much of Germany's public health and health care delivery systems. Allied planes damaged hospitals and the sanitation system, and war conditions increased the incidence of numerous diseases. However, American, German, and NGO efforts after the war were effective. By 1948, three years after World War II ended, the German health system was revived. Most public health and health care delivery indicators improved over the course of reconstruction. Examples include

- Improvement in the nutrition of German children and adults
- Enhancement of sanitation conditions through reconstruction and chlorination of the water supply, as well as rodent and pest control
- Increase in vaccination rates for infectious diseases
- Decline in most disease rates to below pre-war levels
- Improvement in mortality and birth rates
- Increase in the bed capacity of health facilities and in the number of physicians and other medical personnel
- Sufficient production of most medical supplies, such as insulin and penicillin.

Lessons Learned

At least four major lessons emerge from the U.S. effort in Germany. First, the ability to secure health partly depends on the condition of the public health and health care delivery systems *before* the post-conflict phase. This is an exogenous factor and beyond the control of outside actors. However, it is important to recognize that, all else being equal, it is generally easier to rebuild health systems in developed countries with high levels of human capital than in third-world countries. The point is not that governments, international institutions, and NGOs should not try to secure health in undeveloped countries post-conflict. Rather, it is that all parties must understand that there may be limitations, delays, and challenges inherent in third-world countries (such as Somalia) because they lack a developed infrastructure for public health and health care delivery systems. The health system that the United States encountered in Germany after World War II was well-organized, competent, and among the best in Europe—assets that contributed greatly to the success of U.S. efforts to rebuild health. Unfortunately, advantageous conditions such as this do not exist in most health reconstruction efforts.

Second, coordination is critical for ensuring efficient health reconstruction. OMGUS was established to oversee the rebuilding of the U.S. sector in Germany. As such, it coordinated efforts with local, Laender, and national health officials, as well as with such NGOs as CARE, Council of Relief Agencies Licensed for Operation in Germany, Red Cross, and United Nations Relief and Rehabilitation Administration. When an epidemic of typhoid fever occurred in Bavaria in 1946, for example, American, German, and NGO officials effectively coordinated the response. They took such measures as quarantine, hyperchlorination of the water supply, immunization of the population, closing of schools, and prohibition of gatherings to control the epidemic from spreading.

Third, ensuring public safety and security greatly facilitates reconstruction. U.S. efforts to ensure public safety were largely successful in Germany, which is not the case in later U.S. efforts in Somalia, Afghanistan, and Iraq. Despite initial concerns about German "werewolves" and National Socialist guerrilla groups, U.S. forces in the German sector suffered no casualties from hostile attacks. A number of factors probably contributed to the stable security environment: the existence of 1.6 million U.S. soldiers in Germany in 1945, the fact that the German population was exhausted and many German cities had been reduced to rubble by the nearly six years of war, and the clear and unconditional surrender by German leaders. The benign security environment greatly facilitated health reconstruction efforts: There was freedom of movement to health care facilities and hospitals, health facilities were able to rely on steady supplies of water and power because insurgents did not target critical infrastructure, and NGOs faced no security problems in delivering emergency relief.

Fourth, shifting health responsibilities to local authorities, when possible, can improve the development of self-sustaining health care capacities. The Public Health Branch of OMGUS's Civil Administration division initially operated and controlled the German public health and health care delivery systems. But the United States gradually shifted responsibilities to German authorities over the course of reconstruction. By January 1948, German federal and Laender health authorities took over full responsibility for health services. The U.S. Military Government retained responsibilities in connection with narcotics control and the venereal disease control program for the duration of the occupation, and it continued to observe, inspect, advise, and report on health activities. The shift in health responsibilities to German authorities contributed to the establishment of a self-sufficient and sustainable health system.

CHAPTER THREE

Japan

The war in the Pacific ended on August 15, 1945, when the Japanese emperor broadcast a radio address calling for his subjects to "endure the unendurable." The formal articles of surrender were signed aboard the battleship USS *Missouri* by representatives of the emperor and the Japanese military on September 2, 1945, with General Douglas MacArthur and Fleet Admiral Chester Nimitz present.

The stated mission of the Public Health and Welfare section of the allied occupation of Japan was to safeguard the security and health of the occupation forces. But once begun, this mission expanded in scope and import to include responsibility for improving the health and welfare of the local impacted community. As in Germany, the task was monumental. Vast swaths of Japan's urban landscape had been reduced to ash and rubble. Two cities had been utterly destroyed by atomic bombs. Most others, including the capital, Tokyo, had been devastated by incendiary bombings. The health of much of the population was precarious. Also as in Germany, however, the occupation authorities could focus on reconstructing and reforming pre-war institutions and practices rather than creating them from scratch. Pre-war Japan had not attained Germany's levels of public health and health care delivery, but it had strived to do so, basing much of its health infrastructure on German models regarded as Europe's most advanced at the time.[1]

---

[1] See Graig, *Health of Nations,* 1999, p. 97, for a brief history of the foreign influences on the initial development of modern medical care in Japan.

Japan's relatively late entry into the race to modernize had also laid the groundwork for the future success of the occupation efforts. In its attempts to join the elite group of advanced nations quickly, Japan had scoured the globe for the best models to emulate. The government had dispatched several missions to study the most-modern and most-effective forms of governmental organization and administration; it had also imported foreign experts. The combination of overseas missions and invited experts contributed significantly to the development and modernization of Japan, including its health care system. This receptivity to foreign models and to the advice of foreign experts prepared Japan to respond in constructive ways to suggested and required changes during the occupation.

The occupation authorities in Japan had to contend with one other stark difference not faced by other attempts at nation-building. Japan had suffered two atomic bombings: in Hiroshima and in Nagasaki. In many ways, the effects on public health and health care delivery in these two cities were merely magnified versions of the effects in cities hit with incendiary bombs. But the atomic bombings' psychological and physical effects on the affected populations endured far longer.

Despite these challenges, the U.S. effort to rebuild Japan's public health and health care delivery was quite successful. The result of the Japanese occupation is one of the great success stories in America's attempts at nation-building—an achievement once considered singular and now regarded as a model. This chapter focuses on the factors that accounted for this outcome and how it was accomplished.

Historical Context

Japan's pre-war public health administration focused mainly on combating acute epidemics of communicable diseases, tuberculosis, and high infant mortality rates. Following the establishment of a Health Bureau in 1873, the Japanese government took several measures to control and prevent infectious diseases and manage sanitation. For example, the Tuberculosis Prevention Law was passed in 1919 and a

National Health Insurance Law was enacted in 1922.[2] Private social welfare agencies initiated a school lunch program for malnourished children in 1929.[3]

Japan continued to make progress in the area of health care through the 1920s and 1930s. In 1938 alone, the Japanese government organized the Ministry of Public Health and Social Welfare; passed an additional National Health Insurance Law (requiring local governments to offer coverage to those groups not covered under the 1922 law); and opened 50 health centers throughout Japan to provide health education, operate clinics for maternal and child hygiene, and diagnose and treat tuberculosis.[4] In 1931, Japan had 3,710 hospitals with a total of 204,903 beds for a population of 64.5 million. By 1940, that number had increased to 4,732 with almost one doctor and two nurses for every 1,000 Japanese. However, as Figure 3.1 highlights, by 1945 the bed capacity and the number of doctors and nurses had significantly plummeted. Similarly, as Figure 3.2 shows, the number of hospitals and clinics showed a precipitous drop.

There were inadequacies in the system, however. Japan's Ministry of Health and Social Welfare, an arm of the national government, exercised little control over the largely autonomous prefectural governments. At the local level, responsibilities were vested in cities, towns, and village authorities, which could adopt their own local public health ordinances. The Ministry of Health and Social Welfare's authority was further limited by the fact that the Ministry of Home Affairs, through the police, retained supervisory authority over doctors, dentists, midwives, nurses, masseurs, druggists, prostitutes, and the insane. The Ministry of Home Affairs also oversaw the sale,

---

[2] Japanese Ministry of Health, Labor and Welfare, *White Paper: Annual Report on Health and Welfare 1998–1999*.

[3] Crawford F. Sams, *Medic: The Mission of an American Military Doctor in Occupied Japan and Wartorn Korea*, Zabelle Zakarian (ed.), New York: M.E. Sharpe, 1998, p. 63.

[4] Occupation authorities did not rate these centers highly. They found the centers' services rudimentary and the directors ignorant of the health status of the populations they served because their statistics and training were inadequate.

Figure 3.1
Trends of Doctors, Nurses, and Bed Capacity, Japan

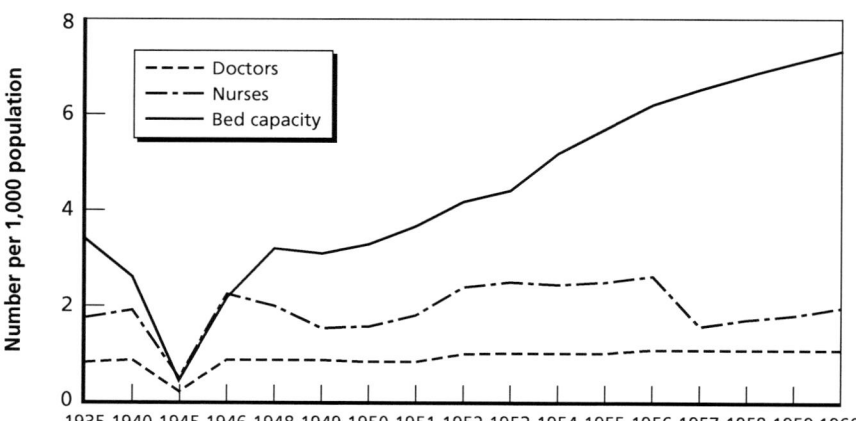

SOURCES: Population information and information on doctors, nurses, and bed capacity for all years except 1935 from Japanese Ministry of Health, Labor and Welfare, *Vital Statistics*. Information for 1935 from United States Strategic Bombing Survey, *The Effects of Bombing on Health and Medical Services in Japan*.
RAND *MG321-3.1*

commercial preparation, and consumption of food. Furthermore, police supervised the biannual cleanup campaigns of private homes and businesses carried out by neighborhood sanitary teams (*eisei kumiai*), and they controlled the collection of vital statistics.[5]

In addition, the health care system remained rigidly stratified. It provided only rudimentary care to the bulk of the population, which continued to follow certain pre-modern practices.[6] Although the graduates of imperial universities and their affiliated medical schools

---

[5] United States Strategic Bombing Survey, *The Effects of Bombing on Health and Medical Services in Japan,* Medical Division, Dates of Survey: 24 October–31 November 1945, Washington, D.C.: War Department, June 1947. p. 2.

[6] For example, before World War II, almost all children in Japan were born at home instead of in hospitals. Since the Japanese historically considered childbirth an unclean event, childbirth often was relegated to dirty, dark, and cold places, such as a shed or a barn. Perhaps unsurprisingly, puerperal fever and infectious diseases in newborns were common neonatal problems at that time.

Figure 3.2
Trends of Hospitals and Clinics, Japan

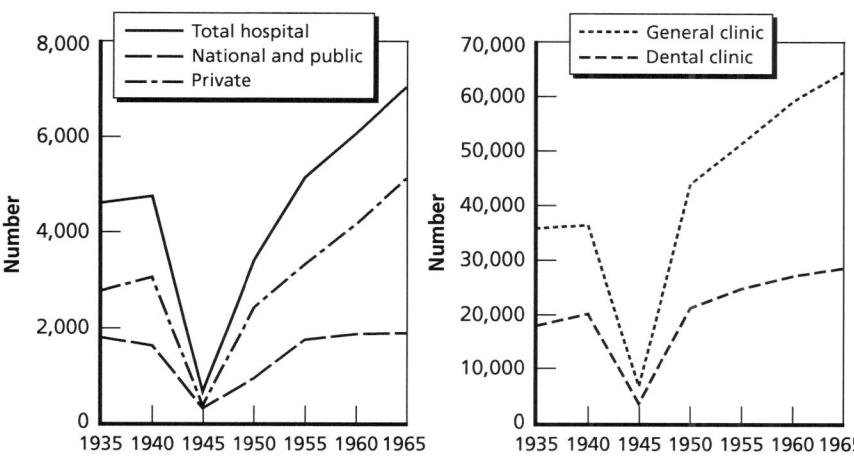

SOURCE: Japanese Ministry of Health, Labor and Welfare, *White Paper: Annual Report on Health and Welfare 1998–1999.*
RAND *MG321-3.2*

were well educated, the large majority of public health officials and public health nurses did not receive adequate training. Thus, even though the numbers of physicians per 10,000 population increased steadily before the outbreak of hostilities, medical care for the general public did not improve accordingly.

Competent care was largely available only in urban areas.[7] Workers in large-scale, modern industries received medical care through their employers. Because small, private hospitals provided the bulk of the care, rural dwellers and unskilled urban workers could often not afford medical care even if it was available nearby.[8] Japan's

---

[7] American experts who examined the local public health system following the war found the local staff incompetent, inexperienced, and unable or unwilling to administer basic health and sanitation. For details on the historical development of health care in Japan, see General Headquarters, Supreme Commander for the Allied Powers, Public Welfare and Health Section, *Public Health and Welfare in Japan,* Annual Summary, 1948.

[8] United States Strategic Bombing Survey, *The Effects of Bombing on Health and Medical Services in Japan,* p. 3.

crude death and infant mortality rates (see Figure 3.3) showed some improvement over the 1930 rates, but even just before the war they were quite high compared with the U.S. rates.[9]

Health Challenges

Crawford F. Sams, who oversaw the reconstruction of Japan's health sector, wrote: "It was a challenge in mere magnitude of numbers and lack of means for meeting the problem that I had not seen equaled in

Figure 3.3
Change in Health Indicators over Time, Japan

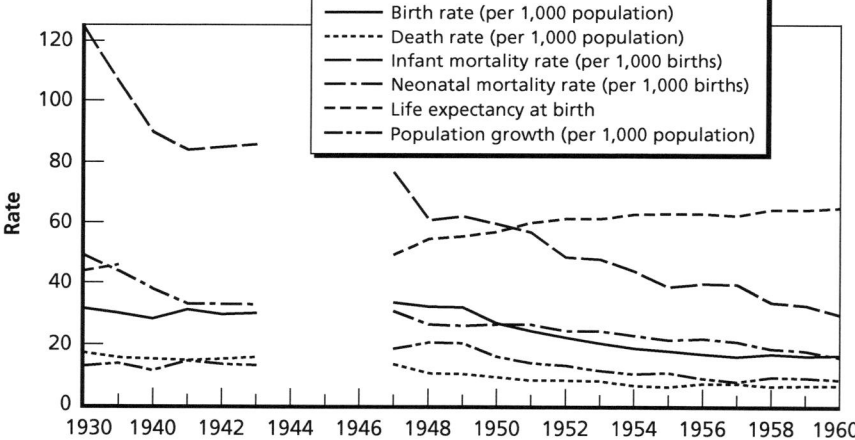

SOURCE: Japanese Ministry of Health, Labor and Welfare, *Vital Statistics*. Data of Okinawa prefecture not included; gaps caused by lack of reliable data for subject years.

RAND *MG321-3.3*

---

[9] For example, Japan's death and infant mortality rates in 1930 were 18.2 and 124.1 per 1,000, respectively, whereas those of the United States were 11.6 and 69 per 1,000. Similarly, average life expectancy in Japan from 1926 to 1930 was 44.82 years, compared with 59.7 years in America. Data on the United States are from the U.S. Census Bureau.

Europe or elsewhere in the world where I had lived and worked."[10]
The occupation was confronted with two immediate public health
challenges: controlling so-called wildfire diseases and providing direct
relief to displaced people. Aid to the victims of the atomic bombings
would also have to be provided.

Public Health

The long conflict had a profound, negative effect on Japan's health
care system and the overall health status of the Japanese people. This
resulted because of lack of maintenance and because of bomb damage
to hospitals, housing, sewage systems, water plants, and other physical
infrastructure. The interruption in vaccination programs and other
public health interventions caused by wartime disruptions and shortages also had a detrimental effect on overall public health. The national food distribution system had collapsed, leaving many without
adequate food. The population's poor nutritional state increased susceptibility to tuberculosis and other endemic diseases. An uprooted
population seeking food and shelter compounded these problems. An
estimated 8.5 million people had lost their homes in the cities because of American bombing raids. Another 6.5 million were to be
repatriated from Japan's former overseas colonies.[11] And 1.2 million
Koreans were attempting to return to Korea. With millions of homeless refugees moving about the country, the conditions were ripe for
the rapid spread of dysentery, typhoid, typhus, smallpox, and parasite
infections. Food, shelter, clothing, and bedding needed to be provided until these refugees and displaced persons could reestablish
themselves.

Yet the public health situation was not as dire as it might have
been had the Americans opted for explosive rather than incendiary
bombs. Those conducting post-conflict surveys reported the damage
from incendiary bombing of most of Japan's major population centers (including Tokyo, Yokohama, Kobe, and Osaka) as having been

---

[10] Sams, *Medic,* p. 31.

[11] Sams, *Medic,* p. 31.

"peculiarly ineffective" in terms of direct effects on Japan's health and sanitation.[12] Although tens of thousands of people died in the firestorms, the destruction by fire of large urban areas effectively "sterilized" them, destroying rats, mice, lice, fleas, and other vectors of disease along with the human victims. Thus, survivors did not suffer from dramatically elevated levels of contagious or enteric diseases.

Fire bombing also had minimal effects on water delivery and sewage disposal. Few Japanese cities, including those with populations over 100,000, were equipped with sewers in the 1930s and 1940s. Instead, the Japanese systematically collected human waste and distributed it to farms for use as fertilizer. This method of disposal caused Japanese water sources to be relatively less polluted than those in the United States and Europe at the time, thus reducing the incidence of waterborne and infectious diseases that could be attributed to wartime destruction during and following the conflict. The high prevalence of dysentery, *ekiri* (infant dysentery), typhoid, and paratyphoid fevers was attributed, instead, to food being contaminated by the use of human excreta as fertilizer and by flies in summer.[13]

Health Care Delivery
During World War II, the military's dominance of all aspects of life in Japan reduced the state's ability to administer and deliver health care services to its citizens. The nation's wartime concentration on military requirements led to the physical deterioration of hospitals and other medical institutions. As an emergency mobilization measure, Japan had set up the Medical Treatment Corporation to oversee and manage all hospitals. One of the challenges for occupation authorities was to dismantle this corporation and either return the hospitals to their original ownership or establish new ownership.

---

[12] United States Strategic Bombing Survey, *The Effects of Bombing on Health and Medical Services in Japan*, p. 4.

[13] United States Strategic Bombing Survey, *The Effects of Bombing on Health and Medical Services in Japan*, p. 6. According to Sams, the Japanese had no DDT at the time and had never attempted modern insect control methods. See Sams, *Medic*, p. 14.

Many factories previously engaged in the production of medical and sanitary supplies had been converted to war material production. The war also cut off Japanese scientists from overseas developments in medicine and other related fields. At the time of the surrender, Japan thus had limited clinical and educational facilities, lacked adequate professional medical personnel to serve the civilian population, and was widely believed to be about a decade behind in terms of modern medical practice. Table 3.1 compares Japan's health care delivery capabilities for 1940 and 1945.

Japan also faced a shortage of serviceable hospitals. Out of 4,000 hospitals, 1,027, including 469 military hospitals, had been destroyed by fire bombs and high explosives.[14] This loss was equivalent to one in every four hospitals. Only 2,852 hospitals with the capacity for more than 20 beds remained in operation. In addition, 320 Army and Navy hospitals were serving 78,000 war casualties. These remaining hospitals were generally filthy and lacked fuel, medical equipment, drugs, and x-ray films. Moreover, it was customary for a hospitalized patient's family to provide nursing services, including meals, so wards were full of family members living, cooking, and sleeping at patients' bedsides. This practice added to the unsanitary conditions.

Table 3.1
Health Care Delivery, Japan, 1940 and 1945

Health Care Delivery	1940	1945
Hospitals	4,732	645
General clinics	36,416	6,607
Hospital beds	204,903	46,924
Doctors	65,332	12,812
Nurses	138,341	35,062

SOURCE: Information on doctors, nurses, and facilities from General Headquarters, Supreme Commander for the Allied Powers, Public Welfare and Health Section, *Public Health and Welfare in Japan*, Annual Summary, 1948.

---

[14] Sams, *Medic*, pp. 28–29.

Another issue confronting the occupation and reconstruction was the devastation in the two Japanese cities that had been subjected to atomic bombing. In Hiroshima, 30 percent of the population had been killed outright, and 30 percent had been seriously injured. Within the city limits, shelter was virtually nonexistent. Only two small hospitals had withstood the bombing and the firestorms that followed, and medical supplies had been nearly totally destroyed. Only 10 percent of the doctors emerged unscathed, and 1,654 of the 1,780 nurses in Hiroshima were killed or injured (Table 3.2).[15] Nagasaki fared somewhat better because of its geography, but medical facilities suffered disproportionately because they were concentrated near the epicenter. Approximately 80 percent of hospital beds were damaged beyond repair, including those at University Hospital, the Medical College, and the Tuberculosis Sanitorium.[16] Exact figures on casualties among medical personnel in Nagasaki do not exist, but it is believed that nearly all the medical students and most of the faculty of Nagasaki Medical College were killed or injured in the bombing.[17] Many of the survivors suffered from severe radiation burns and

Table 3.2
Health Care Delivery in Hiroshima, Before and After Atomic Bomb

	Before August 6, 1945	After August 6, 1945
Doctors	200	30
Nurses	1,780	126
Hospitals	45	3

SOURCE: United States Strategic Bombing Survey, *The Effects of Atomic Bombs*, Chairman's Office, June 30, 1946.

---

[15] United States Strategic Bombing Survey, *The Effects of Atomic Bombs on Health and Medical Services in Hiroshima and Nagasaki*, Medical Division, Washington, D.C.: War Department, March 1947, p. 21.

[16] United States Strategic Bombing Survey, *The Effects of Atomic Bombs on Health and Medical Services in Hiroshima and Nagasaki*, p. 20.

[17] United States Strategic Bombing Survey, *The Effects of Atomic Bombs on Health and Medical Services in Hiroshima and Nagasaki*, p. 21.

radiation-induced illnesses that the Japanese in the afflicted areas were ill equipped to handle.

In sum, the war resulted in a nearly complete breakdown of public health and welfare functions. Bombing combined with shortages and neglect to reduce the health and sanitation infrastructure. According to reports by the General Headquarters of the Supreme Commander of the Allied Powers, the arriving occupation forces found the Japanese public health and welfare activities to be in a very demoralized state.

Health Approach and Assessment

This section first outlines key participants in and donors to the U.S. health reconstruction efforts carried out in Japan after the war. It then examines U.S.-led efforts to rebuild Japan's public health and health care delivery systems and provides an overall assessment of the efforts.

Key Participants and Donors

The final terms of surrender stated that the Japanese government would be subject to the Supreme Commander of the Allied Powers (SCAP), General Douglas MacArthur. The Americans recognized no legal constraint on the range and extent of their authority, with the exception of international law governing the proper treatment of civilians.

General Headquarters SCAP was established in Tokyo on October 2, 1945. Though its name implied it represented the allied powers, SCAP was directed by and reported to the U.S. government from the start of the occupation.[18] The initial directives to MacArthur outlining the scope and conduct of the occupation were prepared by the State, War, and Navy Coordinating Committee

---

[18] Later it became technically responsible to the Far East Commission (FEC), which was made up of members of all the allied powers. But the FEC's location in Washington, D.C., served to limit its power.

(SWNCC) within the U.S. government. Entitled "United States Initial Post-Surrender Policy Relating to Japan" (SWNCC 150/4), the main directive outlined an ambitious program of political and economic democratization.

The Japanese government was left intact, and SCAP was designed as a supervisory overlay. The various staff sections of SCAP were organized to reflect the functions of the ministries of the Japanese government that they would initially oversee. SCAP was staffed largely by American civil servants and by military officers who converted to civilian status. At its peak, in 1948, it employed about 3,500 people, although only about one-quarter of those were actively involved in administering the reform program. The staff for the Public Health and Welfare section never exceeded 150 people.[19]

Colonel Crawford F. Sams, a career army doctor with extensive experience in public health and disease control, was named Chief of the Public Health and Welfare section of SCAP. As such, his duties included preventive medicine, medical care, welfare, and social security. In addition, he had principal interest in the education and training of those engaged in health and welfare fields, such as medicine, dentistry, pharmacy, veterinary medicine, nursing, nutrition, and social work. Sams also retained an interest in the pharmaceutical and medical supply industries, although control fell within the purview of the Economics and Scientific section of the SCAP bureaucracy.[20] During his tenure, Sams's power exceeded that of the Japanese Minister of Health and Welfare (*Kosei Daijin*).[21]

The directive that Washington issued to Public Health and Welfare charged it with safeguarding the security and health of the occupation forces by preventing widespread disease and unrest among the

---

[19] Because of a shortage of medical personnel in the armed forces in 1946, Sams resorted to placing personnel ads, at his own expense, in professional journals to recruit civilian doctors, nurses, and sanitation engineers. See Sams, *Medic*, pp. 35–36.

[20] Sams, *Medic*, p. 34.

[21] Sey Nishimura makes this point in his article, "The U.S. Medical Occupation of Japan and History of the Japanese-Language Edition of JAMA," *Journal of American Medical Association*, Vol. 274, No. 5, August 2, 1995, pp. 436–438.

Japanese populace. Once viewed as an adjunct to the larger and more important occupation goals of democratization and demilitarization, the nationwide provision of health care services came to be seen, under the guidance of Sams, as an integral part of the democratization process.[22] Sams summed up the rationale underpinning this work in a 1951 speech given shortly after the signing of the peace treaty that ended the occupation:

> I know of nothing more important in demonstrating to the people of Japan and other nations of the world—particularly those in the Far East—what we mean by the worth of the individual, which we consider to be the essence of democracy, than the literal gift of life which the occupation has brought some 3,000,000 Japanese who would have died between 1945 and 1951 had these modern programs not been established and had the prewar death rate continued at its normal level.[23]

International aid organizations, still relatively few at the time, played only a minor role in providing relief in occupied Japan. Those that did provide aid did so under the supervision and with the permission of SCAP. The International Committee of the Red Cross provided some immediate medical assistance and aid, especially in Hiroshima and Nagasaki. American relief organizations, religious groups, and other agencies wishing to send food, clothing, and medical aid to Japan were eventually organized within an umbrella organization called Licensed Agencies for Relief in Asia (LARA). Their donations were shipped on government transport to Japan, where the Public Health and Welfare section oversaw distribution. In August 1947, CARE (Cooperative for American Remittances to Europe) was also granted permission to ship packages to Japan under a similar ar-

---

[22] Zabelle Zakarian, the editor of Crawford Sam's *Medic*, points out in her introduction to the book that Sams firmly believed there was no clearer demonstration of the value of individuals—a concept necessary to the functioning of a democracy—than controlling communicable diseases and otherwise improving the health status of individuals.

[23] From a speech given in 1951 by Crawford Sams at a meeting of the American Public Health Association in San Francisco shortly after the peace treaty with Japan was concluded. Quoted in Sams, *Medic*, p. xv.

rangement. Initially, UNICEF (the United Nations Children's Emergency Relief Fund at the time) was prohibited from providing relief in former enemy countries. However, when Sams heard that UNICEF was shipping powdered skim milk to Germany, he immediately set about to obtain shipments for use in Japan's school lunch program.[24]

Public Health

The immediate concerns of Sams and his staff in 1945 were to assess the state of the health care system in Japan, to deal with the humanitarian crisis, and to respond quickly to stem the spread of infectious diseases.

Refugees and Population Movement. Roughly 2.5 million homes were destroyed in Japan during the war. To escape the bombing, 8 million individuals relocated to the relative safety of the countryside. Once hostilities ended, these people began to return to the cities and what remained of their homes. With the breakdown of the food rationing system, there was a nearly constant movement of people from cities to farms in search of food. In addition, 6.5 million Japanese colonists returned to Japan from China and Southeast Asia in the years immediately following the war.

In overseeing the return of refugees, Public Health and Welfare contemplated several approaches, including the establishment of large refugee camps. Sams firmly opposed such camps; he believed they created a permanent class of dependent people. He elected to disburse the refugees throughout Japan in smaller communities where they could grow their own food, the hope being to thereby enable them to achieve self-sufficiency more rapidly. The goal was also to keep them from returning to the destroyed cities before an infrastructure to support them could be rebuilt. To this end, Sams asked MacArthur to issue a population movement order prohibiting the return of refugees

---

[24] Sams, *Medic,* pp. 164–165.

to select cities unless they had employment or a guaranteed residence.[25]

The dispersal of refugees throughout the country was logistically more challenging than setting up a few large camps, because it necessitated that a nationwide relief organization be established for the distribution of food, clothing, medical care, and preventive medicine. The Japanese government was responsible for providing food, clothing, shelter, medical care, and means of subsistence to the indigent population, which numbered about 14.5 million at the end of 1945. Supplies for this effort came initially from food and clothing stocks confiscated from the Imperial Army and Navy.[26]

Atomic Bomb Victims. Because of how severe the effects of the atomic bombs were, the United States was hesitant to send U.S. military personnel into the affected areas, in part due to fears that they might incite mob violence.[27] U.S. scientists associated with the Manhattan Project, however, were eager to visit Hiroshima to assess the effects of the bomb on both property and humans. When the American occupation authorities began to arrive, the International Committee of the Red Cross informed Sams of the dire medical conditions in Hiroshima. He decided to send seven planeloads of surplus medical supplies by troop transport and to allow the scientists, under the direction of General Thomas F. Farrell, to accompany those supplies, ostensibly to aid in their distribution. During the first six months of the occupation, a number of other groups traveled to Japan to survey the bomb damage.[28] Eventually, in November 1946, the Atomic Bomb Casualty Commission (ABCC) was established to study the effects of atomic bombs on humans for all interested agen-

---

[25] The order lasted until 1949. Although Sams believed the public health justifications for such an order had disappeared by 1947, the Japanese government decided to extend the order for two more years.

[26] Sams, *Medic*, p. 159.

[27] See Sams, *Medic,* p. 20. Eventually, troops from the British Commonwealth were used.

[28] They included the Atomic Energy Commission, the Joint Commission on Atomic Effects, the U.S. Public Health Service, the Strategic Bomb Survey, the Army Medical Corps Intelligence, and the Navy Medical Corps Intelligence.

cies. Subsequently, a Japanese counterpart organization was established under Japan's National Institute of Health.

Actual treatment of survivors was left largely to the Japanese themselves, who initially treated the victims with vitamins, liver extract, and blood transfusions.[29] Allied doctors eventually brought in penicillin and plasma, but the slow and inadequate treatment of victims undoubtedly contributed to the high casualty rates in the aftermath of the bombing. Many died of secondary diseases, such as pneumonia and tuberculosis, because of malnutrition and lowered resistance.[30] As was common at the time, those people who took part in ABCC's human subject research did not receive free medical care in return for their participation. Some medical personnel were reported to have provided free medical care anyway; but it was officially discouraged, in part because of concern that it would be equivalent to accepting U.S. responsibility for the victims' suffering.

Water and Sanitation. At the start of the occupation, tuberculosis was the most deadly disease in Japan and enteric diseases were the second most deadly. Enteric diseases, which included dysentery, typhoid and paratyphoid, and poliomyelitis, were taken seriously by the occupation authorities. Only six Japanese cities had modern water supply systems with sewage treatment plants, and bomb damage meant these systems supplied only a part of any given city's population. About 75 percent of the population obtained water from streams or shallow wells that were sometimes contaminated. Flies were another vector of disease.[31] In 1945, 96,500 cases of dysentery were reported, and they led to over 20,000 deaths. In addition,

---

[29] United States Strategic Bombing Survey, *The Effects of Atomic Bombs on Health and Medical Services in Hiroshima and Nagasaki,* p. 19.

[30] Sams reportedly learned that the Japanese believed 80 percent of the 47,000 deaths in Hiroshima in the six months following the bombing resulted from inadequate treatment and lack of supplies. See Sey Nishimura, "Censorship of the Atomic Bomb Casualty Report in Occupied Japan," *Journal of American Medical Association,* Vol. 274, No. 7, August 16, 1995, pp. 520–522.

[31] Sams, *Medic,* p. 92.

58,000 cases of typhoid and 10,000 cases of paratyphoid were re-ported.[32]

Sams believed that the way to combat these enteric diseases was to set up a program to improve the sanitary standards for the entire nation.[33] But occupation authorities were handicapped by the fact that they could locate only two sanitary engineers in Japan at the time, neither of whom was working in his field. The first order of business, therefore, was to institute a training program.

A total of 160 sanitary engineers and 870 sanitarians were trained in SCAP-organized courses. But, more important for the control of dysentery, 360,000 men were trained to serve as members of sanitation teams that Public Health and Welfare organized beginning in spring 1946. The initial plan was to have one six-member team for each 2,000 Japanese that would make weekly visits to everyone in its area. By the end of 1946, 9,000 such teams had been trained in insect control measures (DDT spraying and adult-fly killing) and field sanitary education (food handling and home chlorination of wells). Dysentery rates fell from an average of 138 cases per 100,000 in 1945 to 18.3 per 100,000 in 1948. Subsequent cuts in program funding due to efforts to balance the budget, as well as an emerging insect tolerance for DDT, led to a substantial increase in the incidence of dysentery in subsequent years.

The control of typhoid in Japan was important for two reasons beyond the numbers of lives saved. First, it settled a long-simmering debate over whether a reduction in the incidence of disease should be attributed to improved sanitation or vaccine effectiveness. Second, it exposed as a fallacy the notion that strains of typhoid were culturally distinct and therefore required locally developed remedies. Before the war, Japan had suffered 40,000 to 50,000 cases of typhoid per year, leading to between 6,000 and 12,000 deaths. Japanese scientists' at-

---

[32] These statistics are cited in Sams, *Medic,* p. 278, Notes to Ch. 9.

[33] See Sams, *Medic,* p. 93. Sams had experience with control of insect-borne diseases and with general sanitary standards from his work in Panama and the Middle East. But he admitted he had never attempted anything on the scale of Japan with its 84 million people.

tempts to develop their own vaccine had failed, and all plans to inoculate the population had been abandoned. Sams decided that typhoid and paratyphoid vaccine would be produced in Japan according to U.S. methods. Sixty million people between the ages of 3 and
60 were immunized in Japan by the end of 1948, and the incidence
of disease fell from 80 cases per 100,000 in 1945 to 11.9 cases per
100,000 in 1948. The fact that even as dysentery cases rose again,
typhoid cases continued to fall seemed conclusive proof to Sams that
the typhoid vaccine was effective even in the face of poor sanitary
conditions.[34]

Food and Nutrition. Shortly after the arrival of the occupation
forces, reports of widespread deaths from starvation began appearing
in the Japanese media. Occupation authorities were never able to con-
firm even a single fatality as a direct result of starvation. The poor
nutritional state of many Japanese did put them at risk of contracting
and succumbing to a variety of illnesses, however. Public Health and
Welfare saw its job as twofold: respond to the immediate nutritional
needs of the Japanese through emergency food aid and other programs, and address the nutritional shortcomings inherent in the traditional Japanese diet.

Before initiating either action, Public Health and Welfare began
a cross-sectional nutritional survey of 150,000 Japanese, complete
with home visits and quarterly physical exams. According to Sams,
the survey, which would be conducted during all six years of the occupation, "upset traditional concepts of methods for determining
food requirements in mass feeding programs."[35] The survey indicated
that the Japanese diet, centered on rice or other grains, was high in
carbohydrates and lacking in protein, calcium, and essential vitamins.
Compared with a minimum average requirement of 20 grams of protein per day, rural Japanese were consuming only seven grams and
urban dwellers only 16. This faulty nutrition, rather than a lack of
sufficient calories, was held responsible for the high rates of beri beri

---

[34] Sams, *Medic,* p. 95.

[35] Sams, *Medic,* p. 55.

and tuberculosis in pre-war Japan, as well as the short stature of the Japanese. Sams also believed that malnutrition, in addition to inadequate caloric intake, was responsible for the Japanese susceptibility to disease in the immediate post-war period.

Armed with these data, Public Health and Welfare set out to obtain the necessary food stocks. Sams and his staff faced three obstacles: inadequate food supplies within Japan; international competition for food because of general wartime disruptions and poor harvests; lack of comprehension about the importance of nutrients among those administering the food programs.

Nutritional surveys indicated that food shortages could become acute from May to July because the previous fall's rice harvest would be consumed and the wheat and sweet potato harvests would still be in the future. A release of 100,000 tons of occupation-controlled wheat averted this crisis until "programmed food imports" began to flow in fall 1946. In obtaining these food imports from the Food and Agricultural Organization, which managed worldwide distribution of foodstuff, Sams believed he and his colleagues were at a disadvantage. Their comprehensive surveys allowed them to gauge and accurately report total food consumption in Japan. His colleagues in Germany, however, reported only ration allowances, without reference to food obtained on the black market or elsewhere, thus making the German situation appear direr. The plummeting tuberculosis rate, which was a positive outcome of the effective control program that the Public Health and Welfare staff had implemented, also made Japan's food situation look less critical than it actually was.

Furthermore, Sams struggled to convince bureaucrats in Washington that they should pay attention to more than just total caloric intake when deciding what food to ship. He confronted laymen who saw no reason to ship grain rather than sugar; they thought that if two foods provided equivalent caloric content, one was as good as the other. Sams termed the attempt to convey the notion that a person can be less well-nourished on a 3,000 calorie diet than on a 2,000 calorie diet "one of our most difficult problems obtaining food."[36]

Once the immediate crisis was averted, Sams and his staff attempted to alter Japanese nutritional patterns. Public Health and Welfare launched a nationwide nutritional education campaign, the centerpiece of which was a school lunch program. In December 1946, Public Health and Welfare initiated a pilot program for 250,000 children in the Tokyo-Yokohama metropolitan areas. The goal was to introduce powdered skim milk into the children's diets to increase their protein and calcium intake. The children were also instructed about the importance of a balanced diet. Within one year, the children in the pilot program were taller by one inch on average and weighed more than those not in the program.[37]

Despite this program's clear success, the attempt to expand it nationwide encountered difficulties in three areas: in obtaining fuel and food (especially the 45,000 tons of powdered skim milk needed per year), in locating kitchens and kitchen equipment for the schools, and in obtaining financing. Part of the needed skim milk supply was obtained through Government and Relief in Occupied Areas (GARIOA), an additional supply was purchased through the sale of Japanese products in dollar markets, and the balance was donated by the then newly organized UNICEF. Support among the Japanese population was tremendous. By the end of the occupation, eight million children were benefiting from the school lunch program. To this day, those who benefited recall this program with gratitude.[38]

To have a lasting influence on Japanese nutrition and to sustain the school lunch program, Sams also attempted to alter Japanese land utilization. He believed that less land should be devoted to grain production and more should be used for raising domestic livestock, such

---

[36] Sams, *Medic,* p. 56.

[37] Sams, *Medic*, p. 63.

[38] Most Americans who have spent any time in Japan can relate at least one instance in which someone who was a child during the occupation told them how important this program was to him or her personally.

as pigs, chickens, and goats. A study commissioned by Public Health and Welfare showed that 18 million domestic livestock could be supported on Japan's arable land to supplement grain production. However, attempts to organize an education program on animal husbandry (herding and grazing practices) failed when the U.S. Department of Agriculture showed no interest. Sams did obtain some assistance from the International Dairy Company.

Infectious Diseases and Immunizations. The Public Health and Welfare section saw its mission in reducing the incidence of diseases as threefold: (1) to confront and contain the so-called wildfire diseases, including the highly contagious smallpox, typhus fever, and cholera; (2) to address the sanitation issues underlying the continued prevalence of enteric diseases (those caused by eating food or drinking water contaminated by human feces), such as dysentery, typhoid and paratyphoid, and poliomyelitis; and (3) to deal with the prevention and treatment of diseases such as diphtheria, tuberculosis, and venereal disease.

As part of this comprehensive approach, occupation authorities established a Statistical division within Public Health and Welfare to study vital statistics and to develop from the ground up a nationwide reporting system on morbidity and mortality. The Japanese had been keeping meticulous records on births, deaths, and marriages since 645 AD through their family registers. But because this information was kept by family and recorded in the family's hometown, it was useless for evaluating the geographic incidence of medical problems or confronting outbreaks of disease. Once a new system was established, the number of diseases tracked increased from ten in the prewar period to 35. At the end of the occupation, Japan could boast of the most complete, efficient, and modern health and welfare statistics reporting organization in the world.[39]

Table 3.3 summarizes vaccination and immunization rates for several diseases—smallpox, typhus, diphtheria, cholera, and typhoid

---

[39] Sams, *Medic,* p. 80.

Table 3.3
Vaccination and Immunization Rates, Japan

Vaccine/Immunization	Rate (%)		
	1946	1947	1948
Smallpox	100.00		
Typhus vaccine	0.73	17.79	17.79
Typhus (dusting)	2.33	23.50	9.23
Diphtheria	2.05		
Cholera	47.26		
Typhoid and paratyphoid	27.40		82.19

SOURCE: General Headquarters, Supreme Commander for the Allied Powers, *Public Health and Welfare in Japan*, Annual Summary, 1948, 1949, 1950.

and paratyphoid—in 1946, 1947, and 1948. Smallpox was the most feared of the wildfire diseases. Production of the smallpox vaccine in Japan had ceased by war's end, halting vaccination programs. Some 17,000 cases were reported during the first year of the occupation alone. Controlling this emerging epidemic was the first priority for Public Health and Welfare. To do so required the production of sufficient vaccines to inoculate the entire population of about 72 million people. Though vaccine was produced and 60 million people were vaccinated, the epidemic showed no signs of subsiding. Upon investigation, it was discovered that under conditions of rapid mass immunizations, the use of alcohol to sterilize the arm immediately prior to administering the vaccine rendered the virus in the vaccine inactive. The program was immediately restarted; detailed instructions and close supervision insured it was done without the alcohol swabbing. By May 1946, revaccination was complete and the epidemic subsided. In March 1949, Fukuoka and Osaka reported 124 new cases due to reintroduction from Korea. This validated Sams's belief that the duration of immunity conferred by the vaccine was less than three years in most cases. The entire population was revaccinated. Smallpox was again reintroduced in 1951. This time the numbers exposed were contained and only 13 million people required revaccination.[40]

Americans had heard reports that typhus fever was on the rise in Japan during the war. Since the main centers of outbreak appeared to be among conscripted Korean laborers in Hokkaido coal mines, plans were made to quarantine these groups. But before Sams and his staff arrived in Japan, most of the laborers—carrying lice and rickettsia and spreading typhus—had already traveled the length of Japan to reach the southern port of Shimonoseki and the ferry back to Korea. A delay in shipping what was now needed to combat the disease—DDT, vaccine, and dusting equipment—from the Philippines, where it had been stockpiled, to Japan forced Sams to appeal directly to MacArthur. Between September 1945 and July 1946, 33,500 cases of typhus fever were reported, 48 million people were deloused with DDT, and 5.3 million were inoculated with the typhus vaccine before the disease was controlled.[41]

Cholera had been eradicated in Japan in 1920, but the 6.5 million Japanese repatriating from areas where it was endemic raised fears that an epidemic could emerge. Sams immediately negotiated repatriation agreements with American theater doctors and established quarantine procedures at all ports of embarkation for Japanese returnees. All repatriating Japanese were to be deloused and immunized against smallpox, typhoid, and typhus. At disembarkation in Japan, they were redusted, immunized, x-rayed for tuberculosis, and examined for malaria. Despite these precautions, 14 ships from South China reported passengers sick and dying of cholera in April 1946. By immediately launching a major quarantine of 233,000 people and an inoculation effort in all port cities, Public Health and Welfare was able to contain the number of reported cases to 1,200.[42]

---

[40] Sams, *Medic,* pp. 83–84, 87.

[41] This discussion was drawn largely from Sams, *Medic,* pp. 84–88.

[42] In his book, Sams claims he never forgave the American theater surgeon in China whose failure to enforce the quarantine processing agreement led to this unnecessary loss of life. See Sams, *Medic,* pp. 89–91.

Tuberculosis had been the leading cause of death in Japan since 1932. In 1945 alone, the number of Japanese who died from tuberculosis was greater than the total number who died in all the fire raids and bombings, including the two atomic bombs. Its prevalence was directly related to the overcrowding in Japan, especially the tendency for all family members to sleep in the same room. The lethality of the disease was attributed to the generally poor nutrition of the average Japanese. It was understood at the time that a high-protein, high-calcium diet could help the body ward off the tubercle bacilli; the Japanese diet was low in both. It was assumed that the disruption of the war, combined with the mass movement of people in crowded conditions, would contribute to a massive increase in mortality from tuberculosis during the occupation. That this did not occur served as testimony to the effectiveness of the actions taken by the occupation authorities.

Conditions were certainly ripe for such an occurrence, since the incidence of tuberculosis in 1945 had reached epidemic proportions. At the beginning of the occupation, there were 25,000 hospital beds for tuberculosis patients and an estimated one million to two million clinical cases of tuberculosis. A long-term strategy entailed building more hospitals and training doctors, but a short-term plan to counter the epidemic was also essential. The dramatic reduction in contagious diseases brought about by stringent controls and mass immunizations freed up some hospital beds for tuberculosis patients. But Public Health and Welfare officials, convinced that vaccination was the key, decided to look at the BCG (Bacillus Calmette-Guerin) vaccine. The Japanese had experimented with the vaccine from 1927 to 1943 and had begun an immunization program that had subsequently collapsed. The Public Health and Welfare section revived this program.[43]

Public Health and Welfare started with the 20–24 year age group, which had the highest mortality rates for tuberculosis.[44] Be-

---

[43] Sams, *Medic,* p. 111.

[44] The death rate in this age group was 617 per 100,000.

cause of quality control issues with the liquid vaccine, a switch was made to a dried vaccine developed by Japanese doctors, and the program was reinstated in 1949. A total of 30 million people under 30 were immunized with BCG. Mortality and morbidity dropped among immunized groups, but not until streptomycin was imported and then produced in Japan in 1949 could treatment be offered to those already infected. Tuberculosis was still the leading cause of death in 1950, but it had dropped out of first place by 1960.

Diphtheria was a problem at the end of the war. In 1944, there were 94,274 reported cases; in 1945, the population suffered from the disease at a rate of 122.8 cases per 100,000 population. In the past, the Japanese had produced the diphtheria antitoxin, but they were not familiar with the modern diphtheria toxoid. The occupation authorities aided Japanese pharmaceutical manufacturing companies in learning how to produce the toxoid to support a nationwide vaccination effort. After some initial problems, controls were established and the vaccination program restarted.[45] Eventually, at the urging of SCAP, the Japanese Diet passed a Preventive Vaccination Law providing that all children between the ages of 6 months and 12 months would be immunized against diphtheria. By 1951, all children younger than 10 years of age were immunized, and the rate of disease had fallen 90 percent, to 12.7 per 100,000.

Sexually transmitted infections had been considered diseases of prostitutes, and as a consequence, Japanese physicians were generally unfamiliar with the epidemiological and clinical manifestations of the various sexually transmitted diseases. Control procedures, such as they were, were handled by the police and limited to periodic exams. Pre-war prostitution had been legal in Japan and confined largely to organized brothels. But by the end of the war, many young women were stranded in cities where they had been brought to work in the now-devastated war industries. Many of these women, without skills or family, turned to prostitution. The response of the U.S. authorities

---

[45] One manufacturer failed to detoxify two flasks of the vaccine. Children vaccinated with this batch fell ill, and some of them died. Sams attributed this incident to Communist sabotage. See Sams, *Medic,* p. 179.

veered between acceptance and suppression.[46] In January 1946, SCAP directed Japan to put an end to all practices associated with legal prostitution.

From October 1945, when the occupation forces arrived, venereal diseases were required to be reported. U.S. forces began an education campaign to train medical professionals in the diagnosis and modern treatment of sexually transmitted infections, and 1,700 modern venereal disease clinics were established.

Public Safety and Security. At the time of the surrender, Japan had mobilized over 3.6 million troops to defend against an Allied invasion, and a similar number were stationed overseas. Although American military planners believed that these soldiers would generally obey the Emperor's order to surrender, there were initial concerns about resistance from dissident elements. General MacArthur estimated that he would require between 200,000 and 600,000 troops in the first six months to occupy, pacify, and patrol Japan.[47] By the end of 1945, approximately 350,000 troops were stationed throughout the Japanese archipelago.[48]

This level of troops proved unnecessary and was soon reduced. Even with a level of soldiers per 1,000 inhabitants significantly below that of Germany, Kosovo, Bosnia, and Somalia, no security problems emerged. As in Germany, the unconditional surrender combined with the devastation of defeat produced a population unwilling or unable to continue to resist. U.S. troops suffered no combat deaths during the occupation. Although crime was a problem, the relative safety and stability of occupied Japan allowed the Public Health and

---

[46] Periodically, Military Police would conduct random sweeps of the streets after a certain hour. Telephone operators and female Diet members were among those erroneously arrested in this manner. Such mistakes reportedly contributed to deep resentment among Japanese toward the American military authorities.

[47] For more details on the security situation, see Dobbins et al., *America's Role in Nation-Building: From Germany to Iraq*, MG-1753-RC, Santa Monica, California: RAND Corporation, 2004, pp. 26, 32–35.

[48] United States War Department, Office of the Adjutant General, Machine Records Branch, *Strength of the Army*, Washington, D.C.: U.S. War Department, December 1, 1945.

Welfare authorities to focus on defeating disease and rebuilding the health care infrastructure.

Health Care Delivery

Sams believed firmly in a comprehensive approach to health care. His charge had been simply to prevent disease and unrest, but he argued forcefully that to do so required more than just inoculations and other public health measures. He argued that it required consistently high-quality medical care so that the majority of nonpreventable debilitating diseases could be recognized early and treated effectively. He did not subscribe to the simplistic idea that standards of medical care in underdeveloped countries could be improved by building new hospitals and equipping them with the latest in medical technology. Rather, he insisted that

> The problem must be attacked from many angles . . . through reorganization of professional education, improvement of hospital standards, and other means including education of the public as to their attitude towards the service offered, before a lasting change occurs.[49]

Hospitals and Clinics. The hospital sector faced three main challenges, the most immediate being how to deal with the SCAP policy directive that all Japanese career military personnel be purged from their posts. If this policy were followed, literally all doctors staffing the military hospitals, which were currently treating 78,000 wounded Japanese soldiers, would have to be dismissed. Recognizing the folly in this, Sams applied for and was granted a temporary waiver. He was permitted to retain those doctors below the rank of lieutenant colonel for a year and a half.[50]

The second challenge was rebuilding the physical infrastructure. This was a costly undertaking and could not be attempted all at once. However, because the successful public health campaign had nearly

---

[49] Sams, *Medic,* p. 148.

[50] Sams, *Medic*, p. 146.

emptied the infectious disease hospitals that existed in almost every Japanese community, it was possible to treat infectious diseases in isolation wards in regular hospitals, thereby freeing up buildings for conversion to tuberculosis or general hospitals. An initial success was the expansion in capacity at tuberculosis hospitals from 25,000 to 101,000 beds.[51]

The final challenge was to improve the quality of care provided in all hospitals. This task included making sure that those running the hospitals were well trained. To inculcate modern ideas of hospital administration, Public Health and Welfare set up a school of hospital administration, with Sams and his staff teaching the first courses. They also set up 46 "model" hospitals—one in each prefecture—to serve as the benchmark for standards of cleanliness and good management. In 1948, the Diet passed laws to establish a legal basis for the new, stricter standards and hospitals were re-inspected and classified. Hospitals with fewer than ten beds were downgraded to clinics. Because these clinics lacked operating rooms and laboratory services, patients could not be held in them for longer than 48 hours. As in 1945, hospital occupancy had been hovering around 25 percent. By 1951, however, public confidence in the quality of service had pushed occupancy up to 78.4 percent.[52]

Doctors, Nurses, and Medical Personnel. The biggest challenge Public Health and Welfare faced in the area of medical training was improving the quality of medical care—especially in the rural areas. This involved, among other efforts, an attempt to separate the functions of pharmacy and medicine. Taken together, these reforms were some of the most controversial undertaken by Public Health and Welfare, since they called into question the professional qualifications of current medical professionals and undermined one of their key sources of income.

At the time of Japan's surrender, there were 18 university-level medical schools with what Public Health and Welfare officials con-

---

[51] Sams, *Medic,* pp. 146–147.

[52] Sams, *Medic,* p. 147.

ceded were "fairly high standards." They followed the German system and focused on lectures, paying less attention to laboratory work or clinical methods. Prior to 1945, the numbers of doctors in Japan had been adequate, but about 48,000 of the 77,000 doctors were graduates of second-class medical schools (*semmon gakko*). These graduates had only four years of medical training beyond high school. In 1938, there were ten such schools; but by 1945, this number had increased to 51. Japanese officials believed this level of training was sufficient to meet the needs of rural areas.

Sams found the notion that rural people deserved a lower quality of care repugnant. To remedy this situation, Public Health and Welfare set up a Council on Medical Education. Sams claims he indoctrinated this group in the principles of a first-class medical education. Subsequently, standards were formulated, and all schools were inspected to ascertain how they measured up to these standards. Schools not meeting the new standards were closed. By 1951, there were 45 medical schools in Japan, and all produced first-class doctors.[53]

In his drive to improve the quality of medical care in Japan, Sams tried to rectify existing financial incentives that he believed discouraged doctors from updating their skills. At that time, doctors could make more money from selling drugs to patients than from seeing patients, so Sams revised the fee schedule by raising what doctors were paid for seeing patients and lowering their profits on drugs. This effort precipitated a bruising battle with the leadership of the Japanese Medical Association (JMA), who believed that he was depriving doctors of a lucrative source of income.[54]

---

[53] This discussion draws heavily on Sams's chapter on medicine and dentistry in *Medic*, pp. 120–131.

[54] In particular, he sparred with Taro Takemi, MD, who was at that time vice president of the JMA and a relative of the emperor and the prime minister. Sams won the first battle, forcing Takemi to give up his seat on the JMA. But once the occupation ended, Takemi returned as JMA president, a position that allowed him to be a powerful protector of the pharmaceutical industry. To this day, Japanese doctors earn a share of their income from the sale of pharmaceuticals.

Sams was also an advocate for life-long learning in the medical profession. As part of its effort to improve the quality of professional knowledge in Japan, Public Health and Welfare began a drive to obtain nearly 300 medical journals, textbooks, and manuals that were made available in a reading room for Japanese medical professionals. SCAP had obtained the power to authorize reproduction of any article, regardless of who held the copyright, if it was considered essential for the conduct of the occupation.[55] Sams believed public health qualified under this authorization. Japanese were encouraged to copy and translate any articles that could improve health care and reduce the costs of disease. The policy was widely welcomed, and Japanese medical journals set aside pages for translated articles from American journals. Eventually, this policy put Sams and the Public Health and Welfare section in direct conflict with the Civil Information and Education (CIE) section over what should be given precedence: public health or copyright rules. The CIE section finally did obtain a blanket copyright release for Sams for 17 U.S. medical journals, but the sparring over similar releases for textbooks and manuals continued.[56]

Before the occupation, nursing was not recognized as a profession in Japan. Nurses numbered 166,000, but their training was varied and their roles ranged from doctor's attendants to cleaning women. Families provided much of what is generally considered nursing services. Occupation authorities considered the practice of relying on family members to be unsanitary and a leading cause of the spread of disease. Therefore, Public Health and Welfare undertook a reform of the nursing profession as well. It established a Nursing Education Council and a Model Nursing School at the Central Red Cross Hospital in Tokyo, with American nurses as key instructors. In July 1948, a new Nursing Standards Law was passed. By 1951, there were 116 Class A training schools and 132 Class B schools. By 1954,

---

[55] See Nishimura, "The U.S. Medical Occupation of Japan," p. 436.

[56] Nishimura, "The U.S. Medical Occupation of Japan," p. 437.

two years after the end of the occupation, only those graduating from Class A schools were considered nurses.[57]

Traditional Medicine. Despite the fact that Public Health and Welfare officials were often looked upon as arrogant and authoritarian, they did in some instances take local conditions and culture into account when deciding the most appropriate course of action. Their response to acupuncture and other traditional practices is an illustrative case. Occupation authorities would have liked to completely eliminate acupuncture, moxacautery, and other traditional practices that they termed "quasi medical."[58] However, upon investigation, they discovered that acupuncture was practiced primarily by the blind, and that to outlaw the practice would deprive these people of their livelihood. They thus decided to instead raise the training standards for all traditional medicine and place certain limits on its practice.

Pharmacy. Pre-war Japan had no clear divisions between the professions of medicine, dentistry, and pharmacy. As mentioned above, this created a situation in which some doctors were making a large percentage of their profits from compounding and selling drugs. Likewise, some pharmacists made a living by dispensing questionable medical advice with their drugs. Sams found this blurring of the lines highly objectionable, since he believed it undermined the integrity of both professions. As with other fields, one of the goals of the occupation was to establish a legal framework that would be sustainable in the future. Public Health and Welfare set up a deliberative council of experts and government officials to study the problem and to come up with an alternative economic incentive structure. The Pharmaceutical Affairs Law passed by the Diet in July 1948 established standards for training and licensing pharmacists. A four-year course was set as a prerequisite for the licensing exam. In 1951, after much public discussion in the Diet and the press, and considerable opposition, the

---

[57] See Sams, *Medic,* Ch. 14, "Nursing," pp. 140–143.

[58] Moxacautery is a traditional practice in which a piece of cotton is put on an area where someone is experiencing pain and set afire.

Diet passed amendments to the Medical Practitioners Law, the Dental Practitioners Law, and the Pharmaceutical Affairs Law that gradually shifted the economic incentives in favor of professionalization. As mentioned above, this battle, because it involved confronting powerful, entrenched interests in the JMA, was perhaps one of the fiercest that Sams and his Public Health and Welfare section had to face.

Drugs and Consumables. Approximately 50 percent of the factories engaged in the manufacture of medical supplies and pharmaceuticals before the war had been destroyed or converted to military production. During the war, production and distribution had been centrally controlled, and over 65 percent of the supplies had been diverted to the military. At the end of the war, the civilian sector had very little. Hospital directors and doctors had no supplies, but, as the occupation discovered, there were vast stockpiles of drugs and medical supplies in Imperial Army and Navy depots. Public Health and Welfare subsequently decided, in consultation with the chief of the Economics section, to limit imports of medicine and rely on the stockpiles while trying to revive the domestic industry. The goal was to conserve scarce foreign supplies. Nonetheless, in 1946, over 40 different finished drugs were imported into Japan.

As he had done in the field of medical knowledge, Sams adopted a "copy anything" philosophy with regard to whatever would improve public health in Japan and save U.S. taxpayers money. In 1946, he put on exhibit 4,000 medical and surgical instruments he had borrowed from the U.S. Army hospital in Yokohama. In a speech at the exhibition, he encouraged Japanese manufacturers to ignore the patents and produce similar instruments for medical use in Japan.[59]

The need to save American taxpayers money also drove the rehabilitation of Japan's pharmaceutical industry, especially for those products urgently needed to control disease. For instance, the active ingredients in DDT were initially imported and mixed with talc in Japan. As soon as possible, production of the DDT concentrate was

---

[59] This incident is recounted in Nishimura, "The U.S. Medical Occupation of Japan," p. 436.

shifted to Japan. By the end of the occupation, Japan was producing DDT and dusting equipment to cover its own needs and to export to Korea. It was also producing its total requirements for penicillin.[60] Of the initial 46 drugs that were imported in 1946, only three remained in 1952.[61]

Production was not always easy. Because of spotty refrigeration, the smallpox vaccine had to be produced all over the nation, which meant that buildings and personnel had to be requisitioned, as well as calves and feed for them. Public Health and Welfare officials noticed that the local Japanese officials responsible for procuring the buildings and staff were not always communicating with those responsible for delivering the calves. This resulted in a delay in producing the vaccine, which was only fixed when Public Health and Welfare officials stepped in to serve as intermediaries between these two bureaucratic stovepipes so that smallpox vaccine production could proceed smoothly.[62]

The production of typhus vaccine in Japan was hindered by the food shortage that reduced the quantity of chickens and the availability of chicken feed, both of which were being consumed by hungry Japanese. U.S. government bureaucrats balked at a Public Health and Welfare request for chicken feed under the GARIOA budget, claiming that U.S. taxpayers should not have to pay to feed Japanese chickens. Only a demonstration that this expenditure for chicken feed would actually save $50 million in imported medicines in the future caused them to relent.[63]

Narcotics control was placed under the purview of Public Health and Welfare rather than law enforcement. Before the war, no system of narcotics control existed in Japan, and about 200 farmers

---

[60] Sams reported with pride that when Dr. William H. Draper, the man in charge of Germany's economic rehabilitation, visited Japan he was astounded that Japan was producing its total requirement of penicillin before Germany had even started producing any at all.

[61] Sams, *Medic,* p. 135.

[62] Sams, *Medic,* p. 82.

[63] Sams, *Medic,* p. 87.

were growing opium poppies. The Japanese government had agreed, as a member of the League of Nations, to control narcotics, but there was evidence that heroin production was significantly underreported.[64] In fact, heroin production in Japan and colonial Korea was sufficient at one time to supply the entire world. The occupation authorities first issued a prohibition against planting, growing, and cultivating narcotics seed, as well as against the manufacture and export of narcotics. Subsequently, they established strict, centralized control over processing and distribution. Finally, a reporting and recording system for the dispensation of narcotics for medical use was developed. These regulations were enacted into law in June 1946, and the Ministry of Health and Welfare was given jurisdiction. The U.S. occupation managed narcotics reporting to the UN until the end of the occupation, when Japan assumed this duty.

Overall Assessment

From any objective standpoint, the goals of the Public Health and Welfare section of SCAP were clearly achieved in the fields of both public health and health care delivery.

Public Health. The trends in major indicators show that compared with the pre-war levels, the overall Japanese health status improved significantly during the intervention period (Figure 3.4). The mean crude death rate was reduced from 14.6 per 1,000 population in 1946 to 8.9 per 1,000 in 1952.

Infant mortality rate and neonatal mortality rate were also reduced, from, respectively, 76.7 per 1,000 and 31.4 per 1,000 population in 1946 to 49.4 per 1,000 and 25.4 per 1,000 in 1952. These latter rates were the lowest on record since mortality reporting had begun in Japan. Life expectancy improved dramatically after just three years of intervention, largely because of the application of modern methods in health care and the prevention of diseases on a nationwide scale. Data show that between the years 1895 and 1947, life

---

[64] Sams, *Medic*, p. 154.

Figure 3.4
Trends of Major Indicators for Health Status, Japan

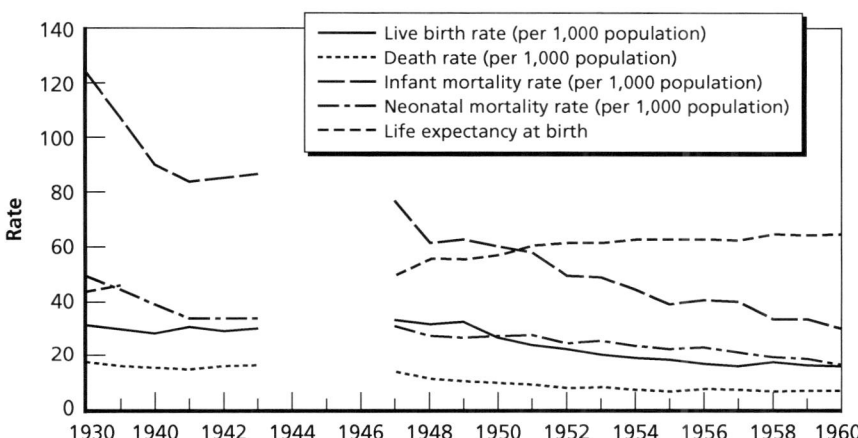

SOURCE: Japanese Ministry of Health, Labor and Welfare, *Vital Statistics.*
RAND MG321-3.4

expectancy increased from 42.8 to 50.6 per 1,000 for men and from 44.3 to 53.96 per 1,000 for women. Between the years 1947 and 1950, life expectancy increased from 50.06 to 58.0 per 1,000 for men and from 53.96 to 61.5 per 1,000 for women.[65]

The increase in life expectancy was achieved through improvements in nutrition and sanitation, as well as reactivation of vaccination programs abandoned during the war. Table 3.4 shows the case rates for smallpox and typhus fever. As can be seen, after an initial rise in cases in 1946, these two diseases were quickly brought under control. There was also a rapid decline in the case rate of diphtheria, a decline attributed to the efforts of occupation officials to make diphtheria toxoid available to the entire population. Similarly, after 1946, a remarkable drop took place in the number of reported cases of such communicable diseases as dysentery, typhoid, and malaria.

[65] General Headquarters, *Public Health and Welfare in Japan,* Annual Summary, 1950, p. 26.

Table 3.4
Case Rates for Smallpox and Typhus Fever, Japan

	Case rates per 100,000 people (%)							
	1940	1945	1946	1947	1948	1949	1950	1951
Smallpox	0.8	2.2	21	0.5	0	0.2	0	0.006
Typhus fever	0.1	3.5	41.5	1.4		0.6	1.1	

SOURCES: Japanese Ministry of Health, Labor and Welfare, *Vital Statistics*; General Headquarters, *Public Health and Welfare in Japan*, Annual Summary, 1948, 1949, 1950, and the data for year 1945.

Tuberculosis seemed to defy the trends, however (see Figure 3.5). In the first years of the occupation, the number of cases reported and the morbidity rate increased, a phenomenon often attributed to an improvement in reporting, a change in the attitude of the majority of Japanese people toward hospitalization, and an increase in diagno-

Figure 3.5
Case Rates of Selected Communicable Diseases, Japan

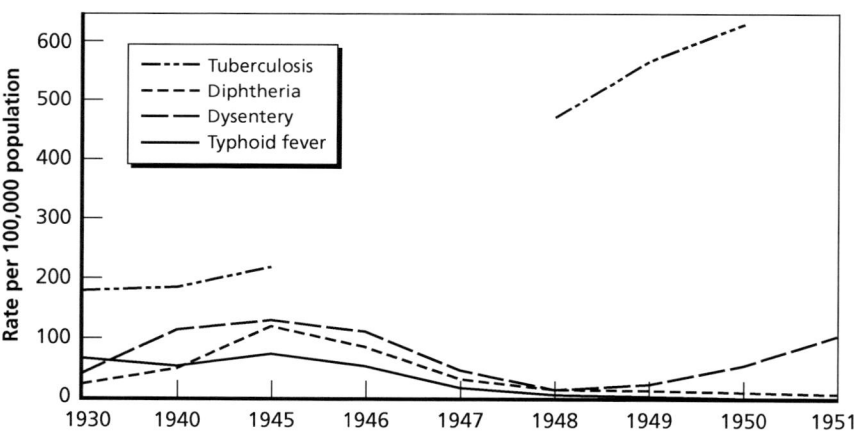

SOURCES: Data for years after 1945 from Japanese Ministry of Health, Labor and Welfare, *Vital Statistics*; General Headquarters, Supreme Commander for the Allied Powers, *Public Health and Welfare in Japan*, Annual Summaries, 1948, 1949, 1950; and Sams, *Medic*, p. 279. Data for 1945 and before from United States Strategic Bombing Survey, *The Effects of Bombing on Health and Medical Services in Japan*.
RAND MG321-3.5

sis. Eventually, even tuberculosis, a disease that before the war had been the leading cause of death among young Japanese men and women (see Figure 3.6), was tamed, due in large part to public health efforts undertaken during occupation. By the end of 1950, a marked reduction also occurred in total venereal diseases.

A concerted public education program brought about dramatic increases in public awareness of proper nutrition and hygiene. During the year 1950, public health nurses made more than 1.7 million home visits, more than one million nutritional consultations, and more than 12 million mass examinations. Similarly, more than 17 million people attended health education activities in 1950.[66] All of this was assisted by a fairly steady increase in the monies available to fund these activities. These monies were first supplemented with U.S. aid. For fiscal year (FY) 1947, the U.S. appropriated about $10 million for medical supplies, equivalent to about 2.5 percent of

Figure 3.6
Death Rates by Cause, Japan

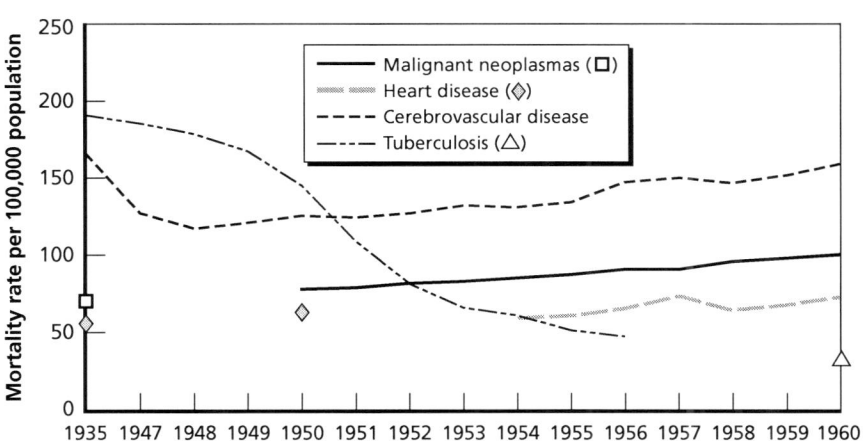

SOURCE: Japanese Ministry of Health, Labor and Welfare, *Vital Statistics.*
RAND *MG321-3.6*

---

[66] General Headquarters, *Public Health and Welfare in Japan*, Annual Summary, 1950, p. 4.

total U.S. aid to Japan. However, in FY 1949, the U.S. appropriation was reduced to less than $3 million for the same purpose, and the Japanese government was required to provide the bulk of the funding. (See Tables 3.5 and 3.6.)

Health Care Delivery. Health care delivery also improved dramatically under the U.S. occupation. Statistics show that by the end of 1950, the number of facilities had nearly returned to the pre-war level (see Table 3.7). Moreover, the hospital system had been reorganized, and medical institutions had been provided with more medical equipment and pharmaceuticals. Eventually, bed capacity surpassed the 1940 level of one bed for every 350 persons; by 1950, there was one bed for every 220 persons.

Table 3.5
U.S. Appropriations for Health Care and Related Activities, Japan

Aid (millions of $US)	Sept 1945– Dec 1946	1947	1948	1949	1950	1951
U.S. aid	193	404	461	535	361	164
U.S. appropriation for medical supplies		10.0		3.0		

SOURCES: Aid information from G.C. Allen, *A Short Economic History of Modern Japan, 1867–1970*, p. 230; U.S. appropriations information from General Headquarters, *Public Health and Welfare in Japan*, Annual Summary, 1948, p. 214.

Table 3.6
Japanese Ministry of Welfare Budget

Budget	1940	1947	1949	1951
Percentage of GDP	0.5	1.0	0.8	0.9
Per capita (in yen)	290.5	289.0	315.55	411.06

SOURCES: GDP information from B.R. Mitchell, *International Historical Statistics: Africa, Asia & Oceania 1750–1993*, 1998; health budget information from General Headquarters, *Public Health and Welfare in Japan*, Annual Summary, 1948, p. 213, and 1950, p. 92.

Table 3.7
Trends in Numbers of Hospitals, Clinics, and Hospital Beds, Japan

	Before and During Conflict				Post-Conflict	
	1930	1935	1940	1945	1949	1950
Hospitals (national, public, private)	3,716	4,625	4,732	645	3,019	3,408
General clinics		35,772	36,416	6,607		43,827
Dental clinics		18,066	20,290	3,660		21,380
Hospital beds			204,903	46,924		376,700

SOURCE: Japanese Ministry of Health, Labor and Welfare, *White Paper: Annual Report on Health and Welfare 1998–1999*; General Headquarters, *Public Health and Welfare in Japan*, Annual Summary, 1948, 1949, 1950.

In addition, the number of doctors and nurses increased as a result of the reorganization and reformation of the Japanese medical education system. By 1952, the number of doctors and the number of nurses had both increased nearly sixfold compared with 1945 levels (Table 3.8). The quality of these medical personnel also increased.

Table 3.9 shows the trend in medical service utilization, or daily average number of patients. For all patient visits (that is, visits of both inpatients and outpatients), utilization increased steadily during the post-conflict period. Of the 514,189 total patients in 1950, 60,000 went to tuberculosis sanatoria, 16,002 to mental hospitals, 8,664 to leprosaria, and the remaining 429,523 to other kinds of hospitals.

Table 3.8
Trends in Numbers of Doctors and Nurses, Japan

	During and at End of Conflict		Post-Conflict						
	1940	1945	1946	1947	1948	1949	1950	1951	1952
Doctors	65,332	12,812	65,301	70,636	72,521	73,195	69,649	71,015	85,374
Nurses	138,341	35,062	164,885	162,857	140,006	126,415	130,272	155,034	208,444

SOURCE: Japanese Ministry of Health, Labor and Welfare, *Vital Statistics*.

Table 3.9
Trends in Medical Service Utilization, Japan

	1946	1947	1948	1949	1950
Total patients	310,809	410,000		460,177	514,189
Inpatients	81,949	100,000		158,470	194,198
Outpatients	228,860	300,000		301,701	319,991
Bed occupancy rate (per 100 beds of rated capacity as of Jan each year)	40.7	44.7	41.8	63.6	73.8

SOURCE: General Headquarters, *Public Health and Welfare in Japan*, Annual Summary, 1948, 1949, 1950.

Sams's series of public health programs achieved his goal of "democracy by demonstration" through the tangible and overwhelmingly positive effect they had on the daily lives of millions of Japanese citizens. However, there was some resentment at the time.

Many physicians found the attitudes of those drafting the new health policies arrogant and offensive. Immediately after the occupation ended, an editorial in the *Japan Medical Journal* included this assessment of the efforts of the Public Health and Welfare section:

> They had no idea what the Japanese national conditions were, and yet they rode on the momentum of military victory; they did whatever they wanted, backed up with the absolute power they had. Burning with anger, we would grind our teeth.[67]

Lessons Learned

An examination of the efforts of the SCAP Public Health and Welfare section highlights a number of important lessons.

- The individual in charge of reconstruction efforts matters tremendously.
- Health care reform, especially if it includes programs that provide tangible and dramatic improvements in the health status of

---

[67] Quoted in Nishimura, "Censorship," p. 456.

the population, can provide the necessary groundwork for building democracy.

- Relatively simple and cheap steps can sometimes be the most effective.
- It is possible to alter traditional nutritional patterns if you can demonstrate the health benefits of the alteration and support the costs of the transition.
- Comprehensive reforms are likely to be the most effective and lasting, but they are also more likely to engender resistance.

One of the principal lessons from the Japan study case is the importance of capable and steady leadership. Colonel Crawford F. Sams, Chief of the Public Health and Welfare section, was uniquely well qualified for his role. Having served multiple tours of duty overseas, he had accumulated extensive experience in public health and disease control in underdeveloped countries. His breadth of experience enabled him to take a comprehensive view of health sector reform, one that encompassed all the elements in a well-functioning system from the training of health professionals to the production of pharmaceuticals.

He was aided in this task by the lack of continued violence in the immediate post-war period. Japanese society was chaotic and life was hard for most citizens, but the hardships were not compounded by continued armed resistance to the U.S. occupation. In addition, like MacArthur, Sams remained in his position as head of the Public Health and Welfare section for the entire occupation. This permitted him and his staff not only to tackle the immediate post-war concerns of refugees and infectious diseases, but also to methodically pursue reforms in the structure of health care delivery in Japan.

Perhaps one of Sams's key contributions as a leader was his belief that the work his Public Health and Welfare section did in Japan was the first, the most tangible, and perhaps the best indication to the Japanese of one of the foremost principles of democracy: the value of the individual. He argued that U.S. investments in the health and physical well-being of Japanese citizens did more than perhaps any other single action to prove that the United States was committed to building a vibrant, functioning democracy out of a former enemy state. In this way, Sams successfully linked the efforts of his staff to the larger goals of the occupation.

Although the costs to the United States of reconstructing Japan's health care system were not insignificant, some of the most memorable and well-received actions were also relatively inexpensive. Securing adequate supplies of powdered milk for the school lunch program, for example, had a positive effect on millions of school children and their families. This simple program created reservoirs of goodwill toward America for decades thereafter. Similarly, investing U.S. taxpayers' funds in chicken feed to enable the domestic production of vaccine not only immunized thousands of Japanese citizens against a potentially deadly disease, but also saved the occupying authorities $50 million.

This case study provides an example of a traditional diet being nutritionally inadequate and needing to be altered to improve the general health of the population—particularly in terms of increasing its resistance to tuberculosis. The idea of introducing dairy products into the Japanese diet was a relatively radical step and one that could have been an utter failure. But occupation authorities recognized that a number of factors might work in their favor: Everyone was suffering from food shortages, and growing children were the most adversely affected; elementary education was free and universal; parents cared about the health and physical well-being of their children; and growth in children was easy to measure. By extending the small pre-war school lunch program to the entire nation and adding one cup of milk a day to these school lunches, the Americans were able to demonstrate a measurable effect of this dietary change. Today, even though Japan's per capita milk consumption greatly lags that of the United States and Europe, Japan is still held up in China as a model to emulate.

The results of the health sector reforms launched during the post-war occupation are now recognized as beneficial by the Japanese—including the Japanese medical community. But at the time, they were not always greeted with approval. U.S. efforts to "democratize" and professionalize the health care system met with resistance from within the Japanese medical elite. They perceived the proposed changes in structure not only as a harsh critique of the system they had largely built, but as being likely to undermine their authority and earning power. Overcoming these entrenched interests required concerted and continued effort, which U.S. occupation authorities were willing to provide.

CHAPTER FOUR

Somalia

In 1992, the UN intervened in Somalia in response to an escalating civil war and humanitarian emergency. It brokered a ceasefire among the warring clans and undertook a limited peacekeeping operation in April 1992. The United Nations Operation in Somalia (UNOSOM I)—a small contingent of 50 UN observers and a 500-person Pakistani security force—was dispatched to monitor the ceasefire agreement. This UN force was followed by two others: a U.S.-led Unified Task Force (UNITAF) in December 1992, and a second UN-led force (UNOSOM II) in May 1993. The UN and a number of NGOs also began efforts to improve the steadily deteriorating humanitarian situation and rebuild the health system. Indeed, the inter-clan warfare that had erupted during the late 1980s and continued with the overthrow of President Siad Barre in 1991 had destroyed much of the country's infrastructure. The combination of the war and a drought-induced famine displaced a large segment of the population. Additionally, Somalia lacked a central government, and civil unrest remained the primary obstacle to the country's economic growth and development.[1] Figure 4.1 shows Somalia and the Horn of Africa.

The health component of the international nation-building effort in Somalia largely failed. Security problems, lack of coordination

---

[1] United States Agency for International Development, *USAID's Strategy in Somalia,* Washington, D.C.: USAID, 2004, www.usaid.gov/locations/sub-saharan_africa/countries/somalia/ (as of December 31, 2004).

Figure 4.1
Map of Somalia and the Horn of Africa

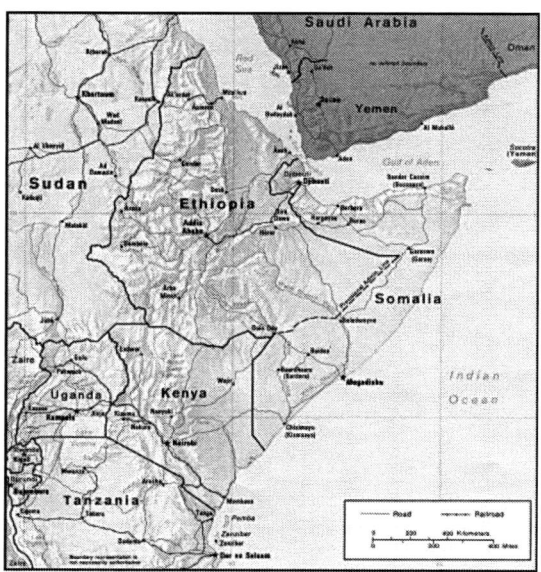

SOURCE: University of Texas, Perry-Castañeda Library
Map Collection.

RAND *MG321-4.1*

among participants, and an expanding UN mission that went beyond
securing relief operations to include disarmament plagued humanitarian relief efforts. Further, the international community failed to
recognize the magnitude of the humanitarian crisis and political
instability, to provide the UN-led mission adequate resources, and to
coordinate the numerous international participants and relief agencies
involved. Additionally, neither the Somali government nor the various warlords that ruled different parts of the country after the civil
war supported development efforts. As late as 2005, the situation in
Somalia remained dire. Lack of security was the most important factor hampering international efforts to provide food aid and humanitarian access, including basic health services. As a result, one of five
children died before the age of five, only one of every six children
was enrolled in primary school, only one of every eight women was

literate, and only one of every four families had access to clean drinking water.[2]

This chapter describes the effect of the Somali civil war and famine on the health sector and the Somali population, examines challenges the international community faced in Somalia, and assesses issues that a "failed state" situation raises about long-term rehabilitation of the health sector. The discussion concludes with a summary of lessons learned from the UN peacekeeping and humanitarian mission in Somalia.

Historical Context

Somalia has had a long history of turmoil and no well-established central government. Early in the 20th century, there were five Somalias, one each under the control of Ethiopia, France, and Italy, and two under the control of the British (one indirectly, through Kenya). The Republic of Somalia gained independence as a new nation in 1960; however, efforts in the 1960s to reunify Somalia were unsuccessful. Most independence leaders of the time became resigned to the fragmentation of the Republic of Somalia.

In October 1969, Army General Mohammed Siad Barre took control of Somalia following a military coup, establishing a new revolutionary government with the assistance of the Soviet Union. The initial vision was hopeful; it included the establishment of a written language and literacy efforts, the promotion of women's rights, and the construction of schools, businesses, and health clinics. Over the ensuing five years, Soviet influence increased, and the government became increasingly more dictatorial and less popular. As a result of these changes, the United States severed ties with the Siad Barre government in 1974. The next two years brought a massive drought to the area, weakening neighboring Ethiopia. Siad Barre invaded Ethiopian Ogaden in an attempt to liberate Somali-speaking people, causing the Soviet Union to terminate its relations with Somalia and sup-

---

[2] United States Agency for International Development, *USAID's Strategy in Somalia*.

port Ethiopia. Somalia was defeated in this effort but reestablished its ties with the United States. The United States Agency for International Development (USAID) returned in 1978, and between 1979 and 1989, the United States provided Somalia over $620 million in assistance, primarily focused on agriculture, health care, and infrastructure projects.[3]

Other international organizations involved before the civil war in health care projects and development work in Somalia included UN agencies and major NGOs. In 1984, the United Nations Children's Fund (UNICEF) began an essential drug program, later on becoming a major supplier of vaccines and other essential drugs. The United Nations High Commissioner for Refugees (UNHCR) and the World Food Programme addressed refugee and food supply shortages in Somalia. Beginning in 1982, the Norwegian Red Cross supported the rehabilitation program for the disabled run by the Somali Red Crescent Society, the only national organization in Somalia.[4] Doctors Without Borders, along with other international NGOs, provided health care services and conducted epidemiological monitoring. CARE International became involved in Somalia in 1983, initially focusing on development projects related to reforestation, agriculture, and refugee self-reliance. In 1991, CARE also became the principal food distributor for the World Food Programme for Mogadishu residents. The International Committee of the Red Cross supported many of the Somali hospitals and was the primary international organization left in-country when the civil war erupted in the late 1980s.

In 1988, an armed struggle began, led by the Somali National Movement (Isaq clan) and other clans, with the aim of overthrowing the Siad Barre regime.[5] The United States responded once again by

---

[3] United States Agency for International Development, *Somalia Strategic Plan 1997*, Washington, D.C.: USAID, 1997.

[4] International Federation of Red Cross and Red Crescent Societies, *Health, Relief and Rehabilitation*, Somalia: IFRC/RCS, 1998.

[5] L.M. Martin, "Somalia: Humanitarian Success and Political/Military Failure," Washington, D.C.: Global Security Organization, 1995, www.globalsecurity.org/military/library/report/1995/MLM.htm (as of December 31, 2004).

withdrawing all aid to Somalia. In response to the growing humanitarian crisis, the UN General Assembly in December 1989 requested that the Secretary General cooperate with the Office of the High Commissioner, World Food Programme, and the donor community to launch an interim assistance program to enable food and other humanitarian supplies to reach the refugee settlements in the northwest districts of Somalia.[6] The UN also appealed to member states, international organizations, and voluntary agencies to provide financial and technical assistance to Somalia to implement projects related to the humanitarian and developmental needs of the refugees.[7]

Nearly three years of civil war culminated in the overthrow of the Siad Barre regime in January 1991.[8] With no national government, the country fragmented, with different parts ruled by various warlords. Two of them, General Mohamed Farah Aideed and Ali Mahdi, competed for control of Mogadishu.[9] Much of the country's infrastructure, especially in the south, was destroyed during the civil war. Agricultural communities in southern Somalia were damaged, and thousands of Somalis sought refuge in the north or in neighboring countries. An estimated one million to two million Somalis were displaced internally or across borders into Kenya and Ethiopia. Hostilities prevented the international donor community from providing food assistance. The widespread famine, drought, and interclan warfare resulted in the deaths of an estimated 240,000 to 280,000 Somalis.[10]

In 1991, the U.S. military initiated airlift of humanitarian relief supplies. It used six C-130 transport aircraft to conduct humanitarian flights from Mombassa, Kenya, into Somalia in support of the Inter-

---

[6] United Nations, *Assistance to Refugees in Somalia*, New York: United Nations General Assembly, 1989.

[7] United Nations, *Assistance to Refugees in Somalia*, 1989.

[8] United States Agency for International Development, *Somalia Strategic Plan 1997*.

[9] Dobbins et al., *America's Role in Nation-Building*.

[10] K. Menkhaus, *Somalia: A Situation Analysis*, United Nations High Commissioner for Refugees, Centre for Documentation and Research, 2000.

national Committee of the Red Cross.[11] As more information became available on the magnitude of the humanitarian crisis and the problems that NGOs were having in delivering aid, it became clear that the humanitarian relief operations required more security. In December 1991, the UN increased the number of forces to provide additional security for the humanitarian relief operations. In spite of the evacuation of relief personnel and the closure of Mogadishu's port between November 1991 and May 1992, the international relief agencies began returning to Somalia. Their immediate focus was on supplying food and providing other basic humanitarian assistance, including health care, to the refugees. For example, CARE International resumed its distribution of World Food Programme food in Mogadishu and expanded its operations into northern and western Somalia.[12] In addition to providing health services, the International Committee of the Red Cross operated mass feeding kitchens.

Although there was not a specific "end" to the civil war, the UN intervened in April 1992, brokering a ceasefire among the warring clans and undertaking a limited peacekeeping operation, UNOSOM I. A small contingent comprising 50 UN observers and a 500-person Pakistani security force was dispatched to monitor the cease-fire agreement. The UNOSOM I mission also included a 90-day action plan for providing humanitarian assistance.

We begin our discussion of nation-building efforts in Somalia at the point of this UN intervention.

The health sector expanded in the 1970s. As Figure 4.2 shows, there was progress in life expectancy during the early 1980s, but Somalia's life expectancy remained among the lowest in the world. The conflict and collapse of the central government brought about a dra-

---

[11] Dan Byman et al., *Strengthening the Partnership: Improving Military Coordination with Relief Agencies and Allies in Humanitarian Operations*, MR-1185-AF, Santa Monica, California: RAND Corporation, 2000.

[12] CARE International, *CARE International in Somalia,* Washington, D.C.: CARE International, 2004, www.careinternational.org.uk/cares_work/where/somalia/ (as of December 31, 2004).

Figure 4.2
Life Expectancy at Birth, Somalia and Selected Countries

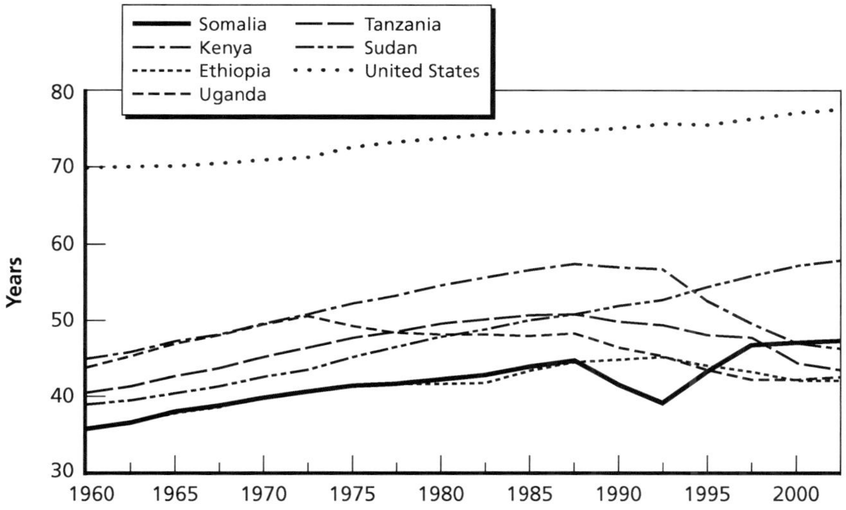

SOURCE: World Bank, *World Development Indicators 2003*.
RAND MG321-4.2

matic deterioration of the infrastructure and a downturn in life expectancy. Somalia also had a high incidence of infectious diseases, including pulmonary tuberculosis, malaria, tetanus, parasitic and venereal infections, leprosy, and skin and eye infections. Health status was severely affected by widespread malnutrition and famine.

In 1990, Somalia's population was estimated to be 7.1 million, with approximately 40 to 60 percent being nomadic. However, the large nomadic population and the displacement of so many citizens during the civil war led to widely varying estimates. From a humanitarian relief perspective, the wide range of population measurements made accurate determination of food supply and security needs difficult.[13]

---

[13] United States Agency for International Development, *Somalia Strategic Plan 1997*.

World Bank estimated that between 1988 and 1990, only 29 percent of the Somali population had access to safe drinking water.[14] This access deteriorated over time due to destruction of the infrastructure.[15,16] Little historical information is available on sewage disposal facilities, particularly before the conflict. The UN estimated a 24 percent literacy rate in Somalia in 1990. The fact that so few Somalis could read hampered relief operations, limiting the ability of the international relief organizations to communicate information about their programs to the Somali population. In 1990, Somalia's maternal mortality rate was estimated at 160 per 10,000 live births—the second highest rate in the world.[17] High maternal morbidity and mortality were related to inadequate prenatal and postnatal services.[18] Selected health indicators (1990) for Somalia are presented in Table 4.1.

The Human Development Index (HDI) is a composite score of life expectancy, education, and standard of living. The UN Development Programme is unable to report an HDI value for Somalia, but data suggest that Somalia's HDI was, and continues to be, among the lowest in the world.

Health Challenges

Public Health

Somalia's public health system was in poor condition before the war, and the conflict made a bad situation worse. Several factors combined to bring public health operations to the brink of total collapse. First,

---

[14] Somalia Aid Coordination Body, *SACB Health Strategy Framework,* 2000, www.sacb.info/commitees/MainHealth.htm (as of December 31, 2004).

[15] Somalia Aid Coordination Body, *SACB Health Strategy Framework.*

[16] World Health Organization, *WHO Somalia Fact Sheet 2002,* www.who.int/disasters/repo/8074.doc (as of December 31, 2004).

[17] World Health Organization, *Somalia Country Profile,* 2001, www.emro.who.int/mnh/whd/CountryProfile-SOM.htm (as of December 31, 2004).

[18] Somalia Aid Coordination Body, *SACB Health Strategy Framework.*

the war displaced a major portion of the population as Somalis fled to the north and to neighboring countries. Food shortages and frequent population movements contributed to malnutrition, especially among children and women, and to outbreaks of disease, such as malaria, cholera, diarrhea, tuberculosis, and measles.[19] Refugees increased the populations in northern towns, straining these communities' health care infrastructures.

Table 4.1
Selected Health Indicators for Somalia and Other Countries, 1990

	Somalia	Kenya	Ethiopia	Uganda	Tanzania	Sudan	U.S.
Fertility							
Crude birth rate (per 1,000 population)	51.9	38.5	50.5	50.3	43.8	38.3	16.7
Life expectancy at birth	40.5	55.5	43.5	46.8	48.6	50.8	75.2
Total fertility rate (births per woman)	7.25	5.64	6.91	6.98	6.25	5.42	2.08
Mortality							
Infant (per 1,000 live births)	133	63	128	100	102	75	9.4
Under-five (per 1,000 live births)	225	97	193	165	163	123	11
Crude death rate (per 1,000 population)	23.2	10.1	19.6	18.0	13.6	13.9	8.6
Adult female (per 1,000 female adults)	432	287	358	461	373	398	91
Adult male (per 1,000 male adults)	508	357	449	526	444	464	173
Immunization							
Measles (% children under 12 mos.)	30	78	38	52	80	57	90
DTP (% children under 12 mos.)	19	84	49	45	—	62	90

SOURCE: World Bank, *World Development Indicators 2003*.

---

[19] International Federation of Red Cross and Red Crescent Societies, "Humanitarian Action," in *International Federation of Red Cross and Crescent Societies Annual Report 1999*, Ch. 1, Geneva: IFRC/RCS, 2000, www.ifrc.org/PUBLICAT/ar/ar1999/arch1.asp.

The second factor moving Somalia's public health sector to the brink of collapse was the destruction from the war, which left cities ill-equipped to handle such dramatic population increases. The electricity distribution system in Mogadishu was destroyed, Somalia's limited road system was in disrepair, and most of the airports and seaports were sufficiently damaged to require extensive rebuilding. Many private businesses were either destroyed or looted.

Moreover, the collapse of the government affected basic sanitation and waste disposal services. During the civil war, the water system in Mogadishu collapsed; residents dug wells to supply water for people and animals. No one had responsibility for maintaining the wells or monitoring their use or the distribution of water. Somalis living in rural areas had to travel in some cases up to six hours to reach a well.[20] Garbage collection ceased, and rubbish piled up in massive dumps around Mogadishu. In some instances, militia claimed ownership of sanitation projects initiated to clean up the dumps. The combination of accumulated trash and poor sanitation created conditions for disease outbreaks.[21]

The third contributing factor was the collapse of the food-production infrastructure, much of which had been dismantled by widespread looting. For example, irrigation pumps were stolen, packing and processing plants were dismantled and sold for scrap metal, and many irrigation canals and flood gates no longer worked. Security concerns led farmers to plant crops only in small plots close to the villages, resulting in reduced crop yields. Farmers often were unable to keep all that they produced, because militias demanded as much as half of a harvest. The end result was a steep reduction in harvests compared with pre-war levels and a sharp increase in malnu-

---

[20] S. Vemuri, and M. Kellerman, *Somalia: A Cultural Profile—Looking at Healthcare*, Toronto: University of Toronto, 2002.

[21] B. Helander, "Getting the Most Out of It: Nomadic Health Care Seeking and the State in Southern Somalia," *Nomadic Peoples*, No. 25/27, pp. 122–132.

trition and chronic hunger among segments of the population. Further exacerbating the situation was a famine in southern Somalia during 1991–1992 that caused malnutrition rates to soar to 80 percent in some areas and several hundred thousand Somalis to die.[22]

The chaotic situation and lack of security effectively halted relief efforts. When the civil war intensified, many of the international relief agencies, including USAID, withdrew their personnel. UNHCR and World Food Programme had suspended their food and other humanitarian assistance programs for refugees in the northwestern districts of Somalia.[23] By 1991, only the International Committee of the Red Cross and a small number of NGOs remained in Somalia to provide food and medical assistance in response to the emerging humanitarian crisis.[24] UN agencies, including UNICEF, closed their Somalia operations.

Health Care Delivery

Even before the war, the Somali government underfunded the health care sector and relied heavily on external donors. The World Bank estimated that 94 percent of the 1989 Somali health budget depended on external aid; following the 1991–1992 war, that fraction rose to nearly 99 percent.[25] The low government investment in health care and the instability of Somalia's finances affected programs set up by international organizations. For example, UNICEF established an essential drug program in the 1980s that eventually was halted due to a lack of foreign exchange in the banking system.[26] The World Bank estimated that in 1988, only 28 percent of the Somali population had

---

[22] K. Menkhaus and R. Marchal, *Somalia 1999 Human Development,* 1999, http:// melting-pot.fortunecity.com/lebanon/254/undp.htm (as of December 31, 2004).

[23] United Nations, *Assistance to Refugees in Somalia.*

[24] U.S. Agency for International Development, *Somalia Strategic Plan 1997.*

[25] Somalia Aid Coordination Body, *SACB Health Strategy Framework.*

[26] Helander, "Getting the Most Out of It, pp. 122–132.

access to formal health care services.[27] In the rural areas, Somalis traveled up to 20 to 30 kilometers to reach the nearest clinic.[28]

Before the war, social services were highly centralized and all health facilities were government owned. The primary health care system's organization at the village level consisted of primary health care posts staffed by a community health worker and a traditional birth attendant.[29] The next higher level was the primary health care unit, which was staffed by a public health nurse, midwife, and sanitarian, and served between 10,000 and 15,000 persons. The district health center, staffed by a senior physician and other physicians, oversaw four primary health care units, thus serving between 40,000 and 60,000 persons. Also part of the primary health care system were maternal and child health centers. In 1990, there were 411 primary health care posts, 50 primary health care units, and 94 maternal and child health centers.

During the civil war, conditions worsened in many areas, and the health care system, along with other government services, collapsed. Of the 18 regions in the country, the primary health care program was working in only nine; the rest had either partial or no coverage before the conflict. By the early 1990s, all regions had only partial coverage. Primary health care in the public sector was further fragmented by international donors' division of the country into primary regions of concern, with each region having its own particular donors and focus.[30]

The secondary health care system comprised district and regional hospitals. Regional hospitals varied in size, from 50-bed to 200-bed capacity. The Bandar Region had two regional hospitals; the other regions had one. Specialized inpatient facilities included ten

---

[27] Somalia Aid Coordination Body, *SACB Health Strategy Framework*.

[28] Doctors Without Borders, *Somalia: Enduring Needs in a War-Ravaged Country*, 2001, www.msf.org/content/page.cfm?articleid=45699808-3D87-4FD5-8C2BA1F84FE072CE (as of December 31, 2004).

[29] World Health Organization, *Somalia Country Profile*.

[30] Helander, "Getting the Most Out of It," pp. 122–132.

tuberculosis hospitals, three psychiatric hospitals, two leprosy hospitals, and one pediatric and obstetric hospital. In 1988, there were 5,857 inpatient beds; by 1990, there were 5,397.

Hospital facilities declined substantially. Before the civil war, Mogadishu had numerous small clinics and four major hospitals in the southern part of the city: the Chinese-built Benadir Hospital for women and children, the European Union–built Digfer Teaching Hospital, the Russian-built Military Hospital, and the Madina Police Hospital.[31] When fighting broke out in 1991, the subclan militia divided Mogadishu in half, and all of the hospitals except for Madina Police Hospital (a 55-bed facility supported by the International Committee of the Red Cross) were looted, destroyed, or occupied by internally displaced persons. As a result of the war, few urban hospitals and no rural hospitals remained functional.[32] The number of hospitals decreased from 96 in 1988 to 20 in 1995.[33] Maternal and child health centers also were destroyed, except for those in the Awdal (Borama) and Sool (Las Anod) regions.[34]

The national emphasis was primarily on hospital and physician care, and less on primary care or public health services.[35] Primary health care and hospital care were not integrated. There was no functioning referral system, which meant that patients self-referred. Before the civil war, health care regulations and codes of practice required all personnel to be certified and licensed by a Ministry of Health board. Following the civil war, controls regulating the health care sector were nonexistent.[36]

---

[31] World Health Organization, *Somalia: A Health System in Crisis*, 2000, www.hartford-hwp.com/archives/33/128.html (as of December 31, 2004).

[32] World Health Organization, *Somalia Country Profile*.

[33] Somalia Aid Coordination Body, *SACB Health Strategy Framework*.

[34] Menkhaus and Marchal, *Somalia 1999 Human Development*.

[35] Somalia Aid Coordination Body, *SACB Health Strategy Framework*.

[36] Helander, "Getting the Most Out of It," pp. 122–132.

Even if the facilities had not been destroyed, few qualified people remained to staff them. Most health care professionals fled the country, except for those working with the NGOs.[37] The only available public or free health care was provided by NGOs such as the Somali Red Crescent Society that had the backing of the International Federation of Red Cross. Training of doctors and nurses also came to a halt. Somalis trained in foreign medical institutions were reluctant to work in the public health sector because of its low salaries; they opted instead to work in the private sector or for the NGOs.[38]

The pharmaceutical sector was only partially regulated. With the collapse of the government and loss of regulatory mechanisms, unregulated pharmacies proliferated. Private pharmacies, although illegal, existed and were operated by individuals with little or no pharmaceutical training.[39] Medications were dispensed without prescriptions, and many drugs had either expired or been improperly stored. This lack of regulation in the pharmaceutical sector raised concerns in the international health community that inappropriate use of antibiotics and lack of appropriate treatment for infectious diseases would contribute to the development of drug-resistant strains in the population.

In terms of health policy, there were few standards and guidelines for the provision of health services. Health care workers were poorly trained; relief agencies implemented training programs in an attempt to remedy the situation. The community did not view provision of health care services as its responsibility. Instead, it saw the responsibility as lying with the central government or international relief agencies. This lack of community ownership would prove to be one of the difficult challenges of the post-conflict phase, when local support for health care reform efforts would become necessary.

---

[37] Doctors Without Borders, *Somalia: Enduring Needs in a War-Ravaged Country.*

[38] Helander, "Getting the Most Out of It," pp. 122–132.

[39] Somalia Aid Coordination Body, *SACB Health Strategy Framework.*

Health Approach and Assessment

The nation-building effort can be viewed in three parts for the purpose of this discussion: UNOSOM I (April 1992 to December 1992), UNITAF (December 1992 to May 1993), and UNISOM II (May 1993 to March 1995). Beyond these efforts, the Somali Aid Coordination Body (SACB) has continued to play a prominent role in efforts to improve conditions in Somalia.

The planning process for UNOSOM I was limited to two short visits. Humanitarian NGOs were represented in the first technical team to visit Somalia, but some of them felt that they were never fully consulted in the final preparations for UNOSOM. When UNOSOM I was unsuccessful in deploying armed guards to protect food supplies, the U.S. military launched Operation Provide Relief in August 1992. This was a limited effort to provide U.S. logistic support by airlifting humanitarian relief supplies from Kenya to NGOs in Somalia.[40] It was clear, however, that a larger UN force was needed to secure the relief operation and enable humanitarian assistance to reach the Somali population. UNITAF, a joint effort primarily of the United States and the UN, began in December 1992. Operation Restore Hope, the U.S. component of UNITAF, was responsible for four of nine humanitarian relief sectors. UNITAF was successful in delivering food and improving agricultural and humanitarian conditions, but the underlying political and military unrest fostered concerns that the gains could not be sustained.[41]

The UN was also pressuring UNITAF to expand its original security mission to include disarmament and to establish a presence in the northern section.[42] In May 1993, UNITAF transferred responsibilities to UNOSOM II, which was charged with focusing on the

---

[40] United States Agency for International Development, *Somalia Strategic Plan 1997*; L.M. Davis et al., *Army Medical Support for Peace Operations and Humanitarian Assistance*, MR-773-A, Santa Monica, California: RAND, 1996.

[41] United States Agency for International Development, *Somalia Strategic Plan 1997*.

[42] Davis et al., *Army Medical Support for Peace Operations*.

immense challenge of restoring law and order. The UNOSOM II mission was more expansive than that of UNITAF. Its mandate was to "make peace," including promoting political reconciliation, coordinating humanitarian assistance, and paving the way for rehabilitation and reconstruction of the country.[43] Although UNOSOM II had an authorized strength of 28,000 troops, it never numbered more than 16,000.[44]

The security situation continued to deteriorate as Somali warlords opposed the UN-led intervention. Tensions rose over the ensuing months, fueled by such events as the ambush of 24 UN Pakistani peacekeeping troops in June and a failed U.S. Army Ranger mission that resulted in 18 American fatalities.[45] In response to growing domestic criticism, the Clinton administration set a March 31, 1994, deadline for withdrawing U.S. forces and pulled U.S. forces out by that date. A smaller UN contingent remained in Somalia. However, after unsuccessful attempts to negotiate with the warlords, the UN finally determined that sustaining an effective humanitarian relief and peacekeeping operation was no longer possible.[46] UNOSOM II forces departed Somalia in March 1995.

In response to the ongoing security problems, the fragmented approach of the NGOs and aid agencies, and the absence of a central government to set a policy framework, the SACB was formed in 1994 to coordinate aid to Somalia. SACB serves as the voluntary forum within which governments, the UN, intergovernmental organizations, and NGOs can share information and develop strategies related to education, health and nutrition, food security, water and sanitation, rural development, governance, and infrastructure. For 2005, SACB's health sector membership included UNICEF, United Nations Population Fund, WHO, the European Commission (EC)

---

[43] United States Agency for International Development, *Somalia Strategic Plan 1997*.

[44] Dobbins et al., *America's Role in Nation-Building*.

[45] Menkhaus and Marchal, *Somalia 1999 Human Development*; Davis et al., *Army Medical Support for Peace Operations*.

[46] Dobbins et al., *America's Role in Nation-Building*.

Somalia Unit, USAID, World Bank, International Federation of Red Cross, the Italian Embassy, and rotating NGO members such as World Vision, Coolerazione Internazionale, and Merlin.

Key Participants and Donors

The international community's prior experience with the role of foreign aid in Somalia influenced its approach following the civil war. Between 1979 and 1989, despite substantial investment by the United States, USAID projects fell far short of achieving their intended objectives. When Siad Barre's government collapsed, achievements from a decade of investments were largely destroyed. In USAID's view, the primary lesson to be drawn from its pre-civil-war experience in Somalia was that true development could not occur if the host government had little or no legitimacy and did not support development efforts.[47]

Figure 4.3 shows foreign aid to Somalia starting in 1960. During the late 1970s and the 1980s, the country experienced a large and rapid increase in foreign aid, largely because of its geographically strategic importance within the Horn of Africa (see Figure 4.1). The increase was then followed by a sharp decline during the civil war. Immediately following the civil war, the major NGOs and international organizations returned to Somalia, and the EC and USAID became the main donors in the health and other sectors. The result was a spike in foreign aid at the height of the humanitarian relief operations and UN intervention in 1994.

Between 1992 and 1994, the United States spent more than $310 million on humanitarian assistance, excluding military expenditures related to humanitarian efforts.[48] Although many lives were saved, the massive external inputs by the United States and other donors ultimately could not stop Somalia's downhill course with respect to humanitarian needs, a problem that still persists today. In retrospect, large-scale investments were not necessarily the right solution

---

[47] United States Agency for International Development, *Somalia Strategic Plan 1997*.

[48] United States Agency for International Development, *Somalia Strategic Plan 1997*.

and may have exacerbated tensions among rival groups competing for control of scarce resources. USAID felt that relatively low-cost, targeted interventions at the local level offered a greater chance of furthering development goals in a failed state situation where there is no centralized government, as was the case in Somalia.

By 1995, donor fatigue had set in, partly due to the unsustainable nature of the interventions and the fact that there was competition for funding for other sectors within Somalia and other parts of the world that required humanitarian assistance.[49] Continuing political instability, security concerns, and the increasing donor requirements and conditions that were placed on relief agencies and NGOs contributed to uncertainty in the funding and long-term commitment of the international community.

After 1995, aid dropped off sharply to pre-1975 levels and has remained at that level, partially as a reflection of the international community's disillusionment with the failed UN intervention and Somalia's declining importance as a strategic interest (Figure 4.3).[50] For example, the United Kingdom's donations fell from $3.2 million in 1994 to $850,000 in 1995. By 1997, combined European Union and U.S. assistance represented 90 percent of all resources flowing into Somalia.[51] Other donor contributions were much smaller and fell rapidly after the initial UN mission.

Coordination among the different international players involved in UNOSOM I and II was problematic for a number of reasons. The military and relief organizations had little prior experience in working together and distrusted one another. In general, the military and humanitarian relief agencies did not understand each other's organizational mandates, structures, operating procedures, and objectives.

---

[49] Somalia Aid Coordination Body, *SACB Health Strategy Framework*, www.sacb.info/commitees/MainHealth.htm (as of September 5, 2005).

[50] United States Agency for International Development, *Somalia Strategic Plan 1997*; Menkhaus and Marchal, *Somalia 1999 Human Development*.

[51] United States Agency for International Development, *USAID Congressional Presentation FY 1997: Somalia*, www.usaid.gov/pubs/cp97/countries/so.htm.

Figure 4.3
Foreign Aid Per Capita, Somalia and Other African Countries

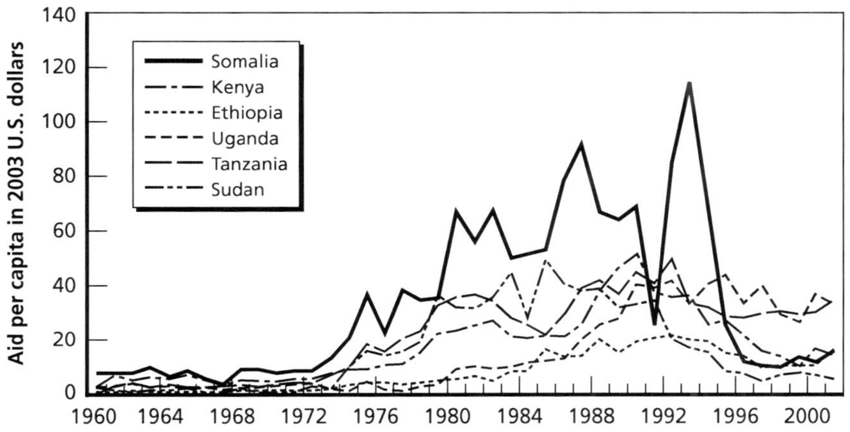

SOURCE: World Bank, *World Development Indicators 2003.*
RAND *MG321-4.3*

Although the relief agencies initially welcomed the military support that was to provide security for humanitarian relief operations, they felt their movements were being restricted unnecessarily and their ability to carry out relief operations was at risk of being compromised.[52] Also, some NGOs were reluctant to coordinate with the military because of their concerns about maintaining neutrality and objectivity; as a result, they resisted being fully integrated into the UN mission.[53]

Yet Somalia proved to be an example of a situation in which the neutrality of the International Committee of the Red Cross and other NGOs did not always afford them protection from warring factions. For example, the International Committee of the Red Cross found itself compelled to employ local guards, but had to hire individuals from all 31 warring clans. This aid directly strengthened the clan-

_____

[52] United Nations, *The Comprehensive Report on Lessons Learned from United Nations Operation in Somalia (UNOSOM),* April 1992–March 1995, 1995.

[53] Byman et al., *Strengthening the Partnership.*

based militias. The chaos that existed also made international organizations prime targets for exploitation, extortion, threats, and violence. Another source of tension between the military and the relief agencies was the issue of information sharing—the type and the amount of information each was willing to share. In the course of their operations, relief agencies acquired information that was of interest to the military. However, the International Committee of the Red Cross refused to reveal information about armed forces that might have intelligence value. The International Committee of the Red Cross also accused the military of not sharing information that might be helpful, such as on interclan fighting in areas where NGOs were operating.[54]

In addition to the coordination problems between the military and the relief agencies, the numerous local and international NGOs in-country were uncoordinated and fragmented in their approaches. The NGOs varied widely in terms of priorities, resources, length of time in-country, and the governing bodies to which they were accountable.[55] The agendas and mandates of donors and aid agencies overlapped, leading to ineffective resource targeting. Whereas the operation's security and political aspects were funded against assessed contributions, its humanitarian, rehabilitation, and development aspects were funded by agencies and NGOs that depended on voluntary contributions, which often arrived late or not at all. This variability impeded the operation's ability to be responsive to changing needs on the ground. UNICEF also commented on the effect that the numerous local and international NGOs had on the health sector, and the importance of UNICEF and other UN agencies in carefully assessing with which NGOs to partner.[56]

The UN experienced problems because of stovepiped communications between the field and UN headquarters and the fact that different aspects of the operation were splintered across several different

---

[54] Byman et al., *Strengthening the Partnership.*

[55] United Nations, *The Comprehensive Report on Lessons Learned.*

[56] United Nations Children's Fund, *Somalia: Programme Evaluation Final Report,* Nairobi: UNICEF, 2002.

UN departments within the Secretariat. High staff turnover also contributed to coordination problems. The lead UN representative in Somalia, the United Nations Secretary-General's Special Representative (SRSG), changed five times during this three-year period.[57] As for the relief agencies, frequent changes among humanitarian coordinators and relief personnel made it difficult to sustain coordination efforts. Another contributor to the coordination problem was the lack of clear roles and responsibilities among the different UN departments and agencies involved in the operation. Security problems also complicated coordination. Senior personnel of some relief agencies were based outside Somalia, in Nairobi; and only junior staff that had little or no authority were based inside.

One change that was made to improve coordination is especially noteworthy. Within the UN-led mission, a humanitarian section led by a senior Humanitarian Coordinator who reported to the SRSG was established. The Humanitarian Coordinator participated in the daily meetings of UNOSOM senior staff and was responsible for coordinating efforts with the NGOs. This was the first time the concept of a humanitarian operations center was put into practice to coordinate relief agencies and military efforts. The Humanitarian Coordinator position changed a number of times during the operation, however, which contributed to coordination problems.

On the military side, the coordination structures, procedures, and policies of the different contingents participating in the multinational force were not uniform.[58] This problem was exacerbated by the fact that not all military contingents were under UNOSOM command and control. Some contingents that were part of UNOSOM chose to follow their countries' orders rather than those of the UNOSOM commander. This made these contingents' actions unreliable and was a key reason for UNOSOM II's inability to maintain a secure environment in Mogadishu after UNITAF's departure. In addition, UNOSOM I and II were plagued by inadequate numbers of

---

[57] United Nations, *The Comprehensive Report on Lessons Learned.*

[58] United Nations, *The Comprehensive Report on Lessons Learned.*

staff, a lack of experienced staff, delays in troop deployment, and a shortage of critical operational equipment (e.g., vehicles, communication equipment, tents, water purification kits, and engineering equipment). These shortages delayed the deployment of military forces into the countryside and the various humanitarian relief sectors.

In addition, UNOSOM's mandate kept changing—for example, protecting the delivery of humanitarian assistance, encouraging and assisting in political reconciliation, and establishing and maintaining a "secure environment." The military's mission expanded under UNOSOM II without a sufficient increase in forces and other resources. All of these factors made it difficult for the SGSR and the Force Commander to implement planned initiatives. They also contributed to misunderstandings with the relief agencies looking toward the military for security protection.[59]

Although the U.S. military provided some direct care to Somali patients, its most significant medical contribution was the security that the UNOSOM forces provided to the NGOs so that they could offer humanitarian aid and deliver medical care.[60] Increased security helped to control crowds, reduced looting, and dampened the threat of violence by individuals demanding care. Security for clinics was nearly 35 percent more effective with the presence of the military than without it.[61]

---

[59] United Nations, *The Comprehensive Report on Lessons Learned*.

[60] Davis et al., *Army Medical Support for Peace Operations*; M.J. VanRooyen and J.B. VanRooyen, "Somalia: Medicine and the Military," *Journal of the American Medical Association*, Vol. 271, No. 12, March 23–30, 1994, pp. 904–905.

[61] Clinic personnel assigned security scores (1 to 5) based on (1) crowd control, (2) the incidence of looting, and (3) threats of violence by individuals demanding treatment. The effectiveness of security measures was scored based on (1) effective crowd control, (2) the lack of theft or threats of violence, and (3) the unimpaired operation of the clinic. When military escorts were provided, the mean security score (4.85 ± 0.46) was 43 percent higher than the mean security score in the absence of military escorts (3.40 ± 0.60) (p<0.001). M.J. VanRooyen et al., "Mobile Medical Relief and Military Assistance in Somalia," *Prehospital Disaster Medicine*, Vol. 10, No. 2, April–June 1995, pp. 118–120.

According to SACB, around the time that UNOSOM II ended in 1995, many international NGOs also ceased operating in Somalia because of security concerns. NGOs operating in the south and central zones were forced to evacuate staff continuously; staff of international agencies were kidnapped, injured, and murdered.[62] By 1996, USAID, UN, and most other international aid operations for Somalia were managed from Nairobi, Kenya, and program activities inside Somalia were limited and were implemented largely by local Somali staff. Activities in Somalia had migrated from emergency and acute care to support for primary care, including the training of community health workers, birth attendants, outpatient dispensaries, village health posts, and immunizations.[63]

USAID and the EC supported the SACB by having members agree to follow the SACB's guidance in their relief and development activities. The international community's recognition of the SACB as an authoritative body, however, was uneven. Because adherence to the SACB's guidelines was voluntary, some relief agencies chose not to follow them.

The lack of a central government continued to hamper the efforts of donors and relief agencies to provide health services based on a policy framework. Without a central government, top-down programming approaches did not work. Instead, assistance needed to be tailored to the diverse organizational structures that existed at the local levels. It was not until 2000 that the SACB produced a final "Strategic Framework in Support of the Health Sector in Somalia" to guide external assistance. The overarching goals were to increase Somali capacity to develop its own health policies, health systems, and plans; improve maternal and child health status; decrease the burden of communicable diseases and other avoidable causes of mortality; improve health status by reducing harmful traditional customs and practices; and increase community participation in the develop-

---

[62] Somalia Aid Coordination Body, *SACB Health Strategy Framework*.

[63] United States Agency for International Development, *Somalia Strategic Plan 1997*.

ment of a sustainable health care system at the local level.[64] Somalia's complex political and social environment called for a mixture of emergency relief and rehabilitation approaches. Many aid agencies continued to focus on emergency relief, and fewer focused on rehabilitation and development.

Public Health

Efforts to improve public health in Somalia were largely a failure for a number of reasons. Lack of security severely hampered humanitarian relief efforts. Two other factors—lack of community ownership of health care systems, and coordination problems among the numerous relief agencies—also limited the effectiveness of public health interventions. In addition, malnutrition remained a chronic problem, one that was exacerbated by droughts and floods, as well as by the civil war.

Reliable statistics on the health status of the Somali population were difficult to obtain before the war, but have been even more so since the civil war and the collapse of the central Somali government.[65] Relief agencies at the local level did collect information, but data comparability is limited because data collection methodologies were not standardized. However, there are data from the World Bank and World Health Organization that provide reasonable approximations of the situation.[66]

In 1999, Somalia ranked at the bottom of the UN's HDI, and its health indicators were among the lowest in Africa.[67] Table 4.2 shows health indicators for Somalia, before and after the interventions. As can be seen, life expectancy at birth in Somalia was still

---

[64] Somalia Aid Coordination Body, *SACB Health Strategy Framework.*

[65] Somalia Aid Coordination Body, *SACB Health Strategy Framework.*

[66] World Bank, *World Development Indicators 2003*; World Health Organization, *Somalia Country Profile*; World Health Organization, *WHO Somalia Fact Sheet 2002.*

[67] Doctors Without Borders, *Somalia: Enduring Needs in a War-Ravaged Country.*

Table 4.2
Selected Health Indicators, Somalia, Before and After Interventions

	Somalia		Kenya		Ethiopia		Uganda		Tanzania		Sudan		USA	
	1990	2000	1990	2000	1990	2000	1990	2000	1990	2000	1990	2000	1990	2000
Fertility														
Crude birth rate (per 1,000 population)	51.9	50.9	38.5	34.5	50.5	43.8	50.3	45.4	43.8	39.4	38.3	34.24	16.7	17.4
Life expectancy at birth	40.5	48.9	55.5	47	43.5	43.3	46.8	42.5	48.6	44.4	50.8	57.5	75.2	80
Total fertility rate (births per woman)	7.25	7.07	5.64	4.42	6.91	5.65	6.98	6.24	6.25	5.3	5.42	4.6	2.08	2.13
Mortality														
Infant (per 1,000 live births)	133	133	63	77	128	117	100	81	102	104	75	68	9.4	6.9
Under-five (per 1,000 live births)	225	225	97	120	193	174	165	127	163	165	123	108	11	8.7
Crude death rate (per 1,000 population)	23.2	17.5	10.1	14.4	19.6	20.1	18.0	18.5	13.6	17.2	13.9	11.1	8.6	8.7
Adult female (per 1,000 female adults)	432	452	287	529	358	535	461	567	373	520	398	291	91	84
Adult male (per 1,000 male adults)	508	516	357	578	449	594	526	617	444	569	464	341	173	147
Immunization														
Measles (% of children under 12 mos.)	30	38	78	76	38	52	52	56	80	78	57	47	90	91
DTP (% of children under 12 mos.)[a]	19	33	84	76	49	56	45	60	—	85	62	46	90	94

SOURCE: World Bank, *World Development Indicators 2003.*
[a]Second-period data reflect 2001 statistics.

among the lowest in the world in 2000, even though it had improved over its 1990 value.[68] Life expectancy at birth dramatically decreased between 1991 and 1992, but it increased thereafter (see Figure 4.2, above). Over the same ten-year period, however, the adult mortality

---

[68] World Bank, *World Development Indicators 2003.*

rates increased, and they were considerably higher for males than for females.

In 1997, Somalia had the second highest infant mortality rate in the world, estimated to be 125.8 per 1,000 live births.[69] Malaria, acute respiratory infections (e.g., pneumonia), and dysentery accounted for more than half of all mortality in children under five years of age.[70] Malnutrition also was a major cause of childhood mortality. Malnutrition remains a chronic problem for Somalis, especially among poorer households in urban and rural areas, and is exacerbated by droughts, floods, and warfare. Poor infant feeding practices, infectious diseases, frequent population movements, and inadequate access to food (especially for those living in conflict or disaster areas) are major contributors to malnutrition.[71] Nutritional surveys have estimated that between 15 and 30 percent of children were malnourished in the south and central zones of Somalia, and 6 to 10 percent in the northern areas. Even in 2000, less than 25 percent of the population had access to safe drinking water.[72] Safe sewage disposal facilities have been estimated at from less than 20 percent to 49 percent in 2000. The 1995 total adult literacy rate was estimated at 24 percent, with female adult literacy at 14 percent.[73] By 2000, the total adult literacy rate had declined to 16.6 percent.[74] High illiteracy rates present significant challenges for international relief operations because they impede the ability to communicate information about programs and services.

In 2000 and 2001, Somalia was still confronted by major infectious diseases, including tuberculosis, communicable diseases

---

[69] World Health Organization, *Somalia Country Profile*.

[70] Somalia Aid Coordination Board, *SACB Health Strategy Framework*.

[71] International Federation of Red Cross and Red Crescent Societies, "Humanitarian Action."

[72] Somalia Aid Coordination Body, *SACB Health Strategy Framework*; World Health Organization, *WHO Somalia Fact Sheet 2002*.

[73] World Health Organization, *Somalia Country Profile*.

[74] World Health Organization, *WHO Somalia Fact Sheet 2002*.

(especially measles), diarrheal diseases (especially in infants), malaria, schistosomiasis, tetanus, sexually transmitted illnesses, respiratory infections, leprosy, acute infectious diseases (malaria, pneumonia, etc.), and chronic communicable diseases.[75] Somalia had one of the highest annual rates of infection, incidence, and prevalence of tuberculosis in the world.[76] Lack of access to treatment for tuberculosis and the unregulated selling of anti-tuberculosis drugs by private pharmacies increased the risk of multi-drug-resistant strains of the disease in Somalia and neighboring countries. Cholera was endemic, particularly in urban areas and the southern part of the country. Other common conditions included obstetrical problems and anemia. A 1999 report estimated that the prevalence of female genital mutilation, which was associated with high rates of tetanus and infection, was 95 to 98 percent in the rural areas.[77]

Somalia also faced infectious disease outbreaks of measles, cholera, dysentery, meningitis, Rift Valley Fever, and Kala Azar. The SACB noted that measles outbreaks in Somalia appear to occur on a cycle of two to four years (there is no comprehensive database on these outbreaks). Before the civil war, about 30 percent of individuals had received the measles vaccine; by 2000, coverage had increased to about 38 percent (see Table 4.2). These vaccination rates were far below those of other developing countries.

Violence (landmines, gunshots, and other forms of trauma) and accidents also were important contributors to morbidity, mortality, and disability in Somalia.[78] Africa is the most heavily landmined continent in the world, and Somalia was among the most severely landmined of African countries, with an estimated one million landmines along Somalia's border with Ethiopia.[79] Physicians for Human Rights

---

[75] World Health Organization, *Somalia Country Profile.*

[76] Somalia Aid Coordination Body, *SACB Health Strategy Framework.*

[77] Menkhaus and Marchal, *Somalia 1999 Human Development.*

[78] Somalia Aid Coordination Body, *SACB Health Strategy Framework.*

[79] African Red Cross and Red Crescent Health Initiative 2010, "Landmines in Africa," www.ifrc.org/WHAT/health/archi/fact/fmines.htm (as of December 31, 2004).

estimated in 1992 that 4,500 Somalis were disabled as a result of landmine accidents.

Health Care Delivery

Health care delivery in Somalia was also a failure because of the lack of security, which resulted in the loss of trained health care workers, hampered the delivery of basic health services, and led to a reluctance of international relief agencies to return to many parts of the country. Further, Somalia remained in a humanitarian crisis phase for some time after the civil war, which kept the focus primarily on public health interventions rather than service delivery. Much of the health care infrastructure was destroyed during the civil war, and many health care workers fled the country. In 1995, only 2.3 percent of Somalia's total GDP was expended on health care, and that figure had declined to 1.3 percent by 2000.[80] Health care and other social services depended almost entirely on external aid. The international community recognized that this dependence was unsustainable over the long term and that a key goal of reconstruction efforts must be to reduce the dependence of the health care system and other social services on external aid.

The private health sector, legalized in 1984, flourished in the aftermath of the civil war, particularly in the cities. Health care workers in the private health care sector were largely the same as those employed by the public health sector, with many workers using their public sector positions to recruit patients for their private clinics. In 1997, WHO estimated that there were only 0.4 physicians and two nurses/midwives per 10,000 people. Given the poor state of the public health sector, it is likely that most government clinics would have closed if health workers had not been able to generate income from the private sector.[81] By 2000, 80 percent of all health services in Somalia were provided by the private sector.[82] A shortage of drugs in

---

[80] World Health Organization, *WHO Annual Report*, 2000.

[81] Helander, "Getting the Most Out of It," pp. 122–132.

[82] Somalia Aid Coordination Body, *SACB Health Strategy Framework*.

public sector health facilities was another reason why Somalis tended to favor private facilities.

In Somalia, where health care is viewed as a responsibility of the central government rather than of the community, relief agencies found it difficult to obtain the support of the local communities and to instill in them a sense of ownership in reconstruction and development projects.[83] There was no central government, so there were no community governance structures or mechanisms for mobilizing local resources for health care development. There was also no community awareness of and training in how to plan for, manage, and evaluate health care services. There were clan-based assistance mechanisms for disasters, but health care was a low priority—especially for women and children.

The Somalia government that existed before the civil war did not support development efforts. During and after the civil war, Somali warlords similarly were unwilling to support the humanitarian relief operations. Too much effort was directed at political bargaining and alliance building, rather than at the development needs of the communities the warlords presumably represented. As a result, health care delivery was sporadic, and security problems prevented most relief agencies from operating in large sections of southern Somalia. Instead, the delivery of health care and other social services was confined to the more secure zones, such as the northwest and northeast, and to the larger towns.[84]

Overall Assessment

Many problems plagued the mission and humanitarian relief operation in Somalia. These problems limited overall effectiveness and caused the international community to fall far short of its objectives. There were some successes, however. The UNOSOM intervention ended the famine and facilitated the return of refugees in some regions. UNOSOM forces, however, departed in 1995, leaving the

---

[83] Somalia Aid Coordination Body, *SACB Health Strategy Framework*.

[84] Somalia Aid Coordination Body, *SACB Health Strategy Framework*.

country still divided, without a central government, and in economic despair.[85]

Problems plaguing the mission in Somalia included the following:

- Policymakers and aid workers did not fully appreciate the magnitude of the humanitarian crisis upfront.
- From the beginning, there was no central government to serve as the focal point for nation-building efforts.
- The Somali warlords did not support the relief efforts or subsequent development efforts.
- UNOSOM II was inadequately resourced to meet its broad mandate.
- The absence of security was a major problem and, along with resource constraints, limited the ability of international relief agencies to provide humanitarian aid and to reach many parts of the country.
- UNOSOM's mandate kept evolving and was open to a number of different interpretations by key participants.

A complex emergency such as Somalia requires a strategy that brings all components together within an integrated structure.[86] Coordination was lacking at many levels, including between relief agencies and the military; between NGOs themselves; and among the UN, the United States, and the other countries contributing troops. The impediments to coordination were numerous:

- The absence of adequate advanced planning that included all relevant players in the planning process impeded cooperation.
- Frequent changes in UN personnel, the humanitarian coordinators, and military and relief personnel made it difficult to sustain coordination efforts.

---

[85] United States Agency for International Development, *Somalia Strategic Plan 1997.*

[86] United Nations, *The Comprehensive Report on Lessons Learned.*

- The desire by NGOs to maintain an appearance of neutrality led to poor coordination with the military.
- Variability in the goals, missions, resources, and time in-country of NGOs made it difficult for the military to determine which ones to support and how best to support their relief efforts.

These impediments spilled over into the health sector. Lack of security was the major reason for relief agencies being severely limited in their ability to reach vulnerable populations so that they could deliver health care services and humanitarian assistance. The international community's pre-civil-war experience in Somalia led some of the major international agencies to conclude that true development cannot occur if the central government has no legitimacy or does not support development efforts. The health sector was almost entirely reliant on donor aid, and without a central government, efforts thus had to focus on the local level. However, the country's lack of community ownership of the health care system created inertia at the local level, hindering attempts to undertake health sector reform or rehabilitation. Further, the humanitarian aid intervention may have exacerbated tensions among rival groups competing for the control of scarce resources. In addition, the absence of a health policy framework led to an uncoordinated approach within the health sector, with efforts focusing primarily on relief instead of development. As observed by USAID, in retrospect and based on the factors just discussed, low-cost, targeted interventions at the local level may have had a greater chance of furthering development goals in a failed-state situation such as Somalia.

The drought that occurred added to the effects of the civil war in worsening the health of the Somali population and increasing the severity of the humanitarian crisis. A report by the United Nations Development Office for Somalia came to the following conclusions:

> In late 1992 and 1993, UN intervention temporarily made dramatic improvements in the supply of high-quality health facilities. This assistance . . . brought more and better health services than the country had ever seen. Consequently, immunization

levels may well have reached an all time high in many parts of the country. Large numbers of MCH [maternal and child health] centres, OPDs [outpatient departments] and hospitals were either rehabilitated or re-established to serve the urban, rural and internally displaced populations. However, after the departure of UNOSOM in 1995, the number of operational NGOs in Somalia dropped to fewer than 40 and funding levels for health declined severely. Many NGOs in the health sector withdrew their staff due to security concerns. Those that remained were limited by security and logistical constraints in terms of where they could operate.[87]

Lessons Learned

Somalia represented a steep learning curve for the international community and was viewed as a test case in how to achieve humanitarian objectives. In June 1995, the UN held a seminar to collect lessons learned at the strategic and operational levels.[88] Attendees included senior UNOSOM and UN officials, representatives from countries that contributed troops, and NGOs working in Somalia. They concluded that the UN-led mission and humanitarian relief operation had failed at the outset to plan adequately and to involve all relevant participants. The seriousness and magnitude of the humanitarian crisis had not been fully appreciated in planning this operation. Further, some seminar participants argued that no one ever raised the question of whether the military's involvement in the humanitarian relief operations might be counterproductive to the long-term humanitarian strategy.

The public health and health care delivery components of this humanitarian effort in Somalia also largely failed. The most significant lessons learned from this failure are:

---

[87] Menkhaus and Marchal, *Somalia 1999 Human Development.*

[88] United Nations, *The Comprehensive Report on Lessons Learned.*

- Security is an essential condition for humanitarian assistance and health sector development.
- In a failed state with no central government, smaller projects at the local or regional levels may have a greater chance of succeeding.
- If the government or political authorities do not support a relief or nation-building effort, little progress can be made in addressing long-term development goals.
- A health policy framework is critical for guiding relief and development efforts and can provide that guidance only if the key participants agree to adhere to it and to let it guide their funding and program decisions.
- A comprehensive planning process is critical for assessing the magnitude of the humanitarian crisis, securing the right resources, and getting buy-in from key participants.
- Resources need to be adequate for the defined mission.

CHAPTER FIVE

Haiti

On September 18, 1994, Haitian General Raul Cédras signed an agreement with the United States stating that he would step down from power in order to avoid an imminent U.S. invasion. The agreement restored to power President Jean-Bertrand Aristide, who had been ousted by a military coup three years earlier following democratic elections. As part of the 1994 agreement, the United States committed to lifting the economic sanctions that had been in place since 1991. A force of 20,000 U.S. troops arrived in Haiti on September 19 to help oversee Haiti's transition to democracy, allowing reconstruction efforts to begin.

Haiti is considered by many to be an example of a failed nation-building effort. Our research concludes that this assessment applies to a large extent to health sector reconstruction. Numerous indicators—such as HIV prevalence, mortality and morbidity rates, and health care delivery systems—either worsened or did not significantly improve, for a number of reasons. First, continuing political instability in the country hampered the international community's efforts to rebuild and reform Haiti's health sector. The instability made it difficult to effect changes and stalled promised reforms. Second, governance problems slowed health reconstruction efforts. The Ministry of Health remained weak and was unable to fully implement its national health policy plan. Haiti's inadequate legal framework hampered the formulation of strategies and the execution of activities to guarantee a minimum set of health services to the population. Third, Haiti remained one of the least developed countries in Latin America, ensuring its reliance on financial support from the international community. For example, it ranked 153 out of 177 countries in the 2004 report that the United Nations Development Programme put out on human development.[1] By 2001, donor countries had withdrawn virtually all support, and Haiti slipped back into crisis. In 2004, violence resurfaced when insurgents seized control of Haiti's fourth largest city and armed groups expanded their control throughout other parts of the country.

This chapter begins by describing the historical context and health status of the Haitian population before reconstruction efforts commenced. We then outline initial challenges to public health and health care delivery faced by the United States and other international actors and describe and assess health efforts during reconstruction. Finally, we outline the major lessons learned from this effort.

Historical Context

U.S. involvement in Haiti dates to as early as 1915, when U.S. Marines were first deployed to Haiti to "counter the German influence." This deployment resulted in a 19-year U.S. presence in the country, during which the American military helped create a Haitian military and a Haitian police force.[2] The next U.S. deployment occurred six decades later.

In the period leading up to the 1994 U.S. intervention, Haiti's health system faced significant challenges. Starting in 1987, the Ministry of Health, with support from the international community, undertook a series of surveys to gather data on mortality, morbidity, and

---

[1] United Nations Development Programme, *Human Development Report, 2004: Cultural Liberty in Today's Diverse World*, New York: UNDP, 2004, p. 142.

[2] Chetan Kumar and Elizabeth M. Cousens, *Policy Briefing: Peacebuilding in Haiti*, New York: International Peace Academy, 1996.

use of services.³ But Haiti lacked surveillance systems at that time for most diseases, with the exception of poliomyelitis, neonatal tetanus, AIDS, and cholera.⁴ In 1991, the United States Agency for International Development (USAID) introduced a sentinel surveillance system that relied on NGOs to provide information on malnutrition and disease indicators. Haiti also lacked a health information system, making it difficult to assess health care needs and the demand for services.

In September 1991, the coup led by General Cédras contributed to a massive exodus of refugees and began a three-year period of sanctions imposed by the international community. The Organization of American States (OAS) and the United Nations Security Council imposed economic sanctions. OAS suspended all aid to Haiti except for humanitarian assistance and called on other members to impose a trade embargo. In fall 1993, UN Secretary-General Boutros Boutros-Ghali sent a joint OAS-UN mission to Haiti to negotiate with the government. He also established the International Civilian Mission in Haiti, a joint OAS-UN civilian mission to monitor human rights. The lack of progress in discussions with the Haitian military triggered another round of sanctions, and the United Nations Security Council imposed an oil and arms embargo on Haiti in June 1993.⁵ The sanctions put UN-affiliated organizations such as UNICEF in a precarious situation in that they were not allowed to interact with the Haitian government but had to maintain programs and continue providing humanitarian aid. The sanctions contributed to a deterioration of health and economic conditions:

---

³ The surveys were conducted by the Haitian Children's Institute (Institut Haitien de l'Enfance); the 2002 survey was financed by United States Agency for International Development, United Nations Children's Fund, Haiti-Canada Cooperation Fund, and the United Nations Development Programme.

⁴ Pan-American Health Organization, *Haiti Country Health Data*, Washington, D.C.: PAHO, 1998.

⁵ International Peace Academy, *Lessons Learned: Peacebuilding in Haiti,* IPA Seminar Report 7, Permanent Mission of Canada to the United Nations, New York: IPA, 2003.

- The Haitian economy experienced a steady decline in GDP and a rise in unemployment. Per capita income also declined precipitously.[6]
- Per capita spending on health decreased from 25 gourdes (approximately US$1.50) in 1990 to 16 gourdes (approximately US$1.00) in 1996, in constant 1990 values.[7]
- The health status deteriorated; serious malnutrition in many parts of the country rose from 6 percent to 32 percent.[8]
- Lack of maintenance and repairs resulted in a further decline in the condition of public health care facilities and medical equipment.
- Ongoing projects in the water supply and sanitation sectors were interrupted.

Health Challenges

Reliable health data on Haiti are limited, especially historical health data. As was the case for several other countries we examined in this study, such as Somalia and Afghanistan, there are significant gaps in the quantitative health data. In public health, for example, this is particularly true for malnutrition, sanitation, and communicable diseases. In health care delivery, it is true for hospitals, hospital facilities, and medical and nursing personnel.[9] Nonetheless, the information available was sufficient to support a tentative assessment.

When reconstruction efforts began in September 1994, Haiti faced significant economic and demographic challenges. Between 1991 and 1995, the inflation rate averaged between 25 percent and

---

[6] Pan-American Health Organization, *Haiti Country Health Data*.

[7] Pan-American Health Organization, *Haiti Country Health Data*.

[8] Frantz Large, *The Health of Children in Haiti: Facing Socio-Economic Realities*, Washington, D.C.: The Panos Institute, 2001.

[9] See, for example, health data sets from such organizations as World Bank, World Health Organization, United Nations, and Pan-American Health Organization.

27 percent. The unemployment rate was an estimated 70 percent, and roughly three-quarters of the population lived below the poverty line. The GDP per capita income and life expectancy declined during this period. Between 1990 and 1995, the population increased by over half a million, giving Haiti, at 260 inhabitants per square kilometer, one of the highest population densities in Latin America. Although most of the population lived in rural areas, most health care resources were concentrated in urban areas. Haiti experienced major migratory movements of its population, first away from the capital following the military coup, and then back after 1995. This second, reverse migration taxed housing in the cities, created unsafe living conditions, and strained public health and health service resources. These factors contributed to public health and health care delivery challenges.[10]

Public Health

The quantitative data on sanitation and malnutrition conditions in Haiti prior to the U.S. intervention are limited, but the information that is available paints a bleak picture. Between 1994 and 1995, only 46 percent of the Haitian population had access to potable water.[11] Safe sewage disposal was available only for 44 percent of the population in urban areas and 18 percent in rural areas.[12] Ongoing projects in the water supply and sanitation sectors, totaling $163 million, were interrupted.[13] Lack of maintenance caused the water supply infrastructure to deteriorate rapidly, with service coverage levels in Port-au-Prince falling by approximately 30 percent between December

---

[10] Pan-American Health Organization, *Haiti Country Health Data*.

[11] Pan-American Health Organization, *Core Health Data Selected Indicators*, 2002.

[12] Pan-American Health Organization, *Health Situation Analysis and Trends Summary*, Haiti Country Profile, Washington, D.C.: PAHO, 1998. Online at www.paho.org/English/DD/AIS/cp_332.htm.

[13] Pan-American Health Organization and World Health Organization, *Health in the Americas*, 1998. Online at http://165.158.1.110/english/sha/prflhai.html.

1990 and December 1994.[14] In addition, serious malnutrition in many parts of the country rose from 6 percent to 32 percent between 1991 and 1994.[15]

Public health care services were integrated into various programs within the Ministry of Public Health and Population. However, this ministry's epidemiology and research unit lacked trained personnel and resources to carry out its programs.[16] Many of these activities were initiated and funded by the international community, which gave high priority to certain programmatic areas, such as AIDS and tuberculosis control. Figures 5.1 and 5.2 show immunization rates, respectively, for measles and for diphtheria, tetanus, and pertussis (DTP). As can be seen, the rates increased in the decade preceding the U.S. intervention but still left Haiti well below other countries in the region.

Figure 5.1
Immunization Rates for Measles, Haiti and Other Countries in Region

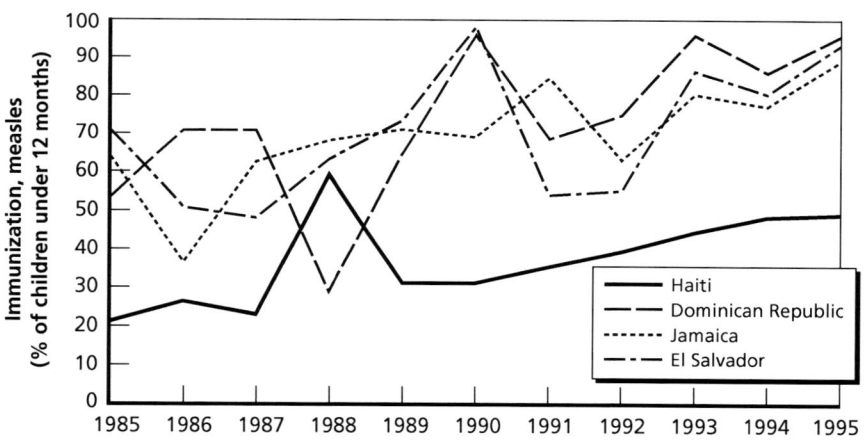

SOURCE: World Bank, *World Development Indicators 2003*.
RAND *MG321-5.1*

---

[14] Pan-American Health Organization, *Haiti Country Health Data*.

[15] Large, *The Health of Children in Haiti*.

[16] Pan-American Health Organization, *Core Health Data Selected Indicators*.

Figure 5.2
Immunization Rates for Diphtheria, Tetanus, and Pertussis, Haiti and Other Countries in Region

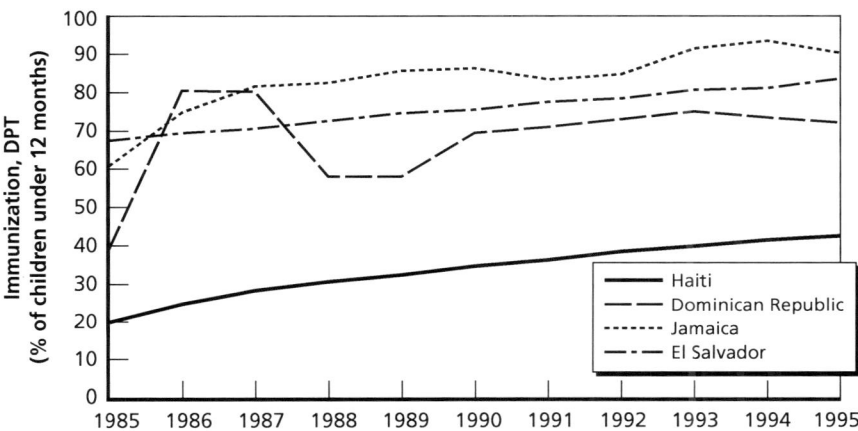

SOURCE: World Bank, *World Development Indicators 2003*.
RAND *MG321-5.2*

Haiti's death and infant mortality rates, which are shown in Figures 5.3 and 5.4, respectively, decreased before the U.S. intervention. From 1975 to 1995, the crude death rate declined from 16.72 to 12.22 per 1,000 people while the infant mortality rate declined from 140 to 91 per 1,000 live births. However, both rates were well above the levels of other countries in the region. Indeed, the United States, international organizations, and NGOs faced enormous challenges during the reconstruction phase because of the extremely poor conditions in Haiti. The country's economic and health indicators were among the worst in Latin America.

Health Care Delivery
In 1994, Haiti had 49 total hospitals and 61 other inpatient facilities, with an estimated 90 beds per 100,000 people.[17] While the number

---

[17] Pan-American Health Organization, *Haiti Country Health Data*.

Figure 5.3
Mortality Rate, Haiti and Other Countries in Region

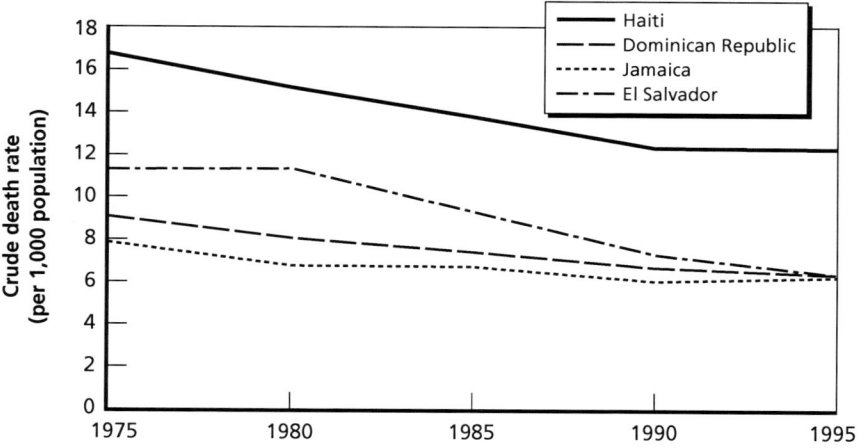

SOURCE: World Bank, *World Development Indicators 2003*.
RAND *MG321-5.3*

Figure 5.4
Infant Mortality Rate, Haiti and Other Countries in Region

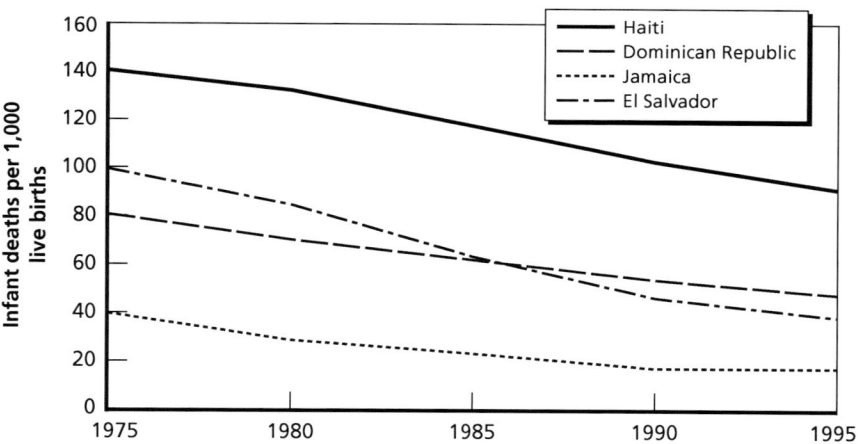

SOURCE: World Bank, *World Development Indicators 2003*.
RAND *MG321-5.4*

of physicians increased slightly, from 0.14 per 1,000 people in 1984 to 0.16 per 1,000 people in 1995, there were significantly fewer physicians in Haiti than in other regional countries (see Figure 5.5). By 1995, the Dominican Republic had 1.5 physicians per 1,000 people, Jamaica had 0.57, and El Salvador had 0.91. The private for-profit sector in Haiti consisted of physicians, dentists, and other health care specialists primarily located in private health care facilities in Port-au-Prince. Access to care was limited, especially for Haitians living in rural areas.[18] Mental health services were not a high priority, with few government institutions providing them within the Port-au-Prince area.[19] A lack of maintenance and repairs resulted in further decline

Figure 5.5
Number of Physicians, Haiti and Other Countries in Region

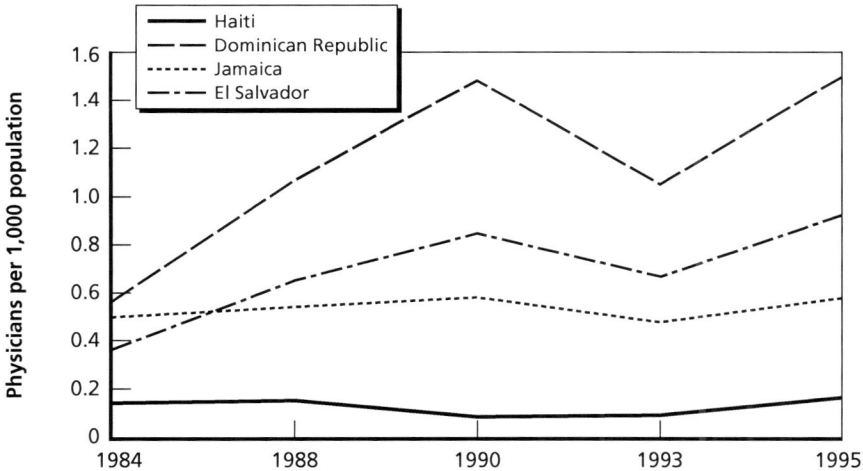

SOURCE: World Bank, *World Development Indicators 2003*.
RAND *MG321-5.5*

---

[18] United States Agency for International Development and World Health Organization, *Haiti Epidemiological Fact Sheet on HIV/AIDS and Sexually Transmitted Infections*, Geneva: UNAIDS and WHO, 2004.

[19] World Health Organization, *Core Health Data Selected Indicators*.

in the condition of public health care facilities and medical equipment.[20]

Hospital equipment and consumables were in short supply. The pharmaceutical laboratories approved to produce pharmaceuticals covered only 30 to 40 percent of the Haitian market. Drugs normally requiring prescriptions were readily accessible and commonly sold by street vendors. Haiti had no drug registration, control of drug imports, or inspections of drug manufacturers. Eighty percent of Haiti's drug expenditures were made by the private sector.

The Haitian health care system comprised several components. One of these was the public sector, which consisted of the Ministry of Public Health and Population and the Ministry of Social Affairs. The Ministry of Health, which was part of the Ministry of Public Health and Population, was organized into central, departmental, and community levels. The central directorates set standards, and the nine departments were responsible for planning, monitoring, and supervision. The Municipal Health Units, under the central directorates, were responsible for carrying out health activities with community participation. Another component of the health care system consisted of the private for-profit sector and the private nonprofit sector, which included donor-financed NGOs, foundations, and associations. There was also a mixed nonprofit sector, which included Ministry of Health personnel working in private institutions or religious organizations. Finally, there was the traditional medicine component. Nearly half of the population relied on traditional medicine, particularly in the rural areas.[21]

Government spending on health ranged between 7.1 percent and 10.7 percent of the national budget between 1990 and 1996, with roughly 90 percent spent on salaries.[22] Per capita health spending—at $12 per person by 1994 and $18 in 1995—was significantly

---

[20] Pan-American Health Organization, *Haiti Country Health Data*.

[21] World Health Organization, *Core Health Data Selected Indicators*.

[22] Pan-American Health Organization, *Haiti Country Health Data*.

lower than that of many other governments in the region (see Figure 5.6). Haiti's $18 in per capita health spending for 1995 compared with $98 in the Dominican Republic, $104 in Jamaica, and $111 in El Salvador. The Ministry of Health was supposed to coordinate all health institutions, but it was unable to assume a leadership role because the economic embargo directed resources toward the nonprofit sector. The public sector was severely affected by the country's political crisis and the economic sanctions imposed by the international community during the three-year period leading up to the 1994 intervention. During that period, all foreign aid was channeled through NGOs. The public and private institutions for the most part functioned independently of one another. NGO and private health care facilities operated without quality standards or oversight and were not coordinated with the public health sector.[23]

Figure 5.6
Health Expenditures Per Capita, Haiti and Other Countries in Region

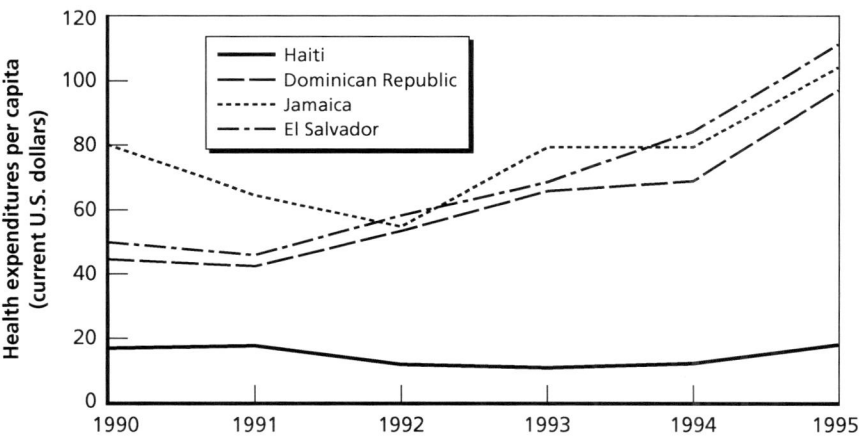

SOURCE: World Bank, *World Development Indicators 2003*.
RAND *MG321-5.6*

---

[23] Pan-American Health Organization, *Haiti Country Health Data*.

Health Approach and Assessment

As mentioned at the beginning of the chapter, the health reconstruction effort in Haiti was largely a failure. Such indicators as HIV prevalence, mortality and morbidity rates, and health care delivery systems either worsened during the effort or did not significantly improve. Continuing political instability, poor governance, and declining economic conditions created significant problems that stood in the way of improving the country's public health and health care delivery systems.

Key Participants and Donors

The United States, through USAID, was Haiti's largest bilateral donor in the areas of health and education. Between 1995 and 2003, USAID provided a total of $850 million in direct bilateral assistance to Haiti. In 2003 alone, USAID contributed $71 million.[24] USAID's efforts in the health sector concentrated on delivering essential child survival and family planning services, as well as food aid supplements.[25] USAID's programs focused on the major causes of infant mortality, maternal health, reproductive health care, HIV/AIDS prevention, and sexually transmitted disease prevention, detection, and treatment.[26]

In addition to USAID, U.S. military medical units supported the various efforts to rebuild and rehabilitate the health sector. The U.S. military helped rebuild hospital and clinic facilities, assisted with rabies control and prevention efforts, aided with vaccination programs, and helped provide equipment to health care facilities. One of

---

[24] USAID planned to provide Haiti with $52 million in assistance in the areas of health, democracy and governance, education, and economic growth in 2004. United States Agency for International Development, *Haiti: Situation Overview*, Washington, D.C.: USAID, 2004.

[25] United States Agency for International Development, *FY 1998 Congressional Presentation on Haiti*.

[26] United States Agency for International Development, *Haiti Country Profile: HIV/AIDS*, 2003.

the challenges the international relief community faced was how to integrate the efforts of U.S. military medical units into the larger humanitarian relief and rebuilding efforts. The Director of the Pan-American Health Organization (PAHO) noted that the frequent turnover in military medical commanders was frustrating because it complicated attempts to coordinate efforts.[27]

Other major donors included PAHO, in the areas of infectious disease and essential drugs, improved maternal and child health, and sanitation; UNICEF, in the areas of micro-nutrients, child health, and STI/HIV; and World Bank, in the areas of tuberculosis drugs and other medical supplies, obstetrical emergency care, and midwife training.

In the initial stages of reconstruction, a clear direction was difficult to identify. The need was overwhelming, numerous organizations were involved in the process, coordination mechanisms were not fully in place, and the national health policy strategy had not been formulated. PAHO viewed its role in Haiti as one of providing technical assistance and serving as a coordinator and spokesperson for affiliated NGOs.[28] The World Bank representative in Haiti in 1996 and several U.S. military medical commanders believed PAHO was the only organization within Haiti with a complete view of the challenges facing the health sector and a solid grasp of what needed to be done.[29]

In October 1994, 12 international organizations, under the auspices of the Inter-American Development Bank, initiated a joint assessment mission to determine how to address Haiti's social and economic problems.[30] The group drafted an Emergency Economic

---

[27] Davis et al., *Army Medical Support for Peace Operations.*

[28] Pan-American Health Organization, *Haiti Country Health Data.*

[29] Davis et al., *Army Medical Support for Peace Operations.*

[30] The organizations involved included Inter-American Development Bank; World Bank (IBRD/IDA); United Nations Development Programme, Food and Agriculture Organization; United Nations HABITAT; United Nations Economic, Social and Cultural Organization; United Nations Family Planning Association; United Nations Children's Fund; United Nations Industrial Development Organization; World Food Programme; European Union;

Recovery Program (EERP) that was to serve as an initial blueprint for Haiti's economic reconstruction. Included in the blueprint was the goal of transitioning from humanitarian assistance to a sustainable and functioning health system. Such a system would foster economic growth and improve living standards.

The strategy laid out by the EERP for rebuilding and reforming the health sector had four key objectives: strengthen the central ministry to fulfill its functions and to guarantee service and quality access to health care; decentralize services to improve quality, accessibility, and efficiency; ensure access to an affordable minimum package of integrated basic health services; and support community participation and coordinate the public sector, NGO, and donor activities to optimize resource use. To reconstruct the health sector's infrastructure and improve services, the EERP recommended several steps:

- Define health priorities, norms, and procedures for supervision, monitoring, and evaluation.
- Strengthen management capacities.
- Develop administrative mechanisms for decentralized management and information systems.
- Retrain health personnel.
- Rehabilitate and re-equip health facilities, and establish mechanisms for ensuring the availability of essential drugs and medical supplies.
- Undertake activities to improve the water and sanitation systems.
- Create a supply storage and distribution system at the provincial and local levels.
- Establish a nutrition strategy.[31]

U.S. Agency for International Development; Organization of American States; Pan-American Health Organization; World Health Organization; and Canadian International Development Agency.

[31] United Nations, "Emergency Economic Recovery Program," United Nations' *International Report*, Vol. 1, No. A1, April 3, 1995.

EERP estimated that the cost to reconstruct the health sector's infrastructure and improve services would be $57.3 million. The participating organizations noted that implementation of EERP's recommendations required that donor agencies commit to long-term development objectives, that strategies be designed at the outset of projects to move them from emergency to medium-term goals, and that capacity-building and the sustainability of projects be emphasized. Given the limited capacity of the Haitian government, much of the work would have to be carried out by contractors, NGOs, and national and international agencies. At the Paris Club meeting of 1995, $2.8 billion was pledged—an unprecedented amount of funding for a country of Haiti's size and ability to absorb aid (see Figure 5.7).[32]

Figure 5.7
Total Aid Per Capita, Haiti, 1960–1999

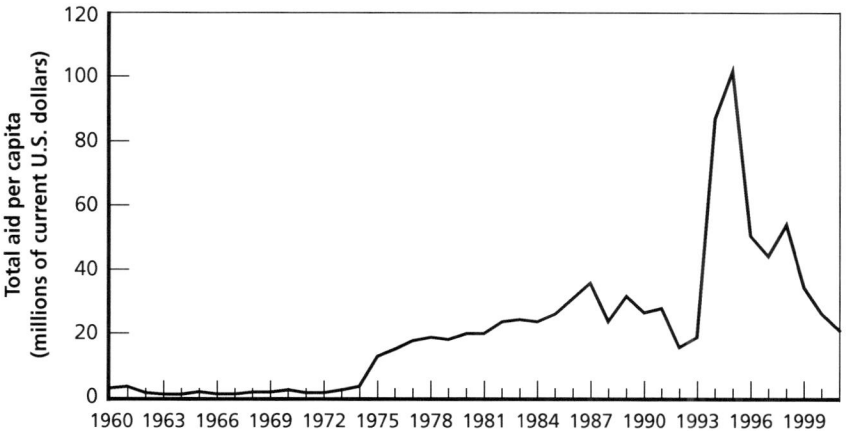

SOURCE: World Bank, *World Development Indicators 2003*.
RAND *MG321-5.7*

---

[32] Patricia Weiss Fagan, "Conflict Reconstruction and Reintegration: The Long-Term Challenges," in Edward Newman and Joanne Van Selm (eds.), *Refugees and Human Displacement in Contemporary International Relations,* New York: United Nations University Press, 2003.

According to the Inter-American Development Bank, official development assistance to Haiti up to 1991 amounted to approximately $150 million per year, including payment support, investment projects, technical cooperation projects, and food aid. Between 75 and 80 percent of this assistance was in the form of grants; the rest consisted of loans.[33] The twelve organizations that developed the EERP noted that development assistance to Haiti had historically had three basic shortcomings: lack of national leadership and control, little measurable effect on basic economic and human development indicators, and no sustainability.[34] They called for these issues to be addressed as part of the effort to rebuild and reform the Haitian economy and government.

Public Health

Public health reconstruction efforts faced numerous challenges, one of the most significant being the lack of health information to inform planning efforts. In September 1996, the Ministry of Health created a committee to design a new National Health Information System.[35] Public health programs and public awareness campaigns about specific health issues were a key focus. Few reliable data existed on the causes of mortality within Haiti. Beginning in 1997, the Ministry of Public Health and Population and PAHO began pushing for death certification.[36]

AIDS, which had become an epidemic in Haiti in the 1980s, had developed into a serious problem. UNICEF had cut back its involvement in AIDS in the early 1990s, but reintroduced AIDS-

---

[33] International Monetary Fund, *Haiti: Selected Issues*, IMF Staff Country Report No. 01/04, January 2001. Online at www.imf/org/external/pubs/ft/scr/2001/cr0104.pdf (as of April 11, 2004).

[34] United Nations, "Emergency Economic Recovery Program."

[35] Pan-American Health Organization, *Core Health Data Selected Indicators*.

[36] Pan-American Health Organization, *Health Situation Analysis and Trends Summary*.

related training in 1995 at the primary health care level.[37] USAID focused on expanding family planning, as well as diagnosis and treatment services for STIs.[38] Over the course of reconstruction, however, the prevalence of HIV in Haiti remained high. Ten years after Aristide was restored to power, Haiti had the highest HIV prevalence in the Western Hemisphere—an estimated 210,000 people in Haiti were living with HIV/AIDS.[39] (With barrier contraception uncommon in Haiti, the virus is mainly transmitted through heterosexual contact.)

Tuberculosis was also a serious problem. NGOs taught health care workers how to diagnose, treat, and do follow-up of tuberculosis patients. In 1995, several cases of drug-resistant tuberculosis emerged, which significantly raised the cost of treatment for such patients. By 1996, 200 health care clinics were diagnosing and treating tuberculosis patients. From 1995 to 2002, the number of patients with tuberculosis declined from approximately 410 to 325 per 100,000.[40]

As part of rabies control efforts, the Ministry of Agriculture undertook a national vaccination campaign with assistance from PAHO, the U.S. Army veterinary teams, and the Ministry of Health. More than 54,000 vaccines were administered between July and August 1995.[41] There are few reliable quantitative data for other diseases. In agreement with PAHO, UNICEF assumed responsibility for purchasing a large portion of the total vaccines and related basic supplies

---

[37] Kate Alley, John Richardson, Jacques Berard, *Country Programme Evaluation 1992–mid-1996: Programme Choices in Political Crisis and Transition,* Haiti Evaluation Team, New York: UNICEF, December 1996.

[38] United States Agency for International Development, *FY 1998 Congressional Presentation on Haiti.*

[39] United States Agency for International Development and World Health Organization, *Haiti Epidemiological Fact Sheet on HIV/AIDS and Sexually Transmitted Infections,* Geneva: United States Agency for International Development and World Health Organization, 2004; United States Agency for International Development, *Haiti Country Profile: HIV/AIDS,* 2004, p. 1.

[40] Pan-American Health Organization, *Core Health Data Selected Indicators.*

[41] Pan-American Health Organization, *Haiti Country Health Data.*

needed for the measles vaccination campaign.[42] As Figures 5.8 and 5.9 illustrate, immunization rates for measles and DPT did not significantly increase from 1995 to 1999, and they remained well below the immunization rates of other countries in the region. A national campaign to eradicate measles that was implemented between 1994 and 1995 resulted in the vaccination of 2.8 million children, representing 98 percent coverage of the target population (children between nine months and 14 years of age).[43] However, subsequent vaccination efforts were discontinued, causing a measles epidemic to break out in various municipalities. About 990 confirmed cases were reported, primarily in the area surrounding Port-au-Prince. This led

Figure 5.8
Immunization for Measles, Haiti and Other Countries in Region

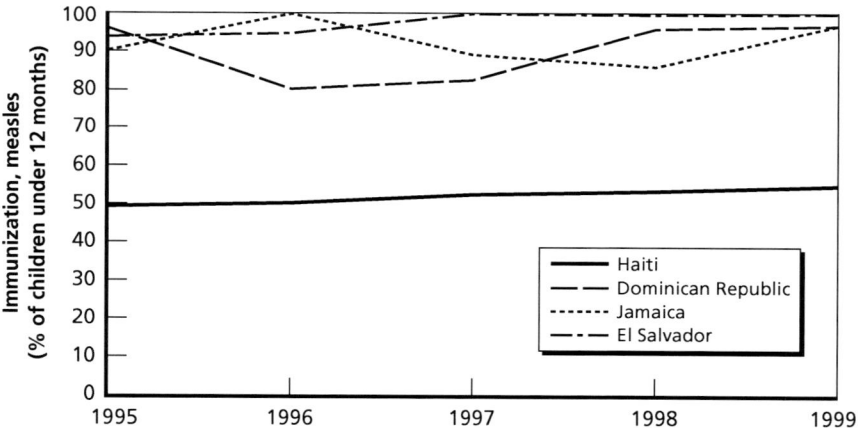

SOURCE: World Bank, *World Development Indicators 2003.*
RAND *MG321-5.8*

---

[42] Alley, Richardson, and Beard, *Country Programme Evaluation.*

[43] Pan-American Health Organization, *Health Situation Analysis and Trends Summary.*

**Figure 5.9
Immunization for Diphtheria, Tetanus, and Pertussis, Haiti
and Other Countries in Region**

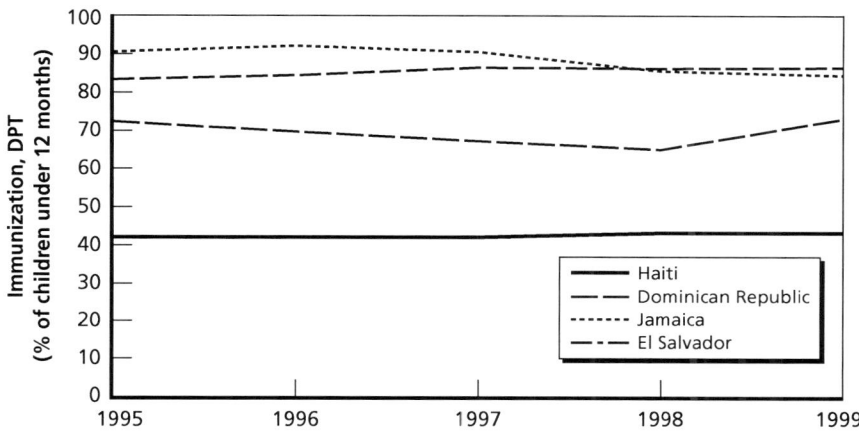

SOURCE: World Bank, *World Development Indicators 2003.*
RAND *MG321-5.9*

to a renewed effort to vaccinate the population in 2000, at the end of
which PAHO reported that measles coverage had reached 75 percent.[44]

Malnutrition and sanitation conditions improved somewhat.
Malnutrition prevalence, defined as height-for-age among children
under five, declined from 34 percent in 1990 to 31 percent in 1995
and 23 percent in 2000.[45] The percentage of the population with
access to sanitation facilities slightly improved, going from 23 percent
in 1990 to 30 percent in 2000, although Haiti still remained
well below other countries.[46] In 2000, approximately 67 percent of

---

[44] Pan-American Health Organization and World Health Organization, *Haiti's Country
Health Profile, Basic Country Health Profiles,* Summary 1999. Online at www.paho.org/
English/DD/AIS/cp_332.htm.

[45] World Bank, *World Development Indicators 2003.*

[46] World Bank, *World Development Indicators 2003.*

the population had access to sanitation facilities in the Dominican Republic, 99 percent in Jamaica, and 82 percent in El Salvador.

Starting in 1995, UNICEF, PAHO, and WHO began working with NGOs to improve the targeting of food aid. In 1994, UNICEF also added the promotion of exclusive breastfeeding for children between birth and 6 months, and in 1995 it began focusing on micro-nutrients, immunization, and control of diarrheal diseases. In its 1998 briefing to Congress, USAID outlined its overall program objectives for Haiti of supporting a long-term sustainable development strategy. It sought to help further reduce rates of malnutrition and fertility by (1) supporting basic health care packages in specific geographic areas; (2) assuring that the food aid program was integrated within existing maternal and child health programs; and (3) assuring that supplementary feeding programs prevent malnutrition in pregnant and lactating mothers and children under three years of age rather than waiting to treat malnourishment. It emphasized family planning programs in the health programs, including programs where food aid was distributed. Goals also included improvements in vaccination rates through support of periodic annual vaccination campaigns.[47]

Mortality and morbidity rates worsened over the course of reconstruction. Infant mortality increased from 73.8 per 1,000 live births in 1996 to 80.3 in 2000. The rise is attributable to a number of factors, such as increased poverty, deficiencies in the health system, and AIDS. By 2000, the leading causes of death among children were intestinal infectious diseases, infections of the perinatal period, malnutrition, and acute respiratory infections. Female mortality rates increased from 291 per 1,000 adult females in 1990 to 348 in 1997

---

[47] United States Agency for International Development, *FY 1998 Congressional Presentation on Haiti.* In 2002, USAID summarized the efforts of the other key international players in the Haitian health sector as follows: "The PAHO (infectious disease and essential drugs, improved maternal and child health, and sanitation), UNICEF (micro-nutrients, child health and STI/HIV), and the World Bank (condoms, TB drugs and other medical supplies, obstetrical emergency care, midwife training) also provide significant levels of assistance." United States Agency for International Development, *Haiti Activity Data Sheet,* Washington, D.C.: U.S. Agency for International Development, 2002.

and 373 in 2000. Maternal mortality rates also substantially increased and have been attributed to such factors as short intervals between births, chronic malnutrition, low antenatal care visit rates, and AIDS. Male mortality rates also increased from 353 per 1,000 adult males in 1990 to 473 in 1997 and 524 in 2000.[48]

Birth rates and life expectancy remained largely unchanged and well below other countries in the region. As Figure 5.10 illustrates, the birth rate dipped from 38 per 1,000 people in 1995 to 37 by 2001. This rate was significantly greater in 2001 than that in the Dominican Republic at 25 per 1,000 people, Jamaica at 21, and El Salvador at 29. Life expectancy slightly decreased from 54 years in 1995 to 52 in 2001. Again, it was also notably lower than others in the region in 2001, such as the Dominican Republic at 67, Jamaica at 76, and El Salvador at 70.[49]

Figure 5.10
Birth Rate, Haiti

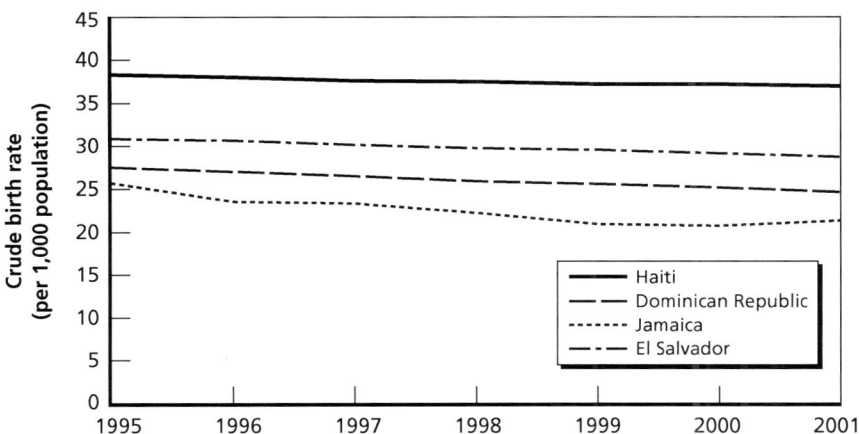

SOURCE: World Bank, *World Development Indicators 2003*.
RAND *MG321-5.10*

---

[48] Pan-American Health Organization, *Haiti Country Health Data*; International Monetary Fund, *Haiti: Selected Issues*.

[49] World Bank, *World Development Indicators 2003*.

Health Care Delivery

Reconstruction of Haiti's health care delivery system also faced serious challenges. Quantitative data are extremely poor regarding the number of physicians and nurses in Haiti following the U.S.-led intervention. However, that which exists shows that the per capita rates are significantly worse in Haiti than in other countries in the region. In 1995, for example, Haiti had 0.2 physicians per 1,000 people, compared to 1.5 in the Dominican Republic, 0.6 in Jamaica, and 0.9 in El Salvador.[50] The geographical distribution of health care personnel varied widely, but was concentrated in the urban areas. Insufficient funding has been a key problem for keeping trained personnel within the public sector. To address this manpower shortage, Haiti signed a bilateral cooperation agreement with Cuba in 1999. Cuba sent approximately 500 healthcare professionals to work in Haiti's municipalities.[51]

To help repair the physical infrastructure of the health sector, approximately $1.3 million was spent on rehabilitation projects undertaken in 46 health care facilities and 5 hospitals between October 1994 and March 1996. An additional $8.3 million was invested for the partial rehabilitation of 88 health care facilities and 5 hospitals, including the Haitian State University Hospital.[52] The U.S. military medical command undertook a comprehensive health care facility assessment in Port-au-Prince to assess the physical and operational status of health facilities in order to guide the military's efforts in helping to rebuild the health sector. The Joint Task Force (JTF) Surgeon presented the facility assessment results to the Director of PAHO, helping to inform PAHO, World Bank, and other relief agencies' efforts in rebuilding the health care infrastructure.[53]

One of the dilemmas the U.S. military's medical command faced was reconciling the inertia of mission expansion with the nu-

---

[50] World Bank, *World Development Indicators 2003*.

[51] Pan-American Health Organization, *Core Health Data Selected Indicators*.

[52] Pan-American Health Organization, *Haiti Country Health Data*.

[53] Davis et al., *Army Medical Support for Peace Operations*.

merous requests for assistance from the NGOs and the need to provide direct medical care. There were strong pressures for the mission to expand as the operation unfolded; medical rules of engagement needed to be clearly defined. There were requests by coalition partners, U.S. agencies, Haitian government officials, and NGOs for the U.S. military medical command to use excess capacity to provide care to Haitians and other civilian personnel. American soldiers sometimes brought in sick or injured civilians they encountered while out conducting patrols or field operations. Other issues, such as patient transfer and evacuation, also had to be addressed. The U.S. military's policy was to transfer civilian patients to local hospitals as soon as possible in order to free up inpatient capacity in the event of a surge in demand—especially U.S. military casualties.[54]

The military's solution to address the demands for medical assistance was to task the JTF Surgeon to serve as the key military medical interface between the U.S. military and the Haitian government, international organizations, NGOs, and other U.S. government organizations such as USAID. In this way, the JTF Surgeon was able to assess which requests legitimately fell within the scope of the medical mission and to establish a mechanism by which injured or ill Haitians treated initially by the combat support hospital could be transferred to local health care facilities for care. The JTF Surgeon was responsible for advising the theater commander on what type of humanitarian assistance was required by the Haitian government and the major relief agencies, and which activities fell outside the scope of the mission.[55]

As Figure 5.11 shows, per capita health spending in Haiti increased over the course of reconstruction. It doubled from $12 in 1994 to $24 in 1999, but remained significantly lower than other governments in the region. Foreign aid accounts for the largest share (50 percent) of the expenditure in health, particularly for capital outlays and operating expenses.[56] In 1996, the government provided

---

[54] Davis et al., *Army Medical Support for Peace Operations.*

[55] Davis et al., *Army Medical Support for Peace Operations.*

[56] Pan-American Health Organization, *Haiti Country Health Data.*

Figure 5.11
Government Health Expenditures Per Capita, Haiti

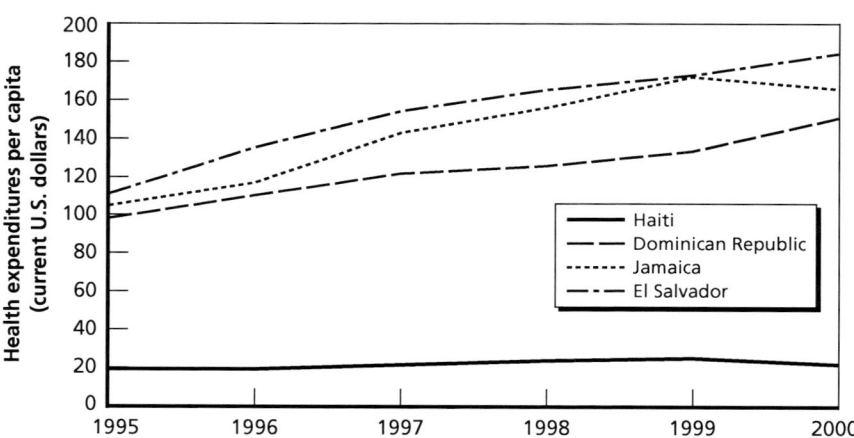

SOURCE: World Bank, *World Development Indicators 2003*.
RAND *MG321-5.11*

only about 16 percent of Haiti's total expenditure on health with external donor agencies, NGOs, and private expenditures accounting for the remainder. Prior to 1996–1997, the main donors in the health sector were USAID, France, Canada, and Japan.

Overall Assessment

Continuing political instability has hampered efforts by the international community to rebuild and reform Haiti's health sector. As part of the conditions for receiving support from the international community, requirements were placed on Haiti to undertake fundamental reforms. Beginning in 1996, the Ministry of Health, with support from PAHO and Inter-American Development Bank, developed a national health policy plan that outlined a strategic plan for reforming the health sector. Although this plan was never instituted, it provided a roadmap for the medium- and long-term reform of the health sector. The strategy called for a reorganization of the health system that included the decentralization of the ministry.[57] The health sector reform strategy also called for a primary health care model to serve as the basis for national health programs. A minimum package of services that included health care for children, adolescents and women, emergency medical and surgical care, communicable disease control, public health education, environmental health, water supply, and the supply of essential drugs was to be adopted. In addition, the Ministry's leadership role in the planning, execution, and evaluation of health programs was supposed to be strengthened.[58]

However, the strategy was not institutionalized. The political instability that continued to plague Haiti, even after the 1994 intervention, led to inertia within the government, making it difficult to effect changes and stalling promised reforms. The Ministry of Health remained weak and was never able to implement fully the new national health policy plan. In addition, Haiti's inadequate legal framework hampered the formulation of strategies and the execution of activities to guarantee a minimum set of services to the population. Although a new law regarding the safety and efficacy of drugs was drafted in 1997, it had not been approved due to the inertia within the government.[59]

USAID identified six key challenges to development in Haiti, all of which were compounded by mounting demographic pressures.[60] The first was a legacy of political and social instability, which circumscribed the actions of the government and threatened to reverse progress. Second, pervasive poverty and poor social services caused suffering, deprived people of opportunities, and contributed to instability. Third, a weak public administration and an overextended public sector, which barely provided services, hampered implementation

---

[57] Pan-American Health Organization, *Core Health Data Selected Indicators*; International Monetary Fund, *Haiti: Selected Issues*.

[58] Pan-American Health Organization, *Core Health Data Selected Indicators*.

[59] Pan-American Health Organization, *Core Health Data Selected Indicators*.

[60] United States Agency for International Development, *FY 1998 Congressional Presentation on Haiti*.

of aid projects. The fourth challenge was a devastated economy. Fifth, uncontrolled population growth degraded the environment and endangered the natural resource base for sustainable agricultural production. Sixth, deteriorated infrastructure in most sectors made private sector development and investment difficult.

Continuing political instability and a lack of progress on required reforms led the international community to withhold aid from Haiti in 2000. The resignation of Prime Minister Rosny Smarth, the failure to replace him for over a year, and Rene Preval's dissolution of the parliament further delayed both the execution of health reforms and the delivery of international aid. Representatives of the U.S. government, International Monetary Fund, and World Bank criticized Haiti's failure to resolve the impasse. Because of the questioned legitimacy of the spring and fall 2000 elections, the international community withheld about $600 million in aid, much of which has expired or been redirected. The UN withdrew from Haiti in February 2001. UN Secretary-General Kofi Annan expressed disappointment about the lack of progress in reforming Haiti's institutions, as well as concern about the Haitians' failure to stem the growing lawlessness and political violence.[61]

The country then lapsed into politically motivated violence in late 2003 as antigovernment demonstrations increased in size and frequency. On February 5, 2004, insurgents seized control of Haiti's fourth largest city, and armed groups expanded their control throughout other parts of the country. On February 29, Jean-Bertrand Aristide resigned from the presidency, and Haiti's seven-person advisory council selected Gerard Latortue to be Haiti's new prime minister.[62]

The 2004 crisis in Haiti underscored the fragility of the health care system and how vulnerable rebuilding and reform efforts remained to political instability within the country. USAID warned

---

[61] Maureen Taft-Morales, *Haiti: Issues for Congress,* Washington, D.C.: Congressional Research Service, 2001.

[62] United States Agency for International Development, *Haiti: Situation Overview.*

that given the chronic nature of Haiti's underdevelopment, the country was susceptible to a rapid deterioration of humanitarian indicators. Both USAID and PAHO expressed concerns that the emergency situation and increase in violence might lead to an increase in the incidence of diseases and result in population displacements.[63] Of particular concern were the following challenges:

- The neutrality of health institutions was violated, and some hospitals became targets of violence that kept staff and patients away from facilities; informal home care replaced hospitalization for some patients;
- It was increasingly difficult to continue distributing drugs and medical supplies, as well as water, propane gas, and diesel fuel;
- Access to services was reduced since some hospitals cut back on services because of a lack of equipment, personnel, or both; those hospitals that remained operational tended to be in the private sector, which limited access to the financially needy;
- Hydraulic pumps in some hospitals and electrical pumping stations in some areas ceased to function because of a lack of electricity;
- Problems in accessing different areas of the country complicated or impeded vaccination efforts, increasing the risk of outbreaks of vaccine-preventable diseases; the national programs for tuberculosis and HIV/AIDS reported problems with patient follow-up;
- Existing emergency services became overloaded with patients injured during the violence; and
- Reporting of data to the health information system was reduced in some areas due to the increase in violence; this decreased the amount of information available on the health needs of the population during this crisis.

---

[63] United States Agency for International Development, *Haiti: Situation Overview.*

In February 2004, PAHO cautioned against allowing the humanitarian crisis to lead to the collapse of the public health system or the creation of a parallel system or a black market for health services and goods. To address immediate health needs, PAHO estimated that a budget of $2,710,000 would be required.[64]

Lessons Learned

The effort to improve public health care and health delivery in Haiti largely failed to accomplish its long-term goals. This leads to a number of important lessons learned:

- The government must have a basic ability to administer aid programs, or aid provided will not achieve short- or long-term goals.
- Funneling aid through NGOs may have immediate health effects, but it may also have perverse long-term effects on the government's ability to establish health programs.
- Involving people with detailed knowledge of the grass roots conditions is crucial to a successful program.
- A long-term perspective is necessary.
- Health programs must match objectives with resources.

Government Capabilities
One U.S. health-related representative in Haiti commented that the initial amount of assistance provided by the international community was never a limiting factor.[65] The problem was the almost complete

---

[64] Pan-American Health Organization, *Humanitarian Crisis in Haiti: Support to the Health Sector*, Washington, D.C.: PAHO, February 2004.

[65] Co-author Lois Davis e-mail communication with Major General Lester Martinez-Lopez, Commanding General, U.S. Army Medical Research and Materiel Command, February 14, 2005.

lack of capacity within the government to implement and administer programs. There was no functioning Ministry of Health or administrative personnel within the ministry who could receive the donor support and oversee its financial administration. Because many Haitian professionals had left the country, the remaining personnel were often poorly trained and educated, with little experience in administration or government.[66] World Bank had a large amount of money to spend on Haiti, but it was unable to spend more than several million due to the lack of capacity and infrastructure.

Use of NGOs in Lieu of Government Agencies

Because the Ministry of Health was unable to move forward with needed services and public health programs, aid organizations funneled resources through the NGO community. This approach had the advantage of enabling the major international health organizations to make progress in key public health areas. The drawback is that it did not develop capacity in the Haitian government to provide needed services on its own. Although PAHO also worked to strengthen the capacities of the Ministry of Health and to put into place a strategy for health sector reform, the process was very slow. The UNICEF experience highlighted the need for international relief organizations to maintain a balance in their partnerships with the NGOs and other civil society actors, as well as with the traditional state partners. Specifically, the UNICEF experience underscored the importance of being able to assess the operational capacities of potential partners in order to develop a realistic assessment of how they might fit into overarching programmatic strategy and goals. In addition, such partnerships should not only involve program delivery but also focus on capacity building of NGOs.

---

[66] Davis et al., *Army Medical Support for Peace Operations*, 1996.

Recruits Knowledgeable About Local Situation

The health effort in Haiti was criticized for not having sufficient local knowledge of the country. The international community and expatriates had an incomplete grasp of the political, social, and economic realities of Haiti, attempting to impose instead a Western European system on the country. One U.S. health-related representative summarized this issue as follows:

> In essence there were two Haitis. There was the Haiti belonging to the well-educated minority elite and the Haitian diaspora who had lived for many years in the U.S. or Europe and had an idealized view of what Haiti needed and could become. Then there was the reality on the ground where the majority of Haitians were poor, with their own set challenges and a different view of what their needs were.[67]

The UN staff also was criticized for not having a sufficient knowledge of Haiti before the operation, and many of the staff initially deployed did not have experience in the country or speak French or Creole.[68]

Long View

Health efforts were not always oriented toward capacity building, but were often focused on achieving immediate results. An example is the Albert Schweitzer Hospital, considered to be the best-run hospital in Haiti. Although Haitian medical personnel worked in the hospital, the key medical staff and management positions were filled by Americans, not Haitians. Part of the problem was a failure by the international community to sustain a long-term perspective in Haiti. The desire for fast fixes that had a quick impact took precedence over long-range building efforts. More attention needed to be given to the management of transition and the transfer of program administration

---

[67] Co-author Lois Davis e-mail communication with Major General Lester Martinez-Lopez.

[68] International Peace Academy, *Lessons Learned: Peacebuilding in Haiti*, IPA Seminar Report 7, Permanent Mission of Canada to the United Nations, New York: IPA, 2002.

to local leaders. Some argued that the intervention in Haiti lacked an overarching vision and a firm commitment to Haiti's transformation.[69] The UNICEF Country Program evaluation team observed that in a complex emergency, the demands for responding to immediate needs can overwhelm any long-term vision or strategies for implementing humanitarian aid or rebuilding the health sector. This makes it challenging for the international players to move from meeting basic needs during a crisis to capacity building and sustained growth.[70]

Objectives Matched to Resources

A final lesson learned from Haiti is the need to match reconstruction objectives with resources. The planning for such a mission needs to consider several factors: (a) What are the baseline health conditions? (b) What is the host nation commitment? (c) What is the time frame? (d) What are the resources? The plan should contain a logical roadmap for accomplishing the objectives, as well as a transition plan for handing over programs to local authorities or actors. One of the classic mistakes of nation-building operations is to try to develop a long-term plan for rebuilding the health care infrastructure if there is only a short-term commitment.

---

[69] International Peace Academy, *Lessons Learned: Peacebuilding in Haiti*, 2002.

[70] Kate Alley, John Richardson, and Jacques Berard, *Programme Choices in Political Crisis and Transition,* UNICEF Latin America and the Caribbean Regional Monitoring and Evaluation Electronic Bulletin, No. 2, New York: UNICEF, September 1997.

CHAPTER SIX

Kosovo

On June 9, 1999, following 77 days of NATO air strikes, NATO and the Federal Republic of Yugoslavia signed an agreement that led to the immediate withdrawal from Kosovo of the Yugoslav army and the Serbian police. The United Nations Security Council subsequently authorized a 50,000-strong NATO-led Kosovo Force (KFOR) and established the United Nations Interim Administration Mission in Kosovo (UNMIK) to oversee the civilian administration of the territory.

The Serbs and Albanians had struggled for control over Kosovo, the southernmost province of the former Federal Republic of Yugoslavia, for years. In 1989, Yugoslav President Slobodan Milosevic revoked Kosovo's autonomous status and imposed direct control from Belgrade. He replaced Kosovar Albanians with Serbs in most official positions and began to dispossess the Kosovar Albanians of their equity in most communally owned enterprises. Albanian resistance to Serbian rule grew, resulting in the emergence of an armed insurgency led by the Kosovo Liberation Army (KLA). Serbian efforts to quell insurgent activity resulted in significant civilian casualties and many refugees and internally displaced persons.[1] By February 1998, the conflict had escalated to clashes between units of the Serbian Ministry of Internal Affairs, the Federal Republic of Yugoslavia Army, and the KLA. The international community intervened militarily in March 1999 with a NATO-led bombing campaign over Kosovo and the rest

---

[1] Dobbins et al., *America's Role in Nation Building,* Ch. 7, p. 111.

of Yugoslavia.[2] An estimated 800,000 persons became refugees, flee-ing to surrounding countries, or were internally displaced.

Efforts to rebuild Kosovo's health sector have been mixed. On the positive side, Kosovo is an important example of how early devel-opment of a health policy framework can guide health sector recon-struction and reform. The fact that the major donors agreed to follow this policy guidance was a significant achievement. Implementation of the action plan for health sector reform, however, was problematic. UNMIK did not take a lead role in implementing the plan, and WHO was reluctant to assume a leadership role and act as the de facto Ministry of Health. The long-term prospects for the health sec-tor hinge on the unresolved political status of the province and secu-rity concerns that continue to hinder economic development and discourage foreign investment.

We begin this chapter by describing the health care system's or-ganizational structure and the health status of the Kosovar Albanians before the conflict. We then examine the conflict's effect on the health care system's functions and the health of the province's popu-lation. Finally, we analyze the challenges faced by the international community in rebuilding the health sector and the key determinants of success.

Historical Context

In the decade prior to the 1999 crisis, the Kosovo health care system was in disarray. This was caused by neglect, poor maintenance, the dismissal of ethnic Albanian employees, and the evolution of parallel health care delivery and medical education systems. While humani-tarian inputs averted a major health crisis, health care indicators (e.g., infant mortality, access to services, and prenatal care) were poor.[3]

---

[2] P. Spiegel and P. Salama, *Kosovar Albanian Health Survey September 1999,* International Emergencies and Refugee Health Branch, Centers for Disease Control and Prevention.

[3] Department for International Development, *Kosovo: Strategy Paper 2001–2004,* Section on organization of the health care system, August 2001.

The formal health care system emphasized secondary and tertiary care, based on the formal socialist model, with less attention to primary care and public health. There were five district hospitals and a tertiary hospital with a collective total of 5,500 beds (Table 6.1). Hospital occupancy was generally under 75 percent.[4] Primary care was provided by specialists in the towns and by general practitioners working in *ambulantas*, or smaller outpatient facilities in villages. At the township level, primary care was organized around a medical facility with multiple subspecialty clinics.[5] Patients self-referred and went directly to specialists of their choosing; there was little coordination of care among specialists. Public health, prevention, and health promotion services were not an integral part of the primary care system.[6]

During the 1990s, Kosovar Albanians were systematically excluded by the Serbian government from the formal health care system and other social services.[7] In 1991, disenfranchised physicians organized a parallel NGO called the Mother Theresa Society (MTS) to improve the access of Kosovar Albanians to social welfare services, including health care. They opened their own *ambulantas* and about

Table 6.1
Characteristics of Formal Health Care System, Kosovo

Hospitals		Health Professionals	
Number of facilities	6	Doctors and dentists	2,300
Number of beds	5,500	Nurses	4,500
Avg. length of stay	12.5	Midwives	200
		Technicians	2,000

[4] Department for International Development, *Kosovo: Strategy Paper.*

[5] World Health Organization, *Operations in Kosovo, Action Plan 2000.*

[6] M.J. Morkiawa, "Primary Care Training in Kosovo," *International Family Medicine*, Vol. 35, No. 6, June 2003, pp. 440–444.

[7] Morkiawa, "Primary Care Training in Kosovo."

120 small private pharmacies. The MTS was supported by many foreign NGOs and by Kosovar Albanians in foreign nations. The private pharmacies were supplied by a number of NGOs and two private wholesalers. Since Kosovar Albanians composed roughly 80 percent of the total population, this parallel health care system was what the majority of the population depended on during the 1990s. When Albanians were denied access to formal medical education, the Kosovar Albanian medical community started its own parallel medical education training through the MTS, graduating 700 doctors and 1,200 nurses during the ten-year period.[8] WHO has questioned the quality of the medical training received under this parallel system. Many graduates had never treated patients in a hospital environment and thus had limited practical experience with direct patient care, management of health care facilities, and treatment of hospitalized patients.[9]

Public health services in Kosovo were organized around the Institutes of Public Health (IPH), which had a central facility and five regional or district facilities. These services included communicable disease surveillance and control, environmental protection, water, sanitation, and food safety. The public health programs were vertically organized and poorly integrated with other sectors. Tuberculosis control included 22 anti-tuberculosis dispensaries, two specialized hospitals for lung diseases, and pulmonary dispensaries in regional hospitals. Urban areas had piped water supplies. However, the distribution systems and pumps were poorly maintained, and the water was not regularly chlorinated. Cross-contamination through pipe breakages occurred. Rural areas relied primarily on well water, and many wells were contaminated.[10]

---

[8] The Mother Theresa Society was supported by many foreign NGOs as well as Kosovar Albanians in foreign nations (Morkiawa, "Primary Care Training in Kosovo"). The private pharmacies were supplied by a number of NGOs and two private wholesalers (P. Mason, "Kosovo After the Conflict: Rebuilding Pharmaceutical Services," *Pharmaceutical Journal*, Vol. 264, No. 7079, January 15, 2000, pp. 98–100.

[9] World Health Organization, *Operations in Kosovo, Action Plan 2000*.

[10] World Health Organization, *Operations in Kosovo, Action Plan 2000*, p. 19.

Before 1991, reporting systems with forms and guidelines written in Serbian and Albanian allowed a summary of demographic, health status, manpower, and service utilization indicators to be produced annually. But the Serbian government in 1991 replaced these forms and guidelines with Serbian-only versions, for the most part omitting the Kosovar Albanians from disease surveillance records for the ten years prior to the conflict. Much of the information on the health status of the Kosovar Albanians prior to the conflict comes from a few disparate sources.

Although incomplete, a 1991 census estimated that Kosovo was home to approximately two million people. Roughly 82 percent were ethnic Albanians, 10 percent ethnic Serbian, and 8 percent from other ethnic groups.[11] Prior to the conflict, Kosovo had approximately two million inhabitants with a population density of about 200 persons per square kilometer and a birth rate around 27.7 live births per 1,000 inhabitants. This was among the highest birth rates in Europe. Population growth averaged 2.1 percent per year between 1981 and 1991.[12] The population was poor, with a 1991 average per capita income of $470 and an unemployment rate estimated at 50 percent.[13]

The IPH reported a monthly crude mortality rate of between 0.29 and 0.36 deaths per 1,000 population between 1990 and 1996. However, WHO questioned the accuracy of the data, and in 1999 the international community undertook a population-based survey of

---

[11] United Nations High Commissioner for Refugees, *Concept Paper on a Proposed Framework for Return of Refugees and Internally Displaced Persons to Kosovo*, Section 3, Planning Figures and Assumptions, UNHCR News, May 12, 1999, p. 2. UNHCR prepared this paper with input from International Organizations for Migration, United Nations Development Programme, United Nations Population Fund, Office of the United Nations High Commissioner for Refugees, United Nations Children's Fund, United Nations Office for the Coordination of Humanitarian Affairs, World Health Organization, and World Food Programme.

[12] World Health Organization, *Operations in Kosovo, Action Plan 2000*, p. 6.

[13] World Health Organization, *Operations in Kosovo, Action Plan 2000*; Department for International Development, *Kosovo: Strategy Paper 2001–2004*, Section on organization of the health care system.

Kosovar Albanians. That survey estimated that the monthly crude mortality rate from natural causes was 0.45 deaths per 1,000 inhabitants, consistent with that of a young population. For adults under 65, heart disease, neoplasms, and stroke were the major causes of death in the pre-conflict phase. For adults over 65, major causes of death included chronic lung diseases, respiratory system neoplasms, and ischemic heart disorders, all related to chronic tobacco use.[14]

In 1989, the infant mortality rate was about 51.2 deaths per 1,000 live births. Major causes of mortality for children under five years of age included neonatal and perinatal conditions, respiratory and gastrointestinal disorders, and congenital abnormalities. In addition, Kosovo had one of the lowest child immunization coverage rates in Europe, estimated at 70 to 75 percent in 1998. UNICEF estimated that in 1996, 93 percent of children between the ages of one and two years had been vaccinated against tuberculosis. Another 75 percent had been vaccinated against DTP and given oral polio vaccines. Of the children between two and three years old, approximately 85 percent had been vaccinated against measles. A July 1999 food and nutrition survey of children under five that was conducted by the NGO Action Against Hunger estimated that 3.1 percent were acutely malnourished and 10.7 percent were stunted—estimates similar to the findings before the conflict escalated.[15]

From 1990 to 1997, 176 epidemics or outbreaks were registered in Kosovo.[16] Hepatitis A was endemic to the region, and sporadic cases of viral hemorrhagic fever (Hanta virus and Crimean-Congo Fever) were reported.[17] New cases of tuberculosis increased from 414 in 1990 to 1,290 in 1996, with an incidence rate two to three times

---

[14] Spiegel and Salama, *Kosovar Albanian Health Survey.*

[15] World Health Organization, *Operations in Kosovo, Action Plan 2000,* pp. 6, 12.

[16] WHO noted that communicable diseases in Kosovo were a major problem, with high case fatality rates for bacterial meningitis, haemorrhagic fever, viral meninogo-encephalitis, shigellosis, and diarrheal diseases.

[17] Spiegel and Salama, *Kosovar Albanian Health Survey,* Background section, p. 15.

that of the entire Federal Republic of Yugoslavia.[18] Surveys conducted in refugee camps in Macedonia found a high prevalence of
chronic conditions such as renal and cardiac disease.[19]

Health Challenges

The conflict significantly impacted the Kosovar Albanian population
and the health sector. The Serbian government's systematic ethnic
cleansing campaign in 1998 and 1999 caused a number of challenges:

- Over 1.5 million Kosovar Albanians were forcibly expelled from
  their homes.
- Over 750,000 people left Kosovo, fleeing to the former Yugoslav
  Republic of Macedonia, to Albania, and to other countries or
  areas within the Federal Republic of Yugoslavia by May 1999.[20]
- Villages and residential areas were systematically destroyed after
  March 1999. An estimated 1,200 residential areas were at least
  partially burned, and over 500 villages were burned.
- Serbian forces killed at least 10,000 Kosovar Albanians.
- The Serbian government systematically stripped Kosovar Albanians of all identity and property documents. At the end of the
  conflict, possibly 50 percent of the population lacked documentation, including records of health care utilization and immunization.[21]

---

[18] World Health Organization, *Operations in Kosovo, Action Plan 2000*, pp. 19, 66.

[19] Spiegel and Salama, *Kosovar Albanian Health Survey*, p. 15.

[20] United Nations High Commissioner for Refugees, *Concept Paper on a Proposed Framework.*

[21] United States Department of State, *Ethnic Cleansing in Kosovo: An Accounting*, Washington, D.C.: Department of State, December 1999, unless otherwise indicated; United Nations High Commissioner for Refugees, *Concept Paper on a Proposed Framework.*

Public Health

The conflict significantly affected Kosovo's public health system. Landmine injuries were a problem. Serbian forces laid landmines between March and May 1999; in the month following the ceasefire, the rate of injuries from mines and other explosives was 10 per 100,000.[22]

The conflict affected the mental health of the population extensively, and there were substantial numbers of victims of violence. For example, refugees were reportedly used as human shields during the conflict. A population-based survey of Kosovar refugees in Albania and Macedonia that was conducted by Physicians for Human Rights found that over one-third of survey respondents reported either witnessing Serb police or soldiers kill someone, or seeing dead bodies they believed were killed by Serb police or soldiers.[23] There were also numerous accounts of organized and individual rape of Kosovar Albanian women. Local human rights associations estimated that between 10 and 20 percent of women and girls had been raped during the crisis.[24] Not surprisingly, the prevalence of post-traumatic stress disorder was estimated at between 15 and 20 percent.[25] Compared to refugees, internally displaced persons in Kosovo during 1999 suffered more traumatic events, such as forced isolation, torture, abuse, lack of shelter, and forced separations from family. Psychiatric morbidity was also prevalent among the Serbian minority remaining in Kosovo after

---

[22] World Health Organization, *Operations in Kosovo, Action Plan 2000*, p. 7.

[23] Physicians for Human Rights, *War Crimes in Kosovo: A Population-Based Assessment of Human Rights Violations of Kosovar Albanians by Serb Forces*, June 15, 1999.

[24] World Health Organization, *Operations in Kosovo, Action Plan 2000*, p. 13; B. Cardozo et al., "Mental Health, Social Functioning, and Attitudes of Kosovar Albanians Following the War in Kosovo," *Journal of American Medical Association*, Vol. 284, No. 5, August 2, 2000, pp. 569–577. A cross-sectional sample survey was conducted from August through October 1999 of 1,358 Kosovar Albanians aged 15 years or older in 558 randomly selected households across Kosovo.

[25] Spiegel and Salama, *Kosovar Albanian Health Survey*, Background section, p. 15.

the war. Defeated Serbs had higher mean scores for depression and social dysfunction than did their Albanian counterparts.[26]

The monthly crude mortality rate for deaths from natural causes was 0.45 deaths per 1,000, with the elderly (those 60 and older) particularly vulnerable. Their rate was estimated at 3.29 deaths per 1,000. The increase in mortality from natural causes was likely an indirect result of the war. It may have been brought about by decreased access to health care for those with chronic conditions or with diseases exacerbated by war-related stress.[27] Other public health challenges included:

- Meeting the basic housing needs of a displaced population, particularly given the impending approach of winter. UNHCR and the International Management Group estimated that of the pre-conflict housing stock of 365,000 units in Kosovo, 34 percent had been damaged or completely destroyed.[28]
- Restoring and improving sanitation and other public works systems. Such basic infrastructure as sanitation, sewage, and waste disposal systems were substandard and neglected before the war.
- Coordinating the relief efforts of the approximately 400 NGOs in-country.
- Implementing immunization programs and re-establishing programs for communicable diseases such as tuberculosis. Tuberculosis incidence was increasing, but the structure for tuberculosis control had disintegrated during the conflict. Of the 22

[26] P. Salama et al., "Mental Health and Nutritional Status Among the Adult Serbian Minority in Kosovo," *Journal of American Medical Association*, Vol. 284, No. 5, August 2, 2000; J. Westermeyer, "Health of Albanians and Serbians Following the War in Kosovo, Studying the Survivors on Both Sides of Armed Conflict," Editorial, *Journal of American Medical Association*, Vol. 284, 2000, pp. 615–616.

[27] Spiegel and Salama, *Kosovar Albanian Health Survey*, Mortality section, p. 23.

[28] The pre-conflict housing stock was estimated to be approximately 365,000 dwelling units. Approximately 125,00 homes had been damaged, 49,000 of them beyond repair. United States Agency for International Development, *Shelter in Kosovo: Challenges and Solutions*, Fact Sheet, Washington, D.C.: USAID, November 10, 1999.

anti-tuberculosis dispensaries existent at the beginning of the conflict, only nine remained by the end.[29]

Because the public health information system had collapsed, there was a lack of basic information on the health status of the population that was needed for the international community's planning and rebuilding efforts. The destruction or looting of *ambulantas*, health houses, and tuberculosis dispensaries affected the reporting centers. Most records were burned or lost.[30] And because the Serbian government had stripped Kosovar Albanians of all documentation, few records of health care needs and utilization remained. In addition, the massive movement and displacement of the population complicated data gathering.

Health Care Delivery

The conflict substantially weakened the health care delivery system. Kosovar Albanian physicians, patients, and medical facilities were systematically attacked, and health care facilities were used as protective cover for military activities. The Physicians for Human Rights and other NGOs estimated that Serbian forces destroyed at least 100 medical clinics, pharmacies, and hospitals.[31] Thus, in the post-conflict phase, the international community had three main tasks: address the immediate needs for food, shelter, water, basic medical services, and safe return; address the new health care and service delivery problems that had arisen as a result of the conflict and the disruption of the population's lives; and rebuild and reform the health care sector.

Kosovar Albanian medical staff needed to be reintegrated and re-trained, either because they had not practiced in ten years or because their MTS training had not sufficiently prepared them.[32] The inter-

---

[29] World Health Organization, *Operations in Kosovo, Action Plan 2000.*

[30] World Health Organization, *Operations in Kosovo, Action Plan 2000.*

[31] U.S. Department of State, *Ethnic Cleansing in Kosovo.*

[32] Morkiawa, "Primary Care Training in Kosovo," pp. 440–444.

national community needed to repair, rebuild, and resupply health care facilities destroyed or looted during the war, and it needed to distribute required medicines and re-establish the pharmaceutical distribution network. Further, it had to face the challenging task of meeting the mental health needs of a severely traumatized population. One percent of the total population had a psychiatric disorder, and 4 percent had psychopathological reactions because of severe emotional trauma. In addition, psychiatric patients had been discharged from facilities in neighboring regions and released into Kosovo, despite Kosovo's limited capacity to meet their health care needs.[33]

Health Approach and Assessment

The early development of a health policy framework for Kosovo was important in guiding the health sector's reconstruction and reform, but unclear participant roles and responsibilities hindered implementation of the action plan for health sector reform. This section outlines key participants and donors, describes the approach taken, and gives an overall assessment of the effort in Kosovo.

Key Participants and Donors

UNMIK was given responsibility for rebuilding Kosovo following the June 1999 peace agreement; UNHCR was designated as the lead agency for ensuring the repatriation and return of the refugees.[34] WHO was to provide major technical support for health to UNMIK, working in an advisory and coordinating role.[35] Under the proposed division of sector responsibilities outlined in a May 1999 concept paper drafted by UNCHR, WHO was to be the lead agency for health. UNICEF and UNHCR were to assist WHO in this effort, as were other key partners from the international and NGO communities:

---

[33] World Health Organization, *Operations in Kosovo, Action Plan 2000*, p. 12.

[34] United Nations High Commissioner of Refugees, *Concept Paper on a Proposed Framework*.

[35] World Health Organization, *Operations in Kosovo, Action Plan 2000*.

EU's Humanitarian Aid Office, International Rescue Committee, Kinderberg International, Pharmacists Without Borders (Pharmaciens Sans Frontieres), Doctors Without Borders (Médecins Sans Frontières), Medair, and Doctors of the World (Médecins du Monde).[36]

On July 28, 1999, a European Commission (EC) task force in Brussels conducted the first major assessment of the Kosovo reconstruction and development costs. The task force estimated that the cost to repair the damage to housing and other village facilities (such as clinics, schools, and water supply) would be $43.9 million. The United States pledged $277.6 million in nonhumanitarian "urgent" aid. This pledge and the U.S. humanitarian assistance pledge together represented 25 percent of all donor pledges.[37]

The EC and World Bank, with broad donor organization support, conducted a more comprehensive conference focusing on reconstruction in November 1999. This assessment included the energy, telecommunications, commercial, and social infrastructure and laid out reconstruction and development objectives for the next five years. The EC and World Bank estimated that $2.3 billion in external financing was required, with nearly half of the funds needed before early 2001. In addition, Kosovo's 2000 government operations were expected to run a $107 million deficit and require external financing. Donors were asked to contribute to the operational budget in addition to the programs outlined in the reconstruction strategy. The EU was to lead reconstruction efforts; it established a European Agency for Reconstruction of Kosovo one month later. The United States Agency for International Development (USAID) established a mission in Pristina to implement the U.S. assistance program. The United States pledged $157 million, 15 percent of the total pledged at the November donor conference. EU member states pledged $759 million, 74 percent of the total requested. At the next donor

---

[36] United Nations High Commissioner of Refugees, *Concept Paper on a Proposed Framework*.

[37] Curt Tarnoff, "Kosovo: Reconstruction and Development Assistance," *CRS Report for Congress*, Updated June 7, 2001, Order Code RL30453.

conference, in February 2001, the United States pledged an additional $94.3 million. Combined with an additional amount for the police force, the total U.S. 2001 contribution for reconstruction and police amounted to $149.7 million.[38]

In Kosovo, the United States provided aid primarily in the form of technical assistance, small grants, and the deployment of civilian police to assume police functions and help train the new police force. USAID's field presence in the Former Republic of Yugoslavia started in 1998, was briefly interrupted during the NATO intervention when all non-emergency U.S. government personnel had to evacuate, and restarted shortly after the conflict ended. USAID's program was implemented primarily through U.S. NGOs working as partners with indigenous NGOs and other local organizations.[39]

USAID was a major player in humanitarian aid, as were other international organizations, including UNHCR, World Food Programme, WHO, and UNICEF.[40] During the crisis, the United States was the major source of food assistance as part of the humanitarian assistance provided to refugees. In 1999, USAID's Office of Foreign Disaster Assistance (OFDA) provided winterization assistance, emergency and nonemergency food distribution, and health care to about 40 percent of the conflict-affected population.[41] OFDA also provided $5.9 million to improve water and sanitation systems, $4.2 million for health care, and $3.5 million for emergency food and nonfood distribution.[42] During 2000, USAID's Food for Peace office and the U.S. Department of Agriculture provided over $90 million in food aid, representing approximately 85 to 95 percent of all food assistance

---

[38] Tarnoff, "Kosovo: Reconstruction and Development Assistance."

[39] United States Agency for International Development, *CP FY 2000: Federal Republic of Yugoslavia*, Washington, D.C.: USAID, 2000.

[40] United States Agency for International Development, *CP FY 2000: Federal Republic of Yugoslavia*.

[41] United States Agency for International Development, *CP FY 2000*.

[42] United States Agency for International Development, *Kosovo CP FY 2001,* Washington, D.C.: USAID, 2001.

distributed.[43] In addition, about $5.2 million in International Disaster Assistance was given to NGOs through an umbrella grant to provide services to conflict-affected populations.[44]

During 2001, OFDA continued to provide housing assistance through its shelter program, deployed mobile medical clinics to the isolated enclaves in Gjilan and Mitrovica, implemented water and sanitation programs for well cleaning and water testing, and supported agriculture programs.[45] USAID Kosovo Assistance Program, an umbrella grant implemented through NGOs, supported priority activities to help stabilize communities, such as women's health projects (e.g., to help develop the maternal and infant health infrastructure) and restoration of community services. In 2002, USAID's infrastructure rehabilitation program funded small-scale rehabilitation projects, including those health facilities, schools, utilities distribution systems, and transport and municipal infrastructure. Other USAID projects included economic policy reform assistance, micro-lending programs to foster small business growth, democratization projects, and efforts to reform Kosovo's judicial system.[46]

The EU was the lead institution in the physical reconstruction of Kosovo's housing sector and major infrastructure. The EC Humanitarian Organization provided assistance in education, water and sanitation, health, and food. Other major donors included WHO; United Nations Fund for Population Activities; UNICEF; EU Agency for Reconstruction of Kosovo; bilateral donors such as Japan, Finland, Canada, Sweden, and the United Kingdom; and nearly 30 international NGOs working in health sector policy, institutional reform, and service delivery.[47]

---

[43] Tarnoff, "Kosovo: Reconstruction and Development Assistance."

[44] United States Agency for International Development, *Kosovo CP FY 2001.*

[45] *Doctors of the World/USA Maternal and Infant Health Project 1998–2002*, Final Report, New York: Doctors of the World/USA, 2002.

[46] Tarnoff, "Kosovo: Reconstruction and Development Assistance," June 7, 2001.

[47] United States Agency for International Development, *Kosovo: Activity Data Sheet*, FY 2003 Program, Washington, D.C.: USAID, 2003.

The EU financed programs for basic power and water infrastructure rehabilitation, provided materials for local housing repair, helped re-establish the customs service, supported village job creation, created a landmine clearance coordination center, and helped repair roads and bridges. Although Kosovo is not eligible for lending, World Bank provided $60 million in grant assistance through a trust fund for Kosovo that supported efforts to reform the health, education, and banking systems; improve agricultural production; and bolster the energy sector.[48]

A contentious issue arose over burden-sharing and the extent of the U.S. role in Kosovo's reconstruction. The position of the Clinton administration, Bush administration, and U.S. Congress was that the EU and its member states should be the principal contributors for reconstruction because the United States had borne the majority of the burden for conducting the war. For this reason, Congress capped the U.S. share of reconstruction activities at 15 percent in the 2000 appropriations bill. This debate was exacerbated by the slowness of European donors in dispensing promised aid to Kosovo in 2000. The EU countered that EU nations had provided 80 percent of KFOR troops and that the EU was providing the majority of reconstruction assistance. Although the November 1999 donor conference yielded sufficient pledges to meet broad spending goals for 2000, the donors were slow in providing the funding, particularly for the health and housing sectors. The issue of how aid should be proportioned among donors continued to be an important one.[49]

Overall Action Plan. One of the initial tasks the international community faced was that of gathering baseline data on the health status of the population, the demand for services, and utilization patterns to inform rebuilding and service delivery planning. Consequently, in September 1999 the international community directed a provincewide survey conducted by the International Rescue Committee (IRC), the Institute of Public Health (IPH), the U.S. Centers for

---

[48] Tarnoff, "Kosovo: Reconstruction and Development Assistance."

[49] Tarnoff, "Kosovo: Reconstruction and Development Assistance."

Disease Control and Prevention (CDC), and WHO.[50] The following month a separate survey of selected remaining Serbian enclaves was conducted.

Given that the health care system prior to the war had been inefficient and that a parallel system of health care had existed, WHO decided, as part of its overarching long-term goal of reforming the health care system, to redirect public health practice toward a primary care model. This was done in part through coordination of the international relief brought into the province and guided by UNMIK's Health Office.[51] A key element was to decentralize the old polyclinic system and establish a primary care system based on the family medicine model. It differentiated primary, secondary, and tertiary care and specified that the majority of medical problems would be treated by primary care providers instead of specialists.[52] In 2000, WHO came out with an action plan for Kosovo that included six core elements:

- Improve and strengthen primary health care.
- Improve and strengthen secondary health care.
- Improve the management system of pharmaceuticals.
- Strengthen the capacity for health policy, planning, and financing.
- Decrease the burden of disease through targeted public and environmental health interventions.
- Coordinate the humanitarian assistance.[53]

The initial planning document for the international community's role in Kosovo stressed the importance of a comprehensive and integrated framework for reconstruction. It also stressed the effect that long-term reconstruction and development assistance would have

---

[50] Spiegel, *Kosovar Albanian Health Survey.*

[51] World Health Organization, *Operations in Kosovo, Action Plan 2000*, p. 32.

[52] Morkiawa, "Primary Care Training in Kosovo," pp. 440–444.

[53] Morkiawa, "Primary Care Training in Kosovo," pp. 440–444.

on Yugoslavia as a whole. A successful effort, UNHCR commented, would aid reintegration of returning refugees and those that had been internally displaced.[54]

The rebuilding of the health sector in Kosovo has been cited as one of the most successful efforts to rebuild health after major conflict.[55] A key lesson from past nation-building efforts in Kosovo was that restoring the original health system, with its vulnerabilities and inequities, was not the right choice.[56] Instead, WHO led a process for developing a health policy framework that addressed the emergency phase and included a plan for long-term health sector reform, summarized in September 1999. Three months after the 1999 conflict ended, an interim health policy document was issued that outlined specific policy goals and organizational principles for reforming the health sector. Elements included promotion of family medicine, specialist consultation through referral, recognition of public and private roles in delivering health services, and an essential drug program.[57]

The interim health policy document specifically stated that humanitarian resources would not be used to expand the health system beyond the limits of national revenue and would only be used to repair damage from the war or due to years of neglect.[58] This document was intended to provide guidance to local health care workers and officials, the humanitarian agencies, and the donor community to help channel the relatively large amount of humanitarian support

---

[54] United Nations High Commissioner of Refugees, *Concept Paper on a Proposed Framework.*

[55] O. Bornemisza and E. Sondorp, *Health Policy Formulation in Complex Political Emergencies and Post-Conflict Countries,* A Literature Review, London School of Hygiene & Tropical Medicine, London: University of London, Department of Public Health and Policy. November 7, 2002, p. 16.

[56] World Health Organization, *The Transition from Relief to Development in the Context of Complex Humanitarian Emergencies and Natural Disasters,* ECOSOC 2002 Humanitarian Segment, WHO technical contribution to the panel, New York: WHO, July 16, 2002.

[57] A. Zwi, *Post-Conflict: Health System Development in Kosovo*, London School of Hygiene & Tropical Medicine, London: University of London, www.lshtm.ac.uk/hpu/post_conflict_kosovo_project.htm (as of January 21, 2004).

[58] Bornemisza and Sondorp, *Health Policy Formulation,* p. 16.

coming into Kosovo in a direction supportive of the long-term reconstruction goals.[59]

Development of the policy framework has been widely cited as a key element in coordinating the external assistance (particularly by major donors and NGOs) to rebuild the health sector in Kosovo. However, problems arose with its implementation. WHO was criticized for not being inclusive in the planning process. The balance between timely emergency efforts and being inclusive clearly created tension.[60] WHO was criticized for not consulting with all relevant players, and thus running the risk of not getting local buy-in and ownership of the plan. Some questioned whether the goal of reform at such an early stage was feasible given the limited local capacity; some also argued that service provision was the immediate priority.[61] Though preliminary drafts of the planning document were not widely distributed, the major health NGOs appear to have used the policy document to guide their own programming. Wider distribution of the policy document might have helped avert the less favorable initiatives taken earlier on by the smaller, less experienced agencies and some of the military actors that were present.[62]

Unfortunately, UNMIK and WHO were unprepared to fill the leadership vacuum in the health sector following the 1999 conflict. Early in the planning phase, there had been discussions of WHO serving as an interim Ministry of Health, but the role had not been clearly defined. Shortly thereafter, the decision was made that WHO would not form the Department of Health (referred to here as UNMIK Health) but would instead provide it and its staff with support to help lead the department. UNMIK Health did not have the capacity needed to take forward the major policy, institutional, and budgetary problems that needed to be addressed for the health sector.

---

[59] C. de Ville de Goyet and E. Sondorp, *Internal Evaluation of WHO Response in Kosovo, June–December 1999*, WHO/EHA, May 2001.

[60] Zwi, *Post-Conflict: Health System Development in Kosovo.*

[61] Bornemisza and Sondorp, *Health Policy Formulation.*

[62] de Ville de Goyet and Sondorp, *Internal Evaluation of WHO Response.*

It maintained only a small central secretariat of three to four international staff and five offices with one or two health officers.[63] WHO criticized UNMIK Health for having low technical and administrative staffing that limited the department's ability to coordinate and regulate the development of health services.[64] WHO, however, was amply funded and grew rapidly. Many of those involved in Kosovo viewed it as the de facto Ministry of Health, with UNMIK Health's role being to "rubberstamp" WHO activities. Confusion as to which entity was the "real" Ministry of Health would persist for a long time in the eyes of most external stakeholders.[65]

Public Health

This section examines two public health issues: the targeted public and environmental health interventions, and the coordination of humanitarian assistance, with particular attention to WHO's role.

Targeted Public and Environmental Health Interventions. One of WHO's most important objectives was to improve the public health and municipal infrastructure services (such as water quality and supply), set health standards for food safety and other areas, undertake immunization campaigns, and re-establish communicable disease control and health information systems.[66] WHO created a Health Commission and implemented a one-year project to revamp public health services, which included changing the IPH organizational structure to focus more on epidemiology, hygiene, social medicine, and health policy and planning. A pilot study was undertaken to create a health information system for outpatients. A tularemia outbreak highlighted deficiencies in the epidemiologist training; WHO subsequently made this a priority area. The Hygiene Department began developing a managerial process for water control and regulation.

---

[63] Department for International Development, *Kosovo: Strategy Paper*.

[64] World Health Organization, *Kosovo Health Sector Situation Report*, January 2000.

[65] de Ville de Goyet and Sondorp, *Internal Evaluation of WHO Response*, p. 23.

[66] World Health Organization, *Operations in Kosovo, Action Plan 2000*, pp. 17–19.

IPH and WHO worked on re-establishing monitoring and inspection of the drinking water supply. WHO took a lead role in introducing health care waste management in the regional hospitals and made re-establishing the waste collection services in the urban areas a priority.[67]

Following the creation of UNMIK, all tuberculosis control activities were to be integrated into a WHO-coordinated tuberculosis commission that eventually was to be administered by the Kosovo Ministry of Health.[68] In 1999, a five-year tuberculosis control partnership program was initiated by the NGOs Doctors of the World (DOW), Médecins du Monde Sweden, WHO, UNICEF, Pharmacists Without Borders, and the IPH in Kosovo to reduce tuberculosis morbidity and mortality, improve treatment completion rates, and support WHO's modified direct observation therapy strategy (DOTS).[69] According to USAID, Kosovo now has 95 percent DOTS compliance and an 84 percent treatment success in new smear-positive patients.[70]

Kosovo's Ministry of Health reported a drop in the incidence of tuberculosis from 78 to 67 per 100,000 from 2001 to 2002. USAID sponsored the HIV/AIDS prevention program supporting Population Services International (PSI) to provide technical assistance, establish three voluntary testing and counseling centers (VTCs), and educate

---

[67] World Health Organization, *Operations in Kosovo, Action Plan 2000.*

[68] UNMIK mandated the formation of a Tuberculosis Technical Commission to advise on the implementation of a tuberculosis prevention and control program. In 2000, the commission published a tuberculosis action plan outlining a strategy for development of a national tuberculosis program, including skill development for all professionals involved, to ensure the supply of essential anti-tuberculosis drugs, strengthen diagnostic support services, and introduce a health promotion and education program. Doctors of the World, *Our Projects: Kosovo*; WHO, *Tuberculosis Action Plan: Kosovo, 2000,* Tuberculosis Technical Commission, WHO, January 2, 2004.

[69] United States Agency for International Development, *USAID Fact Sheet on Special Initiatives: Kosovo,* Tuberculosis Control Partnership Program, Washington, D.C.: USAID, July 17, 2004, www.globalcorps.com/orgs/ngo/dotw/kosovo.html.

[70] United States Agency for International Development, *USAID's Key Achievements: Meeting TB Challenges in Kosovo,* Washington, D.C.: USAID, www.usaid.gov/our_work/global_health/id/tuberculosis/achievements.html#kosovo (as of August 30, 2005).

the public. For 2004, USAID provided support to the Kosovo AIDS Committee and IPH to implement an STI/HIV surveillance system as part of the Kosovo Strategy for HIV/AIDS Prevention.[71]

USAID and the American International Health Alliance (AIHA) supported the formation of a joint partnership between Dartmouth Medical School and the Primary Health Care Authorities in Gjakova/ Djakovica municipality, the goal of which would be to establish a reproductive health partnership with one of the family medicine centers. The aims included creating a system for providing reproductive health services in the family medicine centers, providing evidence-based training to clinicians, increasing the capacity and competency of family physicians and family nurses to provide reproductive health services, and increasing community awareness of these services.[72]

Coordination of Humanitarian Assistance. A near-term goal of the action plan for Kosovo was to provide humanitarian aid and meet the basic needs of the population, and to do so by working in conjunction with the local population, UNMIK, foreign governments, and NGOs. In the period preceding the NATO bombing campaign and continuing until six months after the war ended, humanitarian assistance was needed to take care of the flow of refugees. Assistance was also needed to assist their return, especially during the winter of 1999–2000. The international community provided shelter for 350,000 people and distributed food to more than 900,000. To meet housing needs, nearly 60,000 emergency repair kits and more than 10,000 roofing repair kits were distributed. Thousands of tents and accommodation centers were also made available for those with no other alternative.[73]

---

[71] United States Agency for Independent Development, *USAID Mission in Kosovo: Data Sheet, FY 2004 Program,* Washington, D.C.: USAID, www.usaid.gov/policy/budget/ cbj2005/ee/pdf/167-0410.pdf (as of August 30, 2005).

[72] United States Agency for Independent Development, *Kosovo. Health Issues: Reproductive Health Partnership,* Washington, D.C.: USAID, www.usaid.gov/missions/kosovo/Activities/ Health_initiatives.htm (as of August 30, 2005).

[73] Tarnoff, "Kosovo: Reconstruction and Development Assistance."

The humanitarian assistance mission was one of the major success stories of the initial deployment, with most Kosovar Albanians and displaced persons returning home. UNHCR provided shelter assistance to 700,000 people over the winter. Meanwhile, other relief agencies distributed food aid to 1.5 million people.[74] The U.S. Department of Defense played a key role in the humanitarian response to the refugee situation, helping with the distribution of relief supplies and providing security to relief convoys and the returning Kosovar Albanians and displaced persons. In addition to assisting with the distribution of humanitarian assistance, the U.S. Department of Defense contributed $880,000 in 1999 for 220,000 humanitarian daily rations.[75]

WHO was asked by World Bank and EU to play a humanitarian coordination role in the health sector.[76] It participated in regular meetings of representatives from the donor and NGO communities and sponsored meetings for consultation and consensus-building purposes. In WHO's view, its early and visible presence positioned it to be the lead health agency; WHO was turned to by a number of international health agencies and donors for information, advice, and coordination.

In the early humanitarian phase, UNHCR was the lead agency. To provide relief assistance, UNHCR assigned the responsibility for coordination at the regional level to selected NGOs. However, the international community found that the most pressing need was for rehabilitation and development of the societal systems and infrastructure, including the health sector. Additional challenges included poor water quality, lack of food control, and the potential for disease outbreaks.[77] Because WHO was present in Kosovo before the 1999 crisis

---

[74] Dobbins et al., *America's Role in Nation-Building*.

[75] United States Department of State, *Kosovo Humanitarian Situation Report 1*, Bureau of Population, Refugees, and Migration, Washington, D.C.: Department of State, March 31, 1999.

[76] World Health Organization, *Operations in Kosovo, Action Plan 2000*.

[77] de Ville de Goyet and Sondorp, *Internal Evaluation of WHO Response*, p. 11.

and also at the return of the international community, many expected that WHO would step into an advisory and coordination role and provide critical information about the population's health care needs and status. However, WHO lacked the immediate capacity for such a role.

In the absence of a local government and health authorities to support it, WHO should have been prepared to play a more proactive role from the beginning. It could have adopted a dual-track approach of coordinating the initial transition phase and guiding the early and medium-term development phase. WHO activities during the first six months developed at a rapid pace that outran the planning capacity of the WHO office. The field staff was unprepared to respond to the larger developmental challenge they faced. They were initially oriented toward a relief operation rather than medium- and long-term health planning. WHO was criticized for not having the right mix of technical and support personnel in place, which was seen as leading to delays in program delivery and the recruitment of key personnel, the short duration of the expert missions, and the unsolicited arrival of short-term experts in areas considered of little relevance. The WHO field office was hampered by the initial WHO Mission Head and his team's lack of familiarity with the development side of WHO and with administrative procedures.[78]

The WHO field office was further hamstrung by a cumbersome bureaucracy and the fact that it reported to two different headquarters that had competing agendas. The office's suboptimal functioning stemmed from insufficient logistic and administrative support from higher levels within WHO, a lack of strategic planning, and insufficient internal coordination between various WHO programs providing technical support. Whereas experienced humanitarian organizations empowered local offices to commit large amounts of funds, recruit locally, and compete for local purchases, WHO was handi-

---

[78] de Ville de Goyet and Sondorp, *Internal Evaluation of WHO Response*, pp. 16–17.

capped by its inability to decentralize budgetary and financial management responsibility.[79]

Although WHO was applauded for taking the lead in developing policy guidance, it was viewed as having missed an important opportunity by not directing the humanitarian relief effort in support of that policy and not taking a stronger leadership role. The policy framework alone could not ensure compliance; all issues of authority, mandate, and leadership had to be clarified.[80] WHO, however, saw its role as providing only technical and coordination support. The key players wanted WHO to play a more proactive role in ensuring that the NGO's activities or bilateral initiatives in the health sector would be compatible. The donor community viewed WHO's distribution of guidelines and information as inadequate for ensuring the appropriate direction of the humanitarian and reconstruction effort. WHO, however, did not see its role as enforcing such compliance. An important remaining issue was the question of who would have the authority to enforce the health policy framework and to make relief agencies abide by it.[81] Concerned about the potential long-term damages of inappropriate reconstruction projects, the three main donors—the EU, United Kingdom, and United States—requested WHO's collaboration in reviewing and screening all health projects submitted by NGOs.[82]

De Ville de Goyet and Sondorp, who were commissioned to evaluate WHO's role in Kosovo, concluded that there had not been a full commitment inside WHO to take on such a substantive and proactive role in the early post-conflict phase of the Kosovo operation.[83] In the future, it will be important for UNMIK Health, and other

---

[79] de Ville de Goyet and Sondorp, *Internal Evaluation of WHO Response*, pp. 11, 17.

[80] Zwi, *Post-Conflict: Health System Development in Kosovo.*

[81] World Health Organization, *Kosovo Health Sector Situation Report*, January 2000.

[82] de Ville de Goyet and Sondorp, *Internal Evaluation of WHO Response*, p. 27.

[83] de Ville de Goyet and Sondorp, *Internal Evaluation of WHO Response*, p. 29.

leaders in equivalent situations, to develop some form of enforceable authority to restrain projects not aligned with policy goals.[84]

Health Care Delivery

This section examines the reconstruction efforts carried out in health care delivery by focusing on several areas: primary health care, secondary and tertiary health care, the management system of pharmaceuticals, and the capacity for health policy planning and financing.

Primary Health Care. Over the course of reconstruction, nursing and community services were poorly developed; there was little local capacity in health care planning, policy development, and management; and there was little local responsibility for the development, planning, management, and administration of health services. Health care worker training was a priority, particularly for those trained in the MTS parallel educational system. A near-term objective was to have after six months a primary health care system designed and ready for implementation by UNMIK and other partners. It was to include training programs, the mapping of primary health care facilities, recommended staffing norms, and a defined essential primary health care package per center.[85] By May 2000, WHO established a primary care coordinating group and began developing terms of reference for family health centers. WHO coordinated with the EU task force to obtain support for the capacity-building requirements for doctors and nurses and for common core education programs.[86]

However, WHO's delays in developing policy guidance for health care sector reform and its reluctance to assume a leadership role in enforcing that guidance initially left a vacuum for relief agencies. This had several consequences. First, it caused too much focus on certain areas, such as counseling and post-traumatic stress disorder. Many NGOs lacked the necessary cultural or language expertise. Second, mobile health clinics were deployed even though the 1999

---

[84] World Health Organization, *Kosovo Health Sector Situation Report.*

[85] World Health Organization, *Operations in Kosovo, Action Plan 2000*, pp. 10, 32.

[86] World Health Organization, *Kosovo Activities Update*, May 2000.

population-based survey had showed that few Kosovars relied on these clinics for health services and had suggested that NGO resources might be better directed toward rebuilding the health centers. Third, a strong center-periphery divide in service delivery developed early on. While basic primary care services began, public health programs, such as immunization, were poorly organized.[87]

WHO's action plan for improving primary care also included establishment of a family medicine training program and the rehabilitation of teaching and learning facilities. A top priority was to train general practitioners, including those health care workers trained by the MTS, to function as local family physicians. Major NGOs were to partner with WHO in this endeavor.[88] However, WHO took nearly two years to put the official family medicine training program in place. Plans to establish the program raised concern among the NGOs and Kosovar medical community about whether training received in the interim would be accepted by the new program. There was also widespread anxiety about health workers' job security with the NGOs because of the uncertainty about how long the NGOs would stay to support their training.[89]

By May 2000, WHO gained central policy support for establishing the training program. It also made progress in developing six modules for the family medicine program scheduled to start in two months, as well as in selecting the first two cohorts of Trainers of Trainers. In addition, WHO established a primary care family medicine unit at Pristina University Faculty of Medicine.[90] In October 2000, WHO finally started its two-year family practice training program. By December 2001, there were approximately 300 trainees, and the second-year residents were beginning to function as trainers

---

[87] Department for International Development, *Kosovo: Strategy Paper.*

[88] The NGOs and WHO developed a six-month curriculum that included six modules: orientation to family medicine, child health, reproductive health, management of acute and chronic illnesses, mental health, and community medicine.

[89] Morkiawa, "Primary Care Training in Kosovo," pp. 440–444.

[90] World Health Organization, *Kosovo Activities Update.*

in eight regional health centers. The international NGO community provided the clinical mentors for these trainees. However, several concerning issues affecting the training program's future remained: dwindling financial support from the international relief community, a serious shortage of clinical mentors because of requirements that individuals have a wide range of clinical skills and experience in complex humanitarian emergencies, and delays in offering post-training strategies.[91]

Maternal and child health was another primary care priority. The goal was to make maternal and child health an integral part of primary and secondary health care by incorporating a child health module into the family medicine training program, providing training to 500 health workers on essential newborn care and breastfeeding, and expanding the pool of qualified local Integrated Management of Childhood Illnesses trainers.[92] The NGO community also made headway in this area. In 1998, the NGO Doctors of the World was awarded a grant by USAID to develop the maternal and infant health infrastructure.[93] The goal was to help reduce maternal and infant morbidity and mortality by improving reproductive health knowledge and utilization; addressing poor health infrastructure; improving the skills of health providers in the primary, secondary, and tertiary health facilities; and creating a knowledge base of maternal and infant health status service outcomes. The project initially encountered challenges that included a start-up delay due to interference by Yugoslav authorities, two staff evacuations for security reasons, the need to revamp the project due to changed circumstances after the war, and a compressed implementation time frame. The project established a labor and delivery outcomes database in six regional hospitals and the health house with the highest number of births. Doctors of the World established international health educa-

---

[91] Morkiawa, "Primary Care Training in Kosovo," pp. 440–444.

[92] World Health Organization, *Operations in Kosovo, Action Plan 2000*, p. 12; World Health Organization, *Kosovo Activities Update*, May 2000.

[93] *Doctors of the World/USA Maternal and Infant Health Project 1998–2002.*

tion resource centers in two hospitals to improve the access of medical providers to medical literature. It also established 15 health information centers intended to inform visitors about pre- and post-natal topics and family planning. Doctors of the World provided side-by-side training of Kosovar health professionals, provided and reorganized a hospital maternity module, and established antenatal clinics.[94]

In general, Doctors of the World's experience in implementing its maternal and infant health project highlighted some key challenges that NGOs faced in Kosovo. Although Doctors of the World provided equipment to health care facilities, some of the equipment's utility was hampered by a lack of maintenance resources. Occasionally, NGO resources were duplicated in creating training curricula. And the rigid hierarchy among doctors, nurses, and midwives sometimes limited the effectiveness of the training.[95] Doctors of the World was criticized for not always having a coordinated advocacy and policymaking strategy or role regarding UNMIK and the other UN agencies.

Kosovo did not have an inpatient psychiatric facility. Initial relief efforts focused on stress counseling and post-traumatic stress disorder; NGOs and donors paid less attention to providing services to individuals with severe psychiatric illnesses. Furthermore, there were few local mental health specialists and no community-based mental health care strategies. The priority was to coordinate the numerous relief agencies providing services and to build capacity within the primary care and family medicine teams to diagnose and treat mental health problems. A longer-term goal was to develop community-based mental health services. To improve the management and coordination of mental health service delivery and health policy planning, WHO invited international experts to work with local mental health specialists to develop a regional plan for mental health services. Doctors of the World agreed to establish protected apartments for chronic psychiatric patients, and plans were made to build additional transi-

---

[94] *Doctors of the World/USA Maternal and Infant Health Project 1998–2002.*

[95] *Doctors of the World/USA Maternal and Infant Health Project 1998–2002.*

tional housing. A working group was formed to address training issues for general practitioners and nurses and to develop curricula for the psychiatric residency program. In addition, a training program was to be established for mental health professionals and primary health care workers. By May 2000, 20 Kosovar mental health professionals were sent to community-based mental health services in Trieste (WHO Collaborating Center) for intensive training.[96] Provision of essential drugs for mental health care also was to be addressed.[97]

A related issue was the management, care, and protection of victims of gender-based and sexual violence. This was a sensitive issue in Kosovo, because younger women and girls had been specifically targeted by the Serbian forces. WHO's plan for addressing these needs was to develop protocols for health care workers to follow in identifying and providing services to these victims, to train health care and social services personnel, to help establish mechanisms for referral between different sectors, and to bring all relevant partners together to develop a multidisciplinary plan for providing services to individuals.[98] In August 1999, WHO assessed the situation with respect to violence against women. Between December 1999 and April 2000, it conducted fieldwork to gather additional information in preparation for a strategic workshop with key stakeholders. WHO established an NGO group to coordinate domestic violence issues; conducted focus groups and coordinated skills-building workshops on violence, gender, and HIV/AIDS; and assisted UNICEF in developing a training curriculum for nurses in maternity wards in each hospital. WHO organized a workshop with the major stakeholders to develop a multisectoral public health approach to these issues. UNICEF, Organization of Security and Co-operation in Europe, UNMIK, the

---

[96] World Health Organization, *Kosovo Activities Update*.

[97] World Health Organization, *Operations in Kosovo, Action Plan 2000*, pp. 40–41.

[98] World Health Organization, *Operations in Kosovo, Action Plan 2000*, pp. 43–44.

International Medical Corps, and WHO started a public awareness campaign.[99]

Secondary and Tertiary Health Care. WHO's objective was to develop a plan for reforming the hospital sector that would distinguish between primary, secondary, and tertiary care; correct the overemphasis on specialty care and the unevenness in the distribution of hospital care within the province; outline a strategy for building management capacity within the hospital sector; and determine what administrative systems were needed for monitoring quality. In WHO's plan, the Ministry of Health or another central authority would have the overall responsibility for developing the plan for the hospital sector, and WHO would provide technical guidance and support.[100]

In January 2000, WHO reported that it was developing a business plan for the hospital sector, including recommendations for stepwise changes to improve the effective use of secondary care resources.[101] By May 2000, WHO had established a working group of hospital directors to make recommendations to the Department of Health and Social Welfare on essential and managerial tasks and functions for hospitals. WHO also made headway on gathering information about the health infrastructure needs.[102]

The interim policy document that WHO developed was criticized for providing detailed guidance on how to reform primary care services but only broad guidance on the types of reforms needed for secondary and tertiary care. WHO was viewed as having taken a traditional approach to formulating the plan, one that reflected WHO's strong public health emphasis by overemphasizing communicable diseases and underemphasizing noncommunicable diseases.[103] Furthermore, WHO did not see a key role for itself in strengthening ter-

---

[99] World Health Organization, *Kosovo Activities Update.*

[100] World Health Organization, *Operations in Kosovo, Action Plan 2000*, pp. 46–48.

[101] World Health Organization, *Kosovo Health Sector Situation Report.*

[102] World Health Organization, *Kosovo Activities Update.*

[103] de Ville de Goyet and Sondorp, *Internal Evaluation of WHO Response*, p. 11.

tiary care. As a result of WHO's weaknesses in hospital and emergency care, implementation decisions by major donors such as World Bank and EU ended up being more instrumental in directing practical policy in the health sector. The Department for International Development (DFID) in the United Kingdom concluded that the reform of secondary and tertiary care services deserved greater focus. Efforts so far had been primarily directed at the development of capital plans and site refurbishments, with less attention paid to developing appropriate clinical services and supportive networks.[104]

In mid-1999, when the UN mission assumed administration of Kosovo, a NATO peacekeeping force was deployed. When KFOR entered Kosovo, the majority of the force was from EU nations. However, the United States contributed medical units that provided hospital care to the multinational force. U.S. military medical units were part of the UN task force and took turns with other countries in leading the medical mission for KFOR.

The different countries supporting the KFOR medical mission tended to vary in how broadly they defined that mission.[105] Countries with a long history of peacekeeping and humanitarian relief missions, such as Norway and Canada, tended to define their medical mission more broadly. In particular, this included involvement with the host country and the local community in providing direct medical care, as well as undertaking public health activities and helping rebuild the health sector infrastructure. U.S. policy tended to favor a narrower definition of the medical mission, one that focused on providing medical support to the force and provided care to civilians only in emergencies. According to U.S. policy, military medical units were not to get involved in refugee care or in rebuilding the health care infrastructure.

Differences in coalition partners' medical policies created unrealistic expectations of the U.S. medical units and complicated interactions with government officials, the health NGOs, and civilian health

---

[104] Department for International Development, *Kosovo: Strategy Paper.*

[105] Summary is based on Davis et al., *Army Medical Support for Peace Operations.*

care providers and civilians. Local officials, health NGOs, and some coalition partners criticized the United States for not allowing U.S. medical units to get more involved in health care delivery and in health care reconstruction efforts.

Management of Pharmaceuticals. WHO's short-term objectives included providing support to UNMIK to help ensure the supply of essential drugs for primary and secondary care. Its long-term objectives included assisting the development of an appropriate supply system and providing technical assistance to authorities attempting to develop strategies for improving the rational use of drugs.[106]

Early on, the distribution of medicines was poorly organized. Drug donations included out-of-date stock and half-used, unlabeled boxes. This uncoordinated response at times resulted in chaos, including the stocking and disposing of unwanted drugs.[107]

WHO's pharmaceutical project began in August 1999.[108] Maintaining an ongoing supply of pharmaceuticals and increasing the spectrum of drugs available proved to be a constant challenge. The funds needed to maintain the drug supply were at 50 percent of the budgeted amount, and only a limited range of drugs had been procured for four to six months for the secondary and tertiary level hospitals. WHO started providing support for the development of a cooperative of the former state pharmacies, appointed a WHO hospital pharmacy advisor, placed a pharmaceutical procurement expert in the Department of Health and Social Welfare, and was beginning work on re-establishing a regulatory framework for the pharmaceutical sector.[109]

Capacity for Health Policy Planning and Financing. WHO believed that several health policy issues had to be addressed: whether to reactivate health insurance (and, if so, how) or to introduce co-

---

[106] World Health Organization, *Operations in Kosovo, Action Plan 2000*, pp. 24–36.

[107] P. Mason, "Kosovo After the Conflict," pp. 98–100.

[108] World Health Organization, *Kosovo Activities Update*.

[109] World Health Organization, *Kosovo Activities Update*.

payments for public health care, how to improve donor coordination, and what the public-private mix of health care ought to be. WHO's objective was to prepare a strategy paper that would present UNMIK and major international donors with a set of options in health care financing, for both the short and the long term, that could be tested and implemented.[110] WHO led a process for developing a health policy framework that addressed the emergency phase and included a plan for overall health sector reform. Three months after the end of the 1999 conflict, WHO issued an interim health policy document outlining specific policy goals and organizational principles for reforming the health sector. WHO began providing technical assistance to the Department of Health and Social Welfare on developing a co-payment system; creating a registry of NGO, bilateral, and donor-supported health interventions; and establishing a drug regulatory authority and family health centers.[111]

Human resource issues were complex. Following the crisis, Serbian administrators and officials abandoned their posts. This left a management vacuum not easily filled by the Kosovar Albanians, who had been out of the government and hospital administration for ten years. UNMIK's solution was to assign at each hospital a team of international technical experts with varying levels of responsibility for implementing UNMIK policy. In addition, in the post-conflict phase, medical doctors tended to drift into the hospitals rather than into the health houses or polyclinics.[112]

Most health care workers were Albanian, a fact that raised concerns about Serb and other minorities' access to and reintegration into the health care system. Serbian health care workers feared for their safety. In fall 1999, they took over the Mitrovica hospital, excluding Albanian health care workers. UNMIK's eventual solution was to pursue a policy of co-existence, allowing parallel facilities to be set up to provide services to the different ethnic communities.

---

[110] World Health Organization, *Operations in Kosovo, Action Plan 2000.*

[111] World Health Organization, *Kosovo Activities Update.*

[112] Department for International Development, *Kosovo: Strategy Paper.*

There were shortages in some specialties (such as anesthesiology, radiology, psychiatry, and psychology) and overabundance in others. The issue of accreditation and validation of qualifications was a sensitive one. Many Albanian health workers had received their training in the parallel, MTS system of medical education; many had limited clinical experience; and a number of them had lost the papers documenting their credentials.

Another key issue had to do with the wages paid to health care workers. UNMIK budgeted for 10,500 health care workers. However, by January 2000 there were 13,610 workers registered in UNMIK and WHO's database for health care personnel, including 2,100 physicians, 6,200 nurses and medical technicians, 50 pharmacists, 290 midwives, and 800 Serbian staff thought to be attached to the Mitrovica Hospital.[113] Even though many Albanian physicians were able to resume their previous positions in public office, their salaries were much less than expected, and payment was delayed for several months.[114] WHO felt it was unlikely that salary levels would be able to meet local expectations.[115] In addition, the United Kingdom's DFID augmented the income of Pristina University Hospital staff with payments additional to their UN stipend. This added to the dissatisfaction of health workers with low salaries and sent a message (untrue as it was) that the pay was better in the hospital sector than in primary care.[116]

Overall Assessment

WHO, UNCHR, and key medical NGOs had been in Kosovo before the conflict and knew the health sector and the population's needs. This enabled a rapid assessment of the health care needs and the challenges facing the international community in reconstructing the

---

[113] World Health Organization, *Kosovo Health Sector Situation Report.*

[114] Morkiawa, "Primary Care Training in Kosovo," pp. 440–444.

[115] World Health Organization, *Kosovo Health Sector Situation Report.*

[116] World Health Organization, *Kosovo Health Sector Situation Report.*

health sector. Indeed, Kosovo is an important example of how development of a health policy framework early on in a nation-building process can guide the reconstruction and reform of the health sector. The fact that the donor community and the major NGOs agreed to follow this policy guidance was a significant achievement.

Implementation of the action plan for health sector reform met with some problems, however. Not all relevant parties had been consulted in the plan's development. No strong leader emerged early on to enforce adherence to the policy framework. UNMIK was unable to take a lead role in implementing the plan, and WHO was reluctant to assume the lead role or to act as de facto Ministry of Health. WHO did take the lead in developing the policy framework, and many NGOs turned to WHO for guidance; but WHO saw its role solely as a technical advisor in support of the Ministry of Health. WHO was criticized for not assuming the role of de facto Ministry of Health and for not being more proactive in coordinating and enforcing the policy guidance—in essence, for not filling in the Ministry of Health administrative vacuum.

Many of the social institutions in Kosovo were disrupted, requiring major reconstruction on multiple fronts—not just the health sector. Although there was initially ample donor funding, UNMIK lacked the capacity and the flexibility to use that funding effectively. UNMIK and WHO failed to recognize early on that the mission was primarily one of reconstruction and development, not humanitarian relief. They were thus unable to respond quickly to a rapidly changing situation. The UNMIK staff was small and thus hindered in its ability to meet the nation-building demands. The WHO staff was initially small as well, and it had the wrong mix of expertise. Other impediments included WHO field staff's unfamiliarity with the development side of WHO, a cumbersome WHO bureaucracy, and the fact that the field office staff in Kosovo reported to two headquarters with competing agendas.

Security concerns and uncertainty regarding Kosovo's political status were key factors affecting the long-term prospects for rebuilding the health sector. UNMIK and KFOR largely established a safe and secure environment by 2001,[117] but some security concerns still remained. In April 2004, for example, ethnic tensions erupted in rioting and arson by ethnic Albanian mobs directed against minority Serbs. Hundreds of homes and Serbian cultural sites were destroyed, and approximately 4,000 people were displaced in just two days. These incidents resulted in the death of 19 and the injury of more than 1,000, including civilians, international and Kosovo police, and members of the NATO-led peacekeeping force. According to the SRSG and head of UNMIK, the speed with which the unrest spread overwhelmed the ability of the existing KFOR and UNMIK security forces to respond.[118] A recent report on human rights in Kosovo by the Ombudsperson Institution in Kosovo criticized the UN and local leaders for not achieving a minimum level of protection of rights and freedoms, particularly for the Serbian minority.[119] The report noted that the failure to resolve the province's final status has contributed to distrust between the Kosovar Albanian majority and Serbian minority communities, delays in the return of Serbian refugees, a lack of economic growth, and high unemployment (estimated at 60 percent).

Lessons Learned

The successes and limitations of the nation-building effort in Kosovo provide an excellent opportunity to learn from the experience. First, an overarching health policy framework can be used to guide reconstruction and reform efforts. Second, a comprehensive health policy framework requires buy-in from the major health providers and the

---

[117] Seth G. Jones, Jeremy M. Wilson, Andrew Rathmell, and K. Jack Riley, *Establishing Law and Order After Conflict*, MG-374-RC, Santa Monica, California: RAND Corporation, 2005.

[118] United Nations, *Recent Violence in Kosovo Shook UN Mission 'To Its Core,' Security Council Told*, News Centre, United Nations, May 11, 2004.

[119] N. Wood, "Kosovo Report Criticizes Rights Progress by UN and Local Leaders," *New York Times*, July 14, 2004.

donor community, and strong leadership to enforce adherence. Third, the international community needs to have the leadership and operational capacity to serve as de facto Ministry of Health when a strong central structure is lacking. In such settings the traditional technical advisory role is insufficient. Fourth, WHO's vision for health sector reform must mesh with the local expectations and the vision of the people. Fundamental reorientation of a health care system may not be initially achievable without local acceptance. Fifth, it can be extremely useful to tap into the knowledge of the health sector acquired by those international organizations and health NGOs that were in the country before—and sometimes during—the conflict. Sixth, the health care sector cuts across many other sectors—such as public works, education, and the judicial system—and its reconstruction effort is interdependent with those reconstruction efforts. Finally, health care reconstruction and reform fundamentally depend on a stable security environment and economic growth.

Five years after the signing of the June 1999 peace accord, a health system was in place in Kosovo. There was a training program for family medicine. Kosovo upgraded antiquated systems and moved toward a primary care model. Health clinics and hospitals were restored. But there were still problems. It is too early to judge the long-term success of the efforts carried out to rebuild Kosovo's health sector. Questions about Kosovo's long-term health prospects center on whether the nascent government has the capacity to continue the reforms started under UNMIK. The health policy framework called for a fundamental health care system reorientation to a primary care model. Whether the medical community will embrace such a fundamental change remains to be seen.

CHAPTER SEVEN

Afghanistan

Following the September 11, 2001, terrorist attacks, the United States used a combination of special operations forces, air power, and support from indigenous allies to overthrow the Taliban regime in Afghanistan. While small-scale fighting continued, the United States and the international community began the process of reconstruction. On December 5, 2001, Afghan leaders signed the Bonn Agreement, which detailed a process for moving toward the establishment of an independent Afghan state and set forth rigorous and ambitious benchmarks that included confirmation of an interim government, draft and approval of a new constitution, and national elections.

The post-conflict reconstruction efforts in Afghanistan followed more than three decades of violence and civil war, as illustrated in Figure 7.1. The crisis began in 1973 with a bloodless coup that overthrew reigning King Zaher Shah. His successor, Muhammad Daoud, was removed and killed in 1978 by a partnership of rival Communist groups that soon afterward fell apart as the groups turned on one another in a bloody factional war. Popular opposition to the Communists was significant, and in 1979 the Soviet Union sent in troops to prevent the regime's total collapse. The Soviet invasion triggered civil war, as the United States, Saudi Arabia, Pakistan, and other countries came to the support of the opposition mujahideen, or Islamic guerrilla fighters. The Soviets eventually withdrew in 1989, but Afghanistan again disintegrated into civil war. In 1994, the Taliban—a radical Islamic movement originating among young Afghan refugees who

Figure 7.1
Political History of Afghanistan, 1749–2004

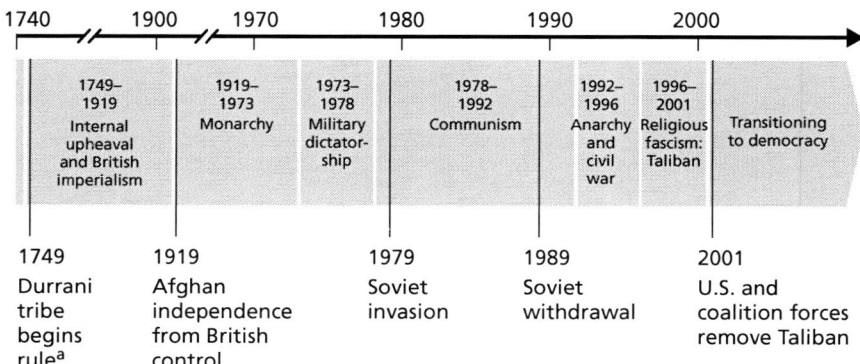

SOURCE: Government Accountability Office, *Afghanistan Reconstruction: Despite Some Progress, Deteriorating Security and Other Obstacles Continue to Threaten Achievement of U.S. Goals*, Washington, D.C.: GAO, July 2005, p. 8.
[a]The Durrani tribe ruled over most of what is present-day Afghanistan—despite domestic turmoil and foreign encroachment—from 1749 through 1978.
RAND *MG321-7.1*

had lived in Pakistani camps and whose ideology was a product of Pakistani madrassas—conquered the capital city of Kabul. Seven years of ongoing warfare ensued, by the end of which, in 2001, the Taliban had succeeded in conquering most of the country and implementing an extremist social and political program.

This chapter examines the U.S., coalition, and Afghan efforts to rebuild Afghanistan's health sector from December 2001 through December 2005. It is not yet possible to conduct a reliable assessment of the health reconstruction efforts, largely because of the absence of dependable data and the short time frame. Nevertheless, some preliminary findings are possible.

Overall, reconstruction efforts have been challenging. Progress might have been more rapidly achieved had the approach been more sensitive to the nature of the crisis and the specific situation. Two somewhat unusual circumstances dramatically affected the reconstruction effort: The setting is essentially a complex political emergency of long duration, and the country was already suffering from substantial poverty and underdevelopment before the recent conflict began. These circumstances created challenges significantly different from those associated with reconstruction efforts in developed societies and led to an experience suggesting that different kinds of conflicts require fundamentally different approaches to health reconstruction.

Historical Context

Reliable health data are extremely limited in Afghanistan, and the most recent census, which was only partial, took place in 1979. At most, rudimentary estimates are possible. Agencies involved in the reconstruction effort, even those with significant resources at their disposal, found that "solid data remain hard to come by."[1] Data that do exist, however, clearly place Afghanistan at or near the bottom of every socioeconomic indicator used to measure human and economic progress.

The successive governments that followed the overthrow of King Zaher Shah in 1973 triggered a destructive round of civil unrest and war. During the war that followed the Soviet invasion, six million to eight million refugees fled to Pakistan and Iran. Among those leaving were a substantial number of the country's health professionals, many of whom emigrated to Canada, Europe, and the United States. They have been reluctant to return. The civil war thwarted reconstruction efforts and discouraged the return of educated professionals.

The Taliban committed atrocities and pushed the country into further decline. Hospitals degenerated into slums or were shut down,

---

[1] James Kunder, USAID Deputy Assistant Administrator for Asia and the Near East, "Reconstruction Situation in Afghanistan," Testimony before the House Committee on International Relations, Washington, D.C.: U.S. Department of State, October 16, 2003, www.state.gov/p/sa/rls/rm/25427.htm. An expert with Management Sciences for Health, whose three tours of duty over several decades have given him a deep familiarity with Afghanistan, put it more bluntly when he asserted that "anyone who talks about Afghanistan and uses numbers is lying through his teeth" (Cheryl Benard communication, Kabul, April 2004).

medicinal supplies were unavailable, and female medical professionals were largely forbidden to work. Women were barred from studying medicine in the universities. This significantly reduced the female population's access to medical care, since the ability of male doctors to diagnose and treat female patients was limited. Preoccupied with its eccentric "cultural revolution" and the ongoing military challenge presented by the Northern Alliance, the Taliban made no serious attempt to govern the country. As a result, the Taliban was too unpredictable to serve as a workable counterpart for even the most persistent donor agencies and international organizations.[2] The remaining medical professionals left the country, and the few NGOs that did not withdraw or were not expelled reduced their operations or had their programs crippled by Taliban obstruction. For example, in May 1997 three female CARE employees working on a project approved by the Taliban government and traveling in an official vehicle were stopped at an intersection, forced to leave the vehicle, and beaten by representatives of the Department of Vice and Virtue.[3]

Even before Afghanistan entered its long period of conflict several decades ago, it was one of the world's most underdeveloped countries. Health indicators were comparatively poor, and the health care system was inadequate. For example, average life expectancy was the lowest in the region, slightly increasing from 35 years in 1960 to 43 years by 2001. Figure 7.2 shows that Uzbekistan, Pakistan, Tajikistan, Iran, and Russia all had higher life expectancy rates than Afghanistan did. In addition, infant mortality rates were high. Afghanistan's poor health indicators remained largely unchanged. One could

---

[2] Anders Davidson and Peter Hjukstroem (eds.), *Afghanistan, Aid and the Taliban*, Stockholm: The Swedish Committee for Afghanistan, 1999; Ahmed Rashid, *Taliban: Militant Islam,, Oil and Fundamentalism in Central Asia*, New Haven, Connecticut: Yale University Press, 2000.

[3] Two particularly insightful reports describing the experiences of NGOs during the Taliban era are Jonathan Bartsch, *Violent Conflict and Human Rights, A Study of Principled Decision Making in Afghanistan*, Peshawar: CARE, October 1998; and Carol Le Duc and Homa Sabri, *Room to Manoeuvre*, Kabul and Islamabad: United Nations Development Programme, July 1996.

Figure 7.2
Life Expectancy at Birth, Afghanistan and Other Countries in Region

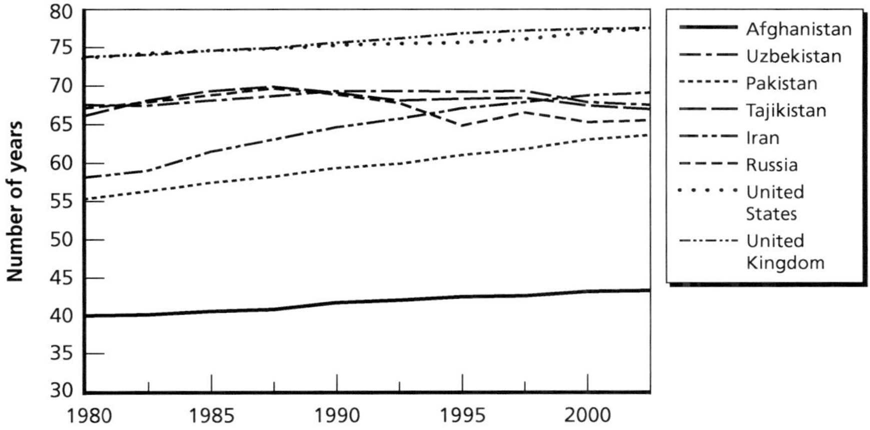

SOURCE: World Bank, *World Development Indicators 2003.*
RAND *MG321-7.2*

argue that the largest effect of the protracted conflict on the health system in Afghanistan was to insulate the country from the social advances and development of its neighbors.

As Figure 7.3 illustrates, fertility rates were among the highest in the region at approximately seven births per woman. The fertility rates of Iran and Pakistan were higher for brief periods, but Afghanistan differed from the other countries in the region by making virtually no progress in lowering the rate in the 1990s. Survival rates for these children were also low. Skilled attendance during childbirth was the exception, occurring only for an estimated 5 percent of births. The country had few trained physicians and few hospital beds. Although the number of hospital beds was already low, the picture is bleaker when corrected for the rural/urban divide. Modern medical practices and facilities were almost exclusively reserved for the elites and a small emerging urban middle class; yet an estimated 89 percent

Figure 7.3
Fertility Rate, Afghanistan and Other Countries in Region

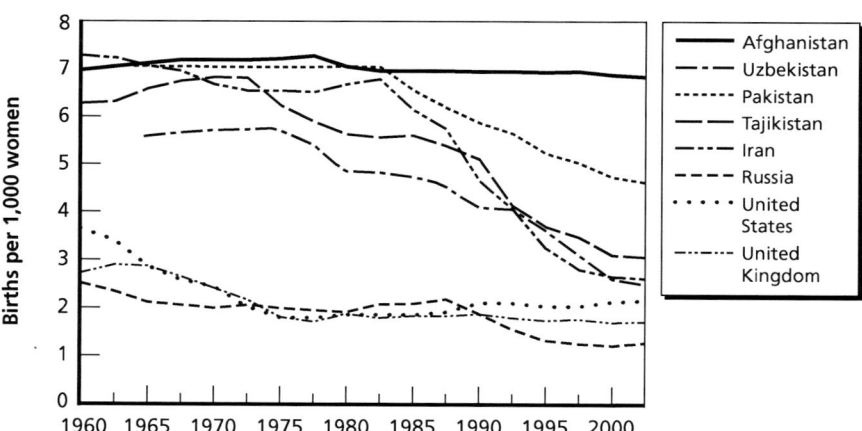

SOURCE: World Bank, *World Development Indicators 2003*.
RAND MG321-7.3

of the population lived in rural areas.[4] A study in Badghis province found 58 percent chronic malnutrition and 7 percent acute malnutrition in children under five.[5] The global acute malnutrition rate for Kabul was 8.7 percent.[6] Improving Afghanistan's poor performance on public health measures and improving circumstances in rural areas have been among the explicit goals of the social reformers, radicals, and revolutionaries in successive upheavals of modern Afghan history.

---

[4] See, for example, Alfred Buck et al., *Health and Disease in Rural Afghanistan*, Baltimore, Maryland: York Press, 1972. The study estimated, on one indicator, an infant mortality rate of 205/1,000 for rural areas.

[5] United Nations Children's Fund, "World Health Day, Plight of Afghanistan's Children Cause for Concern," April 6, 2003, www.unicef.org/media/media_7203.html.

[6] This rate is for children from six to 59 months old. Stephanie Hanouet, *Nutritional, Vaccination Coverage and Mortality Survey*, Kabul Province: Action Contre La Faim, February 1999.

Health Challenges

Afghanistan's health challenges, and its dependency on outsiders to address them, have remained fundamentally unchanged since the 1950s.[7] Four of the reasons for the desolate state of public health and health care delivery in Afghanistan are as follows.

First, poverty has contributed to poor nutrition, a sparse health infrastructure, an absence of services, and a lack of health care professionals. Poverty indirectly links to behavior patterns such as high birth rates, early marriage, authoritarian decisionmaking within the family, illiteracy, and other factors not conducive to improved standards of health.

Second, limits to health care provision have existed on several levels. Poor security made it difficult for health care workers to reach the population and establish facilities in other than a few safe urban areas. And the absence of a transportation infrastructure puts a significant proportion of the population beyond the reach of medical services. Access thus is the reason for the significant regional differences that existed in quality of life and medical care. Whereas there was one basic health center per 40,000 population in the central and eastern regions, there was only one such center per 200,000 population in the south, and 19 districts had no health facilities whatsoever.[8]

Third, culture and tradition have influenced health in two key ways. Traditional beliefs about medicine, nutrition, and hygiene led to mistakes or misinterpretations about what constitutes safe practice. For example, many Afghans believed that any moving water was clean and that liquids should be withheld from children with diarrhea. In addition, prevailing gender attitudes directly impact health, life quality, and life expectancy—especially for women, infants, and children. Included in this value set is a propensity to marry girls off at a very

---

[7] See, for example, Buck et al., *Health and Disease in Rural Afghanistan*.

[8] Ronald Waldman and Homaira Hanif, *The Public Health System in Afghanistan*, Afghanistan: Afghan Research and Evaluation Unit, May–June 2002.

young age, a reluctance to spend money and effort on health care for daughters and wives, inequitable distribution of food within the family, a condoning of physical violence toward women and children, and a reluctance to educate girls and women.[9] Gender attitudes may explain the slow progress in maternal, child, and infant health and mortality.[10] Similarly, female mortality from tuberculosis exceeded that for males because women were less likely to receive medical care.[11]

Fourth, non-health-related agendas have long dominated Afghan health care issues. Strong outside involvement has been pervasive for decades in Afghanistan's health care design, provision, management, and funding. Showcase reform projects in education and health have commonly been part of efforts to gain legitimacy and popular support. Successive regimes and occupying foreign powers regularly embarked on hospital building, doctor training, vaccination, and rural outreach programs. The effect of these programs has in most instances been limited by the short tenure of the regimes. When the current reconstruction began, the remnants of these efforts were seen in Afghanistan's health care system, which was populated by doctors who had trained in India, acquired a degree in Pakistan, or trained in the Soviet Union on Russian scholarships. In addition, most health care facilities were named after the foreign government or NGO that had built and supported them—for example, Turkish Hospital, Indira Gandhi Hospital, Jordanian Field Hospital in Mazar-I-Sharif, Italian Hospital in Kabul, International Security Assistance Force (ISAF) Hospital in Kabul, and the U.S. restored Rabia Balkhi Hospital in Kabul.

---

[9] James East, "Afghanistan: Child Marriage Rate Still High," IRIN (United Nations Integrated Regional Information Networks), July 13, 2004.

[10] Cheryl Benard interview with Deirdre Russo, International Services Office of the American Red Cross, Arlington, Virginia, April 2004. Russo notes that other countries whose profiles are similar to Afghanistan's—in terms of poverty, security, geographic, and infrastructure challenges; prevalence of rural populations; etc.—do not have maternal and infant mortality statistics even approaching those of Afghanistan.

[11] Waldman and Hanif, *The Public Health System in Afghanistan.*

Poverty and cultural factors figured most prominently in impeding progress. Poverty explains the persistence of nutritional and infrastructure problems—the absence of roads, sanitation, and clean water. Most child mortality was caused by diarrhea and respiratory ailments. Maternal and infant deaths were related to unattended births, lack of pre- and post-natal care, and numerous health challenges stemming from cultural factors. These included genetic problems from inbreeding, low levels of maternal health caused by poverty and exacerbated by selective nutritional disadvantaging, early marriage, frequent pregnancies, poor hygiene, physical abuse, and lack of medical care.

Afghanistan's central government had no sustained institutional history of nationally guided and provided health care. Consequently, the country lacked health care leadership, competency, and capacity. Afghanistan was treated as a national reconstruction project when, in reality, it was a development challenge. This misfocused direction—along with the goals, expectations, and instruments chosen to address it—slowed Afghanistan's health care development.

Communicable diseases represented the greatest public health threat in Afghanistan. Most of the population had never had reliable access to safe water or modern sanitation. For as long as there had been medical reporting, digestive and respiratory infections had been pervasive. Afghanistan's first known vaccination program was part of the Intensified Global Eradication Campaign for smallpox in the 1960s. Vaccination programs had been well accepted, resulting in good initial vaccination rates; but completion of vaccination series had been problematic. National immunization days became a recognized annual event beginning in the early 1990s and have even been the cause of ceasefires between warring parties. From 1995 to 2001, ceasefires allowed vaccinator teams to immunize children against polio, coverage for which is now estimated to be between 50 percent and 80 percent of the population. There have also been efforts to supplement the polio vaccinations with measles and DTP immunization.

The vagaries of political conflict clearly affected the ability of health care workers to reach those needing vaccination. In 1997, for instance, 3.7 million children were vaccinated against polio. In 1998, however, when ceasefire negotiations were unsuccessful, only 2.6 million received the vaccine; and the number then rose to 4.0 million the following year.[12]

Health Approach and Assessment

After the overthrow of the Taliban regime in 2001, the United States, UN, and other participants began the process of rebuilding—or, in many cases, building—the health sector. This section outlines key participants and donors, examines efforts to rebuild Afghanistan's public health and health care delivery systems, and provides an overall assessment.

Key Participants and Donors

Through the 1980s, foreign governments and large international organizations provided substantial resources to the Afghan health care system. During the war against the Soviet Union, many of the international NGOs that entered the country were motivated by political reasons. They frequently set up headquarters in Pakistan and assisted Afghan mujahideen. Afghan civilians inside the country and civilian refugees in Pakistan's camps were a secondary concern. Women, children, and the elderly—who together formed the overwhelming majority of the refugee population—were treated on an auxiliary basis, with the bulk of services geared toward combatants. There were some rudimentary programs for tuberculosis, provision of supplemental feeding, and midwife training.[13]

Following the overthrow of the Taliban in 2001, international agencies concerned with improving the health situation quickly embarked on a three-step task: prepare for a potential humanitarian emergency, deliver aid, and transition from aid to reconstruction.

---

[12] "Progress Toward Poliomyelitis Eradication, Afghanistan, 1994–1999," *Morbidity and Mortality Weekly Report*, Vol. 48, No. 37, September 24, 1999, p. 2.

[13] Waldman and Hanif, *The Public Health System in Afghanistan*.

World Bank discussed concerns about the fluidity of Afghanistan's situation but acknowledged the importance of working to secure humanitarian relief even during a period of reconstruction.[14]

U.S. Agencies. The Afghan assistance effort primarily involved ten U.S. government departments and agencies. The United States Agency for International Development (USAID) was the largest of them, followed by the Department of State and the Department of Defense. The health-related contributions of the State and Defense departments focused on support for refugees, humanitarian assistance, food support, and activities of the provincial reconstruction teams. However, these teams were established only in major cities across Afghanistan (such as Kandahar, Mazar-I-Sharif, and Herat) and thus did not reach most of the country, especially rural areas. The U.S. Special Operations Forces (SOF) provided medical care to local villagers at its A-camps in remote villages in Afghanistan, but its resources were limited.

The U.S. GAO was highly critical of the way the U.S. government handled budget and spending information related to Afghanistan, since there was no single, consolidated source of expenditure data. In June 2004, GAO reported that the unavailability of obligation and expenditure data was making it difficult to determine the extent to which funds were used to achieve measurable results in Afghanistan.[15] GAO was also dissatisfied with the degree of interagency collaboration and information sharing. As Figure 7.4 shows, U.S. health and nutrition assistance in 2004 was approximately $100 million, which is considerably less than the amounts for several other areas: improving Afghan livelihoods by encouraging income generation, rebuilding transportation, improving economic management, and building the police and Afghan National Army.

---

[14] World Bank, Afghanistan: World Bank Approach Paper, November 2001, Washington, D.C.: World Bank Group, November 29, 2001, www.reliefweb.org.

[15] Government Accountability Office, *Afghanistan Reconstruction: Deteriorating Security and Limited Resources Have Impeded Progress—Improvements in U.S. Strategy Needed*, Washington, D.C.: GAO, June 2004, p. 5.

Figure 7.4
U.S. Support to Afghanistan, 2004

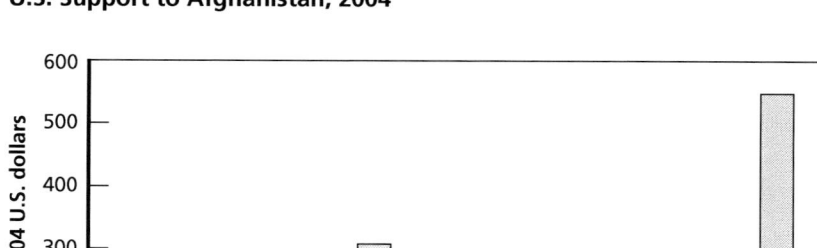

SOURCE: *Afghanistan Development Update*, United States Mission to Afghanistan.
RAND *MG321-7.4*

UN Agencies. In March 2002, the United Nations Assistance Mission in Afghanistan (UNAMA) was created by United Nations Security Council Resolution 1401 for an initial period of 12 months. UNAMA managed, planned, and conducted all UN humanitarian relief, recovery, and reconstruction activities in Afghanistan, and it continues to be the lead UN agency for Afghan reconstruction in 2006. However, the bulk of its mandate involved rebuilding the country's government and judiciary, establishing mechanisms for the rule of law and human rights, and preparing for national elections.

Non-Governmental Organizations. Afghanistan's health care system was overwhelmingly supported by NGOs and international organizations. As Table 7.1 indicates, over 80 percent of health care was in the hands of NGOs. The Asian Development Bank conservatively reported that as many as 80 NGOs worked in the health sector; most

Table 7.1
Support for Health Care Facilities, Afghanistan

Health Care Support	Number	Percent
NGO only	410	45.0
Government/NGO	149	16.3
Government only	102	11.2
Government/NGO/UN	90	9.9
NGO/UN	60	5.6
Government/UN	43	4.8
UN only	23	2.5
Private	21	2.3
Other community	6	0.7

SOURCE: Asian Development Bank, *Improving Primary Health Care in Afghanistan Through NGOs*, December 23, 2002, www.adb.org/Documents/News/2002/nr200228. asp.

operated a few clinics or provided specialized support. For example, Population Services International distributed contraceptives beginning in 2003 and insecticide-treated mosquito nets beginning in 2004. It also prepared health messages for broadcast on Voice of America. Christian World Services, an NGO based in New Zealand, constructed shelters. Numerous other NGOs (such as the World Assembly of Muslim Youth, Intersor, and the Islamic Relief Agency) were involved in focused projects.

Smaller NGOs routinely operated outside government oversight. The interim government was not in a position to monitor or interdict when programs and activities were outside Kabul. Further, the government would have been reckless to turn away assistance when the country's needs were so enormous, so it did not seriously try to do so. Finally, Afghanistan has a tradition of accepting the delivery of social services by foreigners. This developed during the mujahideen era, when countless groups, committees, and organizations operated in Peshawar and ran their programs with no supervision except that of their own external sponsors.

The policy emerging in Afghanistan enshrines the role of the NGOs. A $3 million NGO grant from the Asian Development Bank was specifically designed to permit the Ministry of Health to contract rural basic health care to NGOs. The Performance-Based Partnership Agreement system assigned official responsibility for health delivery in a sector or a geographic region to international organizations and NGOs and was embraced within the basic health services package. Not all believed this was the optimal approach. Doctors Without Borders, which withdrew from Afghanistan in July 2004, was outspoken that this course contributed to weaknesses within the Afghan system.

U.S. and Coalition Military Forces. The U.S. military and coalition forces focused on establishing and providing security in their attempt to establish basic conditions for a functioning health system. The provincial reconstruction teams engaged in community-based activities that more directly affected health, such as safe water provision, clinic structural repair, and emergency food aid.

Japan and EU countries maintained a strong presence, both through state-run development agencies and through national NGOs. While they stressed Afghan sovereignty, this emphasis was more fiction than fact. The interim national government had little ability to plan, implement, or enforce health efforts, and it had little reach outside of Kabul. High-ranking officials were inexperienced— or at best under-experienced—and lacked competent staff and an effective infrastructure. Though nominally in charge, they commanded no resources beyond what they received from foreign agencies and governments. There is no evidence that the Ministry of Health opposed any recommendation made by an external donor or agency or that it put forward any independent ideas. This situation not only accurately reflected the country's dependency on outside sources, it also highlighted the need to build internal capacity in Afghanistan.

Finally, the private sector's health provision role in Afghanistan was small. There were, however, a number of privately practicing physicians and small private clinics, as well as a flourishing pharmaceutical business.

Public Health

A joint donor mission in April 2002 initiated the design of a basic health services package, the outlines of which were made public later that year. As Table 7.2 highlights, the package addressed seven key programs that formed the backbone of public health planning.

This package was overly ambitious and initially included no benchmarks, no cost budgeting, and no approach for dealing with HIV/AIDS. In response, over 100 international experts compiled a report to help rectify these shortfalls. The report provided costs for all goals listed in the plan, a schedule of milestones for 2006 and 2015, an amended plan that added mental health and care for the handicapped and those with HIV/AIDS as second-tier issues, and thoughts on how to make the health sector sustainable in the future. The report suggested that there was a large gap between the requirements ($87.4 million) for the basic package of health services and the

Table 7.2
Basic Health Services Package, Afghanistan

Programs	Components
Maternal and newborn health	Antenatal care Delivery care Postpartum care Family planning Care of the newborn
Child health and immunization	Expanded Program on Immunization services (routine and outreach) Integrated Management of Childhood Illnesses
Public nutrition	Micronutrient supplementation Treatment of clinical malnutrition
Communicable diseases	Control of tuberculosis Control of malaria
Mental health	Community management of mental health problems Health facility–based treatment of outpatients and inpatients
Disability	Physiotherapy integrated in the Public Health Care services Orthopedic services expanded to hospital level
Supply of essential drugs	

SOURCE: Ronald Waldman and Homaira Hanif, *The Public Health System in Afghanistan*, p. i.

$42.9 million available. Funding and other constraints left 60 percent of the problems outside the package's reach.[16]

Another product published under the official auspices of the Ministry of Health was the report *Public Nutrition Policy and Strategy 2003–2006.*[17] This report provided objectives through 2006 (such as ensuring that waste was reduced and increasing the prevalence of exclusive breastfeeding from 35 percent to over 60 percent for infants from birth to six months of age). It also proposed targets for 2004 to 2015.

Water and Sanitation. A safe water supply was a goal for both urban and rural areas. Well-digging projects in the rural areas, which were conducted by the provincial reconstruction teams, were one of the items that communities could choose within World Bank's "menu" of rural reconstruction projects. Communities received an allotment of funds based on the size of their population and contingent on their ability to organize a representative, democratically elected village council. Using the menu, they could then decide how to spend this money. Most water and sanitation efforts were concentrated in Kabul, where UNICEF, WHO, and the World Food Programme reported the chlorination of 17,500 shallow wells and 20 water reservoirs. Still, only 13 percent of the population had access to safe water by 2004.[18]

Infectious Diseases and Immunization. Immunization campaigns piggybacked on the tradition of "national immunization days." According to UNAMA, six million children were immunized against polio in 2002. Polio is rare in Afghanistan; there were 11 confirmed cases in 2001, four in 2002, and seven in 2003. A measles campaign reached nine to ten million children and was estimated to have saved

---

[16] *Securing Afghanistan's Future: Accomplishments and the Strategic Path Forward, Health and Nutrition Technical Annex,* Prepared at the request of the Transitional Islamic Government of Afghanistan, January 2004, www.af/resources/mof/recosting/draft%20papers/Pillar%201/Health%20and%20Nutrition%20-%20Annex.pdf.

[17] *Public Nutrition Policy and Strategy 2003–2006,* Final draft for comment, Ministry of Health, October 30, 2003.

[18] *Securing Afghanistan's Future,* p. 20.

30,000 lives. According to UNICEF, 700,000 women were immunized against neonatal tetanus during 2003. Given the variation in
vaccination numbers reported, there is some question about the reliability of the immunization data. A 1999 Action Contre La Faim
(Action Against Hunger) study in Kabul found that when the in-
validity of doses was corrected for, the assumed coverage rate of 62.3
percent dropped to 24.3 percent.[19]

Tuberculosis accounted for around 15,000 annual deaths, most
of them women. A national tuberculosis laboratory was established,
but it did not have the staff needed to properly perform the testing.
The Afghan Ministry of Health estimated that there were between
200 and 300 AIDS cases in the country, but virtually no screening
was done for HIV/AIDS. Sterilization and safe needle use were
poorly understood, and visiting experts repeatedly observed multiple
use of needles. Prostitution and drug use were additional risks.
UNICEF and WHO attempted to increase the administration's and
the public's HIV awareness. UNICEF conducted workshops for religious leaders, who frequently serve as community leaders, to make
them aware of the problem.

Food and Nutrition. In the early phase of reconstruction (late fall
2001 to spring 2002), food provision was the primary focus of aid.
Afghanistan's agriculture had been disrupted by the flight of rural
populations, the presence of landmines, and drought-like conditions.
Even during the Taliban era, organizations such as CARE maintained
food programs, most notably the network of bakeries operated by
widows in Kabul. This program continued during reconstruction, as
did other emergency food provision programs for widow-headed
households. Doctors Without Borders and other NGOs ran supplemental feeding programs, especially in camps for returnees and internally displaced persons, where malnutrition was prevalent. UNICEF
provided vitamin A supplementation in some schools and ran a program to iodinate salt. Indeed, iodine deficiencies were prevalent in

---

[19] Hanouet, *Nutritional, Vaccination Coverage and Mortality Survey*, p. 40.

Afghanistan, causing a high incidence of goiter and contributing to miscarriages, stillbirths, and mental and physical retardation.[20]

Mortality Indicators. The statistical indicators for Afghanistan continue to be grave, although pre-conflict figures are too unreliable to provide a benchmark for comparison.[21] Forty percent of childhood deaths are preventable, and chronic malnutrition is estimated to be 50 percent. As Figures 7.5 and 7.6 indicate, the mortality rates for infants and children under five were much higher than in neighboring countries. The unanticipated return of large numbers of refugees,

Figure 7.5
Infant Mortality Rate, Afghanistan and Other Countries in Region

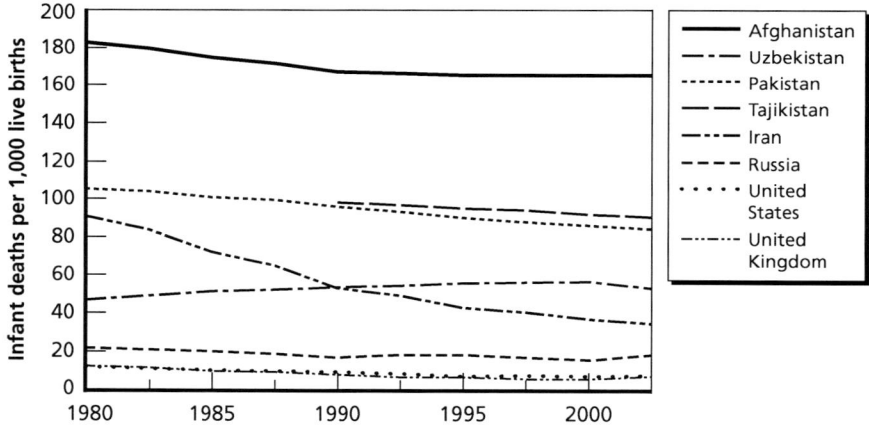

SOURCE: World Bank, *World Development Indicators 2003*.
RAND *MG321-7.5*

---

[20] Iodine deficiencies are prevalent in Afghanistan, causing a high incidence of goiter and contributing to miscarriages, stillbirths, and mental and physical retardation. Carlotta Gall, "Afghans Lack Even the Basic Ingredient Needed to Cure a Disease," *The New York Times*, October 7, 2003.

[21] L. Hjelm-Wallén, *Mother and Child Health Care in Desperate Need of Funds*, Kabul: Swedish Committee for Afghanistan, 2003.

Figure 7.6
Mortality Rate for Children Age Five and Under, Afghanistan and Other
Countries in Region

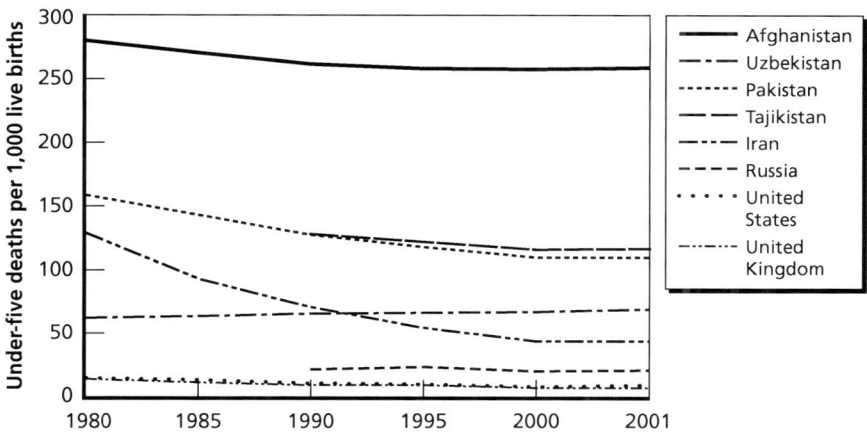

SOURCE: World Bank, *World Development Indicators 2003*.
RAND *MG321-7.6*

predominantly from Pakistan but also from Iran, posed particular challenges. In July 2002, Doctors Without Borders, UNICEF, and the Centers for Disease Control and Prevention reported the crude mortality rate in the Maslakh camp for refugees and internally displaced persons at 15 per 1,000 people per day. They also reported the under-five mortality rate at 61 per 1,000 per day, exceeding emergency thresholds. Most alarming of all, however, was the fact that morbidity and mortality were believed to be caused mainly by preventable communicable diseases.[22]

Security and Personal Safety. Security remained an ongoing concern, affecting the ability of international organizations and NGOs to conduct their health care programs and forcing them to close down their operations either temporarily or for longer periods of

---

[22] International Development Project, "Survey of Maslakh Camp Shows Alarming Levels of Mortality," Global IDP Database, July 2002, www.db.idpproject.org/Sites/idpSurvey.nsf/ wViewCountries. Data are from United Nations Children's Fund and Centers for Disease Control and Prevention.

time. A number of aid workers were killed, including five members of Doctors Without Borders who were shot in Badghis in northwestern Afghanistan in June 2004.[23] As Figure 7.7 illustrates, insurgent attacks steadily increased between January 2002 and July 2005.

Continued flare-ups of violence, a weak state with insufficiently consolidated central power, the proliferation of opium cultivation and drug-trafficking, and an international security force that many observers consider too small—all of these have hampered the Afghanistan reconstruction efforts in all sectors, including health. Consider what the Afghanistan National Security Council said four years after the reconstruction efforts began: "Non-statutory armed forces and their commanders posed a direct threat to the national security of Afghanistan. They are the principal obstacle to the expansion of the rule of law into the provinces." In addition, the council argued that

Figure 7.7
Terrorist Attacks, Afghanistan, January 2002–July 2005

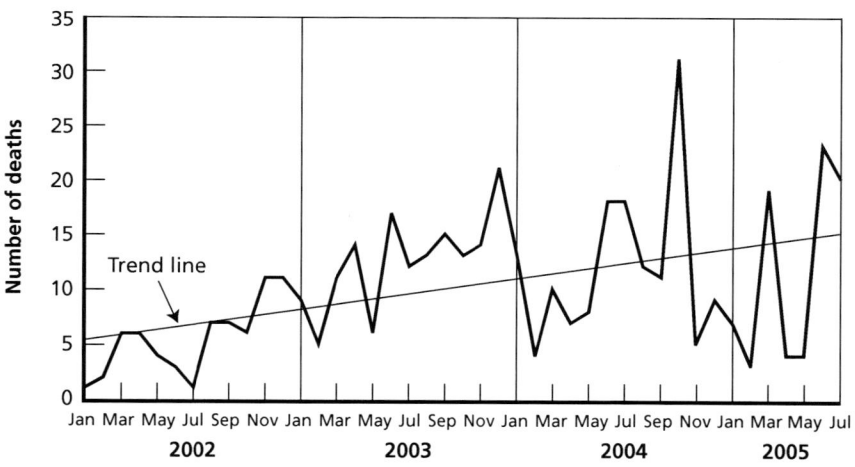

SOURCE: RAND-MIPT Terrorism Incident Database.
RAND MG321-7.7

---

[23] Cheryl Benard, "Afghanistan Without Doctors," *The Wall Street Journal*, August 12, 2004.

"continued growth of the heroin and opium-producing poppy remains a major threat to the security of Afghanistan."[24]

Over the course of reconstruction, the reports of international organizations and NGOs were replete with tales of health-related programs that had to be suspended, canceled, postponed, or significantly scaled back because of security issues. USAID was scheduled to rebuild 121 health clinics and birth centers in 2004, but by March of that year it had downgraded the plan to 72 facilities. Afghan women employed by international NGOs have been the focus of particular threats by supporters of the former Taliban regime. On July 28, 2004, following a fatal attack on one of its vehicles in Badghis, Doctors Without Borders announced that it would close all medical programs in Afghanistan. Efforts to demobilize private militias, construction of an Afghan national police force and an Afghan national army, and national elections invited resistance as much as they served as benchmarks for progress toward a new Afghan nation.

Personal safety for the average Afghan was far from being established, with children and women at particular risk. There have been persistent rumors of child abduction and child trafficking, along with allegations that these are linked to organ theft. UNICEF instituted programs in cooperation with the Afghan police, Ministry of the Interior, UNAMA, Afghan Independent Human Rights Commission, and others to investigate these claims and develop responses.[25]

Attempts to provide security for women faced continuing challenges. Amnesty International and Human Rights Watch examined such women's issues as forced marriage, underage marriage, abduction of girls and women, rape, honor killings, domestic violence, and intimidation of women and girls to prevent their presence in public

---

[24] Afghanistan Office of National Security Council, *National Threat Assessment*, Kabul, September 2005, pp. 4–5.

[25] United Nations Children's Fund, "UNICEF Expresses Concern over Reports of Child Abduction and Trafficking in Afghanistan," Kabul, 25 September 2003, www.unicef.org/media/media_14783.html. On coercive restrictions, see Human Rights Watch, "'We Want to Live as Humans': Repression of Women and Girls in Western Afghanistan," HRW Index No. C1411, December 17, 2002.

spaces.[26] Amnesty International found that women were threatened with violence in every aspect of their lives. Hospitals interviewed by Amnesty International reported frequent treatment of fractures and other injuries to women caused by domestic violence. Suicide rates were so significant that they have become the subject of international inquiries. Most suicides appear to be in response to forced marriages and untenable domestic situations. An Amnesty International survey found that the typical age at marriage in rural areas was between ten and 16, in spite of the fact that 16 is the legal minimum.[27]

Health Care Delivery

Reconstruction of Afghanistan's health care delivery system also faced serious challenges. Although the quantitative data were extremely poor, our qualitative assessment showed that there were significant challenges in rebuilding the health care delivery system. Progress might have been quicker if the approach had been more sensitive to the nature of the crisis and Afghanistan's particular situation.

Hospitals and Clinics. By 2005, NGOs operated more than 160 facilities throughout Afghanistan and built or repaired an additional 140 health facilities. Hospitals were restricted to urban centers, however, and even they were in poor condition. Clean running water was not routinely available; beds, incubators, bandages, medicine, and other basic instruments were lacking; and the facilities were severely understaffed. Almost half of all health facilities had no female staff, making it unlikely that women would be permitted to receive treatment. Only 30 percent of primary care clinics offered basic maternal and child services, and only 10 percent of hospitals could perform cesarean sections. Of 31 provinces, only 11 had essential obstetric care.

---

[26] On ongoing incidents of rape by armed groups, see especially Human Rights Watch, "Killing You Is a Very Easy Thing for Us: Human Rights Abuses in Southeast Afghanistan," HRW Index No. C1505, July 29, 2003.

[27] Amnesty International, "Afghanistan: Justice Denied to Women," Amnesty International, 2003, www.web.amnesty.org/library/print/ENGASA110232003.

Doctors, Nurses, and Medical Personnel. *Securing Afghanistan's Future*, the report put out in 2004, established benchmark targets for 2015. Given the state of Afghan health and health care at that time, the assumption that measurable progress would require this amount of time might have been realistic—provided that the plan was appropriate and that realistic implementation strategies could be found for its most important goals. Even in its developed and expanded form, the plan did not include solutions for some of Afghanistan's most pervasive problems, such as the difficulty of training health care workers and deploying them to the parts of the country and the sectors of the population that needed them most. Figure 7.8 shows the ratio of medical doctors to population by region; Table 7.3 provides an overview of the 2004 distribution of health care professionals.

Figure 7.8
District Population per Medical Doctor, Afghanistan

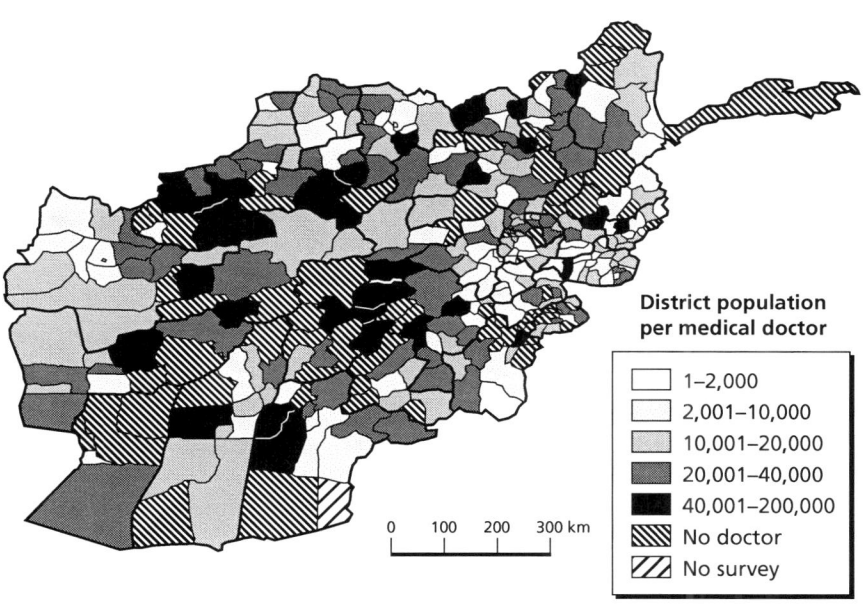

SOURCE: *Securing Afghanistan's Future: Accomplishments and the Strategic Path Forward, Health and Nutrition Technical Annex,* 2004.
RAND *MG321-7.8*

Table 7.3
Health Staffing in Afghanistan, by Job and Gender

Job Category	Male	Female	Total
Total professional staff	8,865	2,955	11,820
Total health sector staff	13,898	4,468	18,366
Physicians	1,598	605	2,203
Physician specialists	557	90	647
Dentists	130	29	159
Nurses	2,034	566	2,600
Midwives	22	467	489
Pharmacists	489	88	577
Laboratory technicians	685	62	747
Vaccinators	803	205	1,008
Community health workers	859	467	1,326

SOURCE: *Securing Afghanistan's Future.*

Opinion was divided on the matter of mental health. Some experts argued that mental health, though important, could not realistically be included in the first few years of reconstruction while resources were so limited. The expanded plan foresaw mental health being addressed by approximately 2010.[28] In 2002 and 2003, the total amount contributed by international donors for programs not related to security was $3.7 billion, 38 percent of which came from the United States and other large donors, such as Japan and the EU. World Bank, Asian Development Bank, and United Nations Development Programme conducted a preliminary needs assessment, projecting a $14.5 billion cost for the reconstruction of Afghanistan over ten years. The first two and one-half years were estimated at $4.9 billion, excluding humanitarian assistance and emergency relief. A donor conference held in January 2002 in Tokyo obtained pledges for nearly that amount.[29]

---

[28] Cheryl Benard communication with Amr Bhat, U.S. Department of Health and Human Services, October 17, 2003.

[29] Executive Board of the UNDP and of the UNPF, "Assistance to Afghanistan," U.N. DP/2003/36, New York, July 30, 2003; "International Conference on Reconstruction Assistance to Afghanistan Held in Tokyo January 21–22, 2002." For country and organization pledges, see www.brookings.eduj/dybdocroot/fp/projects/terrorism/images/todkyo.htm.

In June 2003, World Bank approved a $59.6 million grant for a "Health Sector Emergency Reconstruction and Development Project" to reduce rates of infant, child, and maternal mortality; childhood malnutrition; and fertility. The project included capacity building for ministerial administrators and water treatment; implementation was to occur through Performance-Based Partnership Agreement contracts. In 2003, one and one-half years after the official start of reconstruction, UNICEF budgeted $35 million for its health programs in Afghanistan, with a $4 million shortfall in maternal health program funding.[30] In December 2003, Asian Development Bank approved a $3 million grant to enable the Ministry of Health to contract community-based primary health care to NGOs, the goal being to reduce child mortality rates by 30 percent within three years. Part of that money was earmarked for physical infrastructure.[31]

Overall Assessment

To assess the achievements of the health reconstruction effort in Afghanistan since December 2001, one must rely largely on descriptive and anecdotal evidence. Reliable quantitative data are scarce, inaccuracies are common, and existing statistics are not calibrated finely enough to identify progress. Other problems with the health data were as follows:

- Many Afghanistan statistics were rough estimates and projections rather than actual measurements. Even the size of the population and its current pattern of geographic distribution were unknown.
- The reporting of agencies and organizations suffered from redundancy. The larger agencies and the smaller ones to which they subcontracted tasks sometimes reported the same activities.

---

[30] United Nations Children's Fund, "World Health Day, Plight of Afghanistan's Children."

[31] Asian Development Bank, "Improving Primary Health Care in Afghanistan Through NGOs."

- There were large discrepancies in the data (e.g., immunization rates varied by as much as one million children).
- Reports often failed to reflect the gap between what was intended and what was accomplished. Due to security and budget restraints, planned programs were delayed by as much as a year, reduced to a fraction of the original intent, or scrapped altogether.
- Even large and experienced agencies found themselves unable to do reliable accounting and reporting in Afghanistan. GAO was sharply critical of USAID, not only because it failed to monitor and oversee its projects in Afghanistan, but also because it did not even know where those projects were located.
- Reports contained major inaccuracies. For example, despite reports that the Rabia Balkhi Hospital in Kabul had been restored with U.S. government funds, we found it to be unrenovated and in extremely poor condition during a RAND visit in April 2004.

Regardless of these drawbacks, however, a tentative assessment is still possible. This leads us to ask, Were health reconstruction efforts in Afghanistan the best that could be expected after a relatively short time, given the difficult operating conditions and the starting point? Some knowledgeable observers think not and have expressed disappointment at the level of achievement. Doctors Without Borders concluded in 2003: "People are not prospering. Many have returned to find they lack even basic access to health care, shelter, or economic opportunities. The promised reconstruction is not as widespread as hoped."[32]

Our judgment is less severe. The reconstruction challenge in Afghanistan is complicated. Effective measures are not possible yet,

---

[32] Doctors Without Borders, "Afghanistan, Neither Safe nor Stable," *Field News*, October 15, 2003, www.doctorswithoutborders.org/news/2003/10-15-2003.cfm. See also Sharon Schmickle ("Afghanistan to Get Help in Launching a Blood Bank," *Times Record News*, November 3, 2003), who, after interviews with the U.S. Agency for International Development, International Committee of the Red Cross, World Health Organization, and the Red Crescent Society, concluded that "gains in health care have been slower than was hoped because of security problems and funding shortages."

given the baseline, the chronic nature of many of the most severe health challenges, the need to build a human and physical infrastructure, and the need to change behavior and values in order to fix the root causes of Afghanistan's health challenges. In addition, the continued insecurity and localized conflict hamper health efforts. However, the approach could have been more effective in several areas.

First, international organizations misjudged the humanitarian threat to the population. By October 2001, they had three primary concerns: famine, epidemics, and a projected 1.5 million new refugees.[33] Yet none of the concerns ensued. Neither a famine nor any epidemics occurred. And quite the reverse happened with the refugees: an unanticipated number of Afghans returned to Afghanistan following the overthrow of the Taliban. To avert a famine, between 100,000 and 200,000 tons of wheat were trucked into Afghanistan during the fall and early winter of 2001. When a famine did not occur, the World Food Programme and USAID stated that a catastrophe had been averted through this effort. Other experts believe that the predictions were initially incorrect or exaggerated.[34]

While it is better to prepare for a catastrophic contingency than to be caught unprepared and risk significant loss of life, this approach entailed important opportunity costs. The emergency food operation consumed $320 million from the United States alone; resources were diverted from alternatives. Information available to the agencies was at best equivocal. During 2000 and early 2001, repeatedly issued warnings of imminent famine for Afghanistan were the subject of careful on-the-ground investigation by expert teams sent by the World Food Programme. These surveyor teams heard reports of ongoing acute starvation, but they were never able to substantiate any of them.[35]

---

[33] A. S. Natsios and J. Kreczko, "Special Press Briefing on Humanitarian Assistance to Afghanistan," Washington, D.C.: U.S. Department of State, 2002.

[34] See, for example, David Rieff, *A Bed for the Night, Humanitarianism in Crisis*, New York: Simon and Schuster, 2002, p. 256.

[35] See, for example, Relief Web, "Afghanistan: WFP Team Investigating Famine Reports," March 19, 2001, www.reliefweb.int. In that instance, the agency had received reports of

Even if the danger of famine was high, wheat shipments, whose volumes were only 20 percent of the calculated need, would not have been likely to avert disaster. Distribution was minimal. Expatriate NGO staff were evacuated before the U.S. bombing, and the security situation was tenuous. The more likely interpretation is that these organizations geared up for the wrong contingency. Afghanistan had a chronic food shortage but was not on the brink of famine.[36] This is not the first time that international organizations misjudged the nature of the threat to a population. Affected populations are sometimes more resilient and resourceful than initially thought by aid workers and UN officials, particularly when these populations have been forced to accommodate to the low and unreliable availability of essentials such as food.[37] Chronic conditions may be a greater threat than acute conditions, since the populations accommodate to a low standard at or below subsistence.

Second, the start-up was slow. Despite much publicized donor conferences, funding was delayed, often significantly. Large organizations were slow to focus on the design of strategies. In the second half of 2003, the major players were still discussing the allocation of resources for planned programs. For example, World Bank announced the funding of a $59.6 million grant to support the three-year Afghanistan Health Sector Emergency Reconstruction and Development Project. Not until the third year of reconstruction was there "a rapid expansion of health services to rural areas where hundreds of thousands of people, mainly women and children, die every year due to the absence of such services."[38]

---

widespread deaths from starvation, but its field team was unable to find any supporting evidence.

[36] For a more detailed analysis of whether or not there was a serious threat of famine, and why the aid organizations may have mistakenly presumed one, see Seth Ackerman, "Afghan Famine on and off the Screen," *Fair*, May/June 2002, www.fair.org/extra/0205/afghans-famine.html.

[37] Rieff, *A Bed for the Night,* p. 256.

[38] World Bank, "World Bank Helps Afghanistan Meet Urgent Health Needs," News Release 2003/388/SAR, web.worldbank.org/WBSITE/EXTERNAL/NEWS/0.

Third, agencies underestimated the degree of operational difficulty. Jack Bell, head of the U.S. State Department's Afghanistan Reconstruction Group, wrote in 2004 that "the most important programs—including roads, schools, and clinics—are in serious trouble. The health program was well on its way to becoming a disaster."[39] It took time for international agencies to grasp the setting that confronted them and its implications for their work. There were no banks to transfer money; cash had to be transported into the country in suitcases, sometimes needing to be carried overland in convoys vulnerable to bandits. There were no telephone lines, and electricity was sporadic, so organizations had to import generators. Satellite phones, at $8 per minute, represented an unanticipated and burdensome expense. Business equipment—such as fax machines, e-mail, the Internet, and photocopy machines—was simply unavailable during the first year and only began coming in slowly after that. Outside-world coordination with Afghan counterparts was extremely difficult. It was not uncommon for a ministry to rely on one cell phone, owned by the minister, for all of its communications. Practical coordination and vertical follow-up were thus rendered nearly impossible. Every matter, large or small, had to be dealt with at the highest level.

In late 2003, James Kunder, who had reopened the USAID mission to Kabul in January 2002, described the situation to the House Committee on International Relations. He acknowledged that Afghanistan provided one of the most complex reconstruction challenges the U.S. government had encountered anywhere: "When our USAID team arrived . . . we found . . . a place where all the basic trappings of a nation-state had been obliterated."[40] This statement accurately portrays the magnitude of the challenge. However, it also implies that the complexity came as a surprise, and that the USAID team was scouting out a new and unknown setting. In fact, Afghanistan and its degraded condition were well known in the international

---

[39] Joe Stephens and David B. Ottaway, "A Rebuilding Full of Cracks," *Washington Post*, November 20, 2005, p. A1.

[40] Kunder, "Reconstruction Situation in Afghanistan."

aid community. A number of NGOs, including the Swedish Committee for Afghanistan, CARE, and several UN agencies, had operated in Afghanistan throughout the Taliban and previous periods. The international community had all the information it needed about the environment it would encounter.

Lessons Learned

The basic lesson in Afghanistan is that in severely degraded environments, sophisticated planning may be unrealistic and premature. International agencies spent significant effort designing "joint" plans, strategies, and policies with the Afghan Ministry of Health. Most of the studies did not produce significant new insights, but merely repeated what was already known about Afghanistan: there were too few skilled health care workers, especially in rural areas. As for the national plans, their recommendations were either obvious—that maternal deaths needed to be reduced and maternal and child health needed to be the focus—or they were overly ambitious and unlikely to be implemented for several years.

The basic health services package, for example, was extremely elaborate in some regards and extremely vague in others. One table listed 12 monitoring bureaucracies that were to review the program's success at the "central national level," with additional reviews at other levels. Some reviews were to be annual, others biannual. It is difficult to imagine that this sort of oversight would be either feasible or desirable given the state of total disarray in delivery mechanisms, central government reach, and reporting capacity. Meanwhile, there was no comparably elaborate design for implementing the program that presumably was to produce the outcome all of these bureaucracies were to evaluate.[41]

Instead of devising largely fictitious or abstract "grand plans," agencies should focus on assessment, oversight, and coordination of

---

[41] Cheryl Benard communication with Dr. Ellyn Cavanaugh, Rabia Balkhi Hospital.

actual activities. Several consultative and planning mechanisms at-tempted to coordinate donors and NGO activities and keep them aligned with the goals of the government. International organizations and NGOs did not successfully communicate or coordinate either with each other or with the Afghan agencies that theoretically were in command.[42] There were exceptions at both extremes. Entire pockets of the country, including Herat, were effectively autonomous and implemented their own programs. In other places, such as Kandahar, more-effective consultation mechanisms appeared to be working well, in part because a smaller number of agencies were involved.

Even within single agencies, troubling defects in oversight, in-formation, and evaluation were common. GAO found that USAID's program in Afghanistan generally lacked "measurable goals, specific time frames, and resource levels"; did not "delineate responsibilities"; had not "identified external factors that could significantly affect the achievement of its goals"; and did not "include a schedule for pro-gram evaluations" to assess progress against such goals."[43] In a setting like the one presented in Afghanistan, international agencies may be better off focusing on effectively monitoring their own efforts rather than assisting the Afghan ministry in designing an unwieldy and purely hypothetical monitoring structure.

It is essential that the nature of the conflict be correctly deter-mined and taken into account. Afghanistan properly falls into the category of a "complex political emergency." This is a specific type of conflict that commonly has a severe impact on the health of the population and the provision of health care, as well as a strong nega-tive effect on post-conflict reconstruction efforts. This category has all or many of the following characteristics:

- The conflict is within as well as across state boundaries.
- The conflict is protracted, lasting many years.
- The country experiences institutional collapse.

---

[42] Government Accountability Office, *Afghanistan Reconstruction*, p. 38.

[43] Government Accountability Office, *Afghanistan Reconstruction*, p. 38.

- Civilians and civilian structures are targets of the violence.
- Groups experience many social cleavages, which are manipulated by the parties to the conflict.
- Normal accountability mechanisms are absent because there is no legitimate government.[44]

One feature of complex political emergencies is that the conflict often fails to have a distinct ending. Continuing flare-ups of violence and a weak state with insufficiently consolidated central power and legitimacy cause persistent insecurity and impede reconstruction. Civil wars also degrade aggregate measures of national health performance, the degradation manifesting most strongly in the elevated mortality rates and degraded health of women and children.[45] The curve of decline and recovery for complex political emergencies is likely to differ from those of other types of conflicts. Countries emerging in such a setting are affected by long-term degradation of health. Challenges are deeper, and progress should be expected to be slower. There may never have been a health infrastructure. Such situations require a reconstruction—or, perhaps, a construction— effort strongly shaped by the goal of development. In Afghanistan, the international community geared up for a standard post-conflict reconstruction effort instead of acknowledging that what it actually faced was a development challenge.

If development is the goal, several questions arise with respect to Afghanistan: Was the Performance-Based Partnership Agreement system truly the best approach? Did it perpetuate a tradition of national dependency on the external design, delivery, and financing of health care that has not served the country well in the past?

---

[44] J. Goodhand and D. Hulme, "From Wars to Complex Political Emergencies: Understanding Conflict and Peace-Building in the New World Disorder," *Third World Quarterly*, Vol. 20, 1999, pp. 13–26.

[45] Adam Ghobarah Hazem, Paul Huth, and Bruce Russett, "Civil Wars Kill and Maim People—Long After the Shooting Stops," *American Political Science Review*, Vol. 97, No. 2, May 2003.

Afghanistan has certainly not been a failure. Important activities were implemented to address each of the four basic challenges noted earlier: poverty, geography, culture/tradition, and political agendas. These activities included efforts to stimulate the economy, build a school and education system, invigorate agricultural production, control the drug trade, and provide small loans and vocational training. Road building projects, most notably the Ring Road, and development of rural areas extended the central government's ability to provide services to more distant areas. Obstacles grounded in tradition and culture were addressed by building a nationwide education system. In only a few years, about half of the school-age population was in school, a third of them girls. This is a respectable achievement in so short a time, particularly when one considers the 180-degree change this represents from education under the Taliban. In addition, various agencies conducted multiple public education campaigns to address such issues as family violence and women's health. For example, the media organization AINA prepared short films about core issues related to values and behavior. In one of the films, a man urges his brother to take his sick wife to a clinic, confessing that he himself had refused his wife such care when she fell ill and she had subsequently died. While the effect of such public education efforts is hard to measure, we do know that film and radio are well accepted in Afghanistan and thus may be effective as vehicles for education.

The main health challenges in Afghanistan are not amenable to quick fixes. The population must become stronger and healthier through improved nutrition, access to clean water and sanitation, and other health efforts. A new generation of health care professionals must be recruited, trained, and motivated to work in rural areas. Some long-standing habits and attitudes, particularly related to marriage, family, and the status of women, must change. And the country needs some decades of stability and security for these changes to occur and to take hold. The reconstruction effort, meanwhile, must define the challenge correctly and set appropriate goals and benchmarks.

CHAPTER EIGHT

Iraq

On March 19, 2003, military forces led by the United States invaded Iraq to remove Saddam Hussein from power. A U.S. Disaster Assistance Response Team simultaneously deployed to the region to assess and coordinate humanitarian relief, emergency reconstruction, and civil administration efforts. After limited air strikes and ground force operations, President George W. Bush declared major combat operations over on May 1, 2003. The U.S.-led Coalition Provisional Authority (CPA) took over as the official interim governing body until June 28, 2004, when it transferred sovereignty back to Iraq.

The reconstruction effort followed more than two decades of conflict and international sanctions. Iraq was involved in a bloody war with Iran from 1980 to 1988, invaded Kuwait in August 1990, and was expelled from Kuwait by the United States and coalition forces in 1991. For most of the 1990s, the United Nations Security Council insisted that Saddam Hussein's government allow UN weapons inspectors into the country and demanded that the government destroy all weapons of mass destruction.[1] The resulting multilateral sanctions that were enforced against Iraq placed an enormous strain on the Iraqi health system and created a series of chronic and communicable disease challenges.

This chapter examines U.S., coalition, and Iraqi efforts to rebuild the health sector from May 2003 through December 2005. Al-

---

[1] Central Intelligence Agency, *World Factbook,* Washington, D.C.: CIA, various years, www.cia.gov/cia/publications/factbook/geos/iz.html#Intro; Center for Economic and Social Rights, *The Human Costs of War in Iraq,* Brooklyn NY: CESR, 2003, www.cesr.org/iraq/.

though the figures needed for basic health indicators are not yet available, making it impossible to properly assess the results of these efforts, a partial picture has emerged. This picture suggests that the deteriorating security environment had a detrimental impact on health reconstruction efforts. Progress has been slow in sectors that have a crucial influence on the population's health, such as water and sanitation. Two successful outcomes, which stem from the early response effort, are that a major epidemic and starvation—both of which were considered likely—did not occur.

Historical Context

In the mid-1980s, Iraq had one of the most effective and modern health systems in the Arab world. It provided primary, secondary, and tertiary health care to 97 percent of the population in urban areas and 79 percent of the population in rural areas.[2] By 2000, however, Iraq's health indicators dramatically deteriorated. This evolution is partially shown in Figure 8.1, which depicts changes in infant mortality (deaths per 1,000 live births) and life expectancy at birth for Iraq and some nearby Middle Eastern countries from 1985 to 2000. As can be seen, Iraq is the only country that experienced both an increase in infant mortality and a decrease in life expectancy during that period.

The turning point for Iraq was the 1991 Gulf War and the ensuing UN-imposed economic sanctions. United Nations Security Council Resolution 687 barred all trade with Iraq, except for medical supplies, foodstuffs, and other humanitarian items subject to UN approval. The country was hard hit by the trade embargo. After several years of sanctions and little apparent progress in eliminating Iraq's weapons of mass destruction program, the UN modified the sanctions. In 1996, the United Nations Security Council passed Resolution 986, establishing the Oil-for-Food Program. Iraq was allowed to

---

[2] Center for Economic and Social Rights, *The Human Costs of War in Iraq.*

Figure 8.1
Infant Mortality Rate Versus Life Expectancy at Birth, Iraq and
Other Countries in Region, 1985–2000

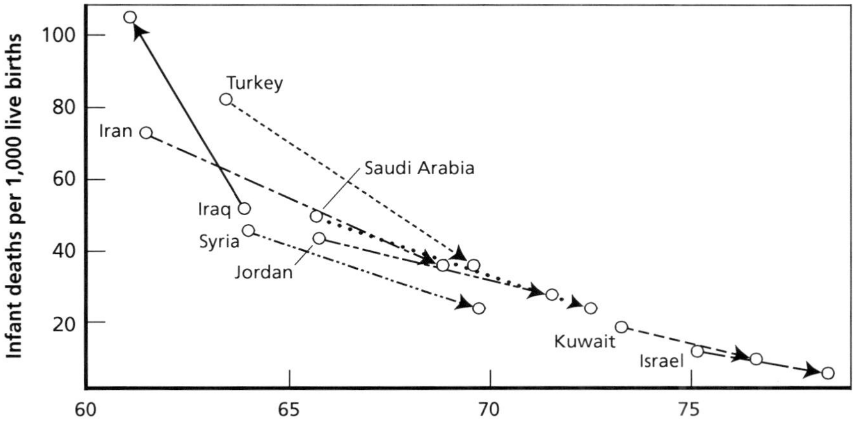

SOURCE: World Bank, *World Development Indicators 2003*, Washington D.C.:
World Bank, 2003.
RAND *MG321-8.1*

export $2 billion worth of oil every 180 days in exchange for food
and medical supplies.[3] The UN-operated program in the north region of Iraq allowed for a cash component, which was unavailable for
the central and south regions until December 2000.[4]

As a result of the Oil-for-Food Program, health conditions
started to improve in 1997, albeit slowly. But the program was not
designed to replace Iraq's national development planning process and
therefore could not meet all of the health system's needs. In particular, the absence of a cash component for central/south regions of Iraq
limited the government's ability to provide services, rebuild and repair the water and sanitation infrastructure, and compensate health

---

[3] United Nations, www.un.org/Depts/oip/background/index.html.

[4] United Nations Children's Fund, *The Situation of Children in Iraq*, 2003, www.unicef.org/
publications/index_4439.html.

care workers.[5] The north region recovered much more quickly than the rest of the country after the 1991 Gulf War, as illustrated in Figure 8.2. However, the figure suggests that the recovery started earlier than the Oil-for-Food Program and its cash component. Several factors may have contributed to the north's better outcome: the northern three governorates' partial autonomy from the central government, their relative stability (which allowed a higher flow of NGOs to the area), and their porous borders with Turkey, Iran, and Syria, which allowed smuggled goods to be imported.

The absence of a cash component in the central/south regions and the large unmet health care needs prompted government changes in health care financing. In 1999, the Ministry of Finance adopted a partial fee-for-service system after years of offering fully subsidized

Figure 8.2
Infant Mortality Rate in Iraq's North and Central/South Regions

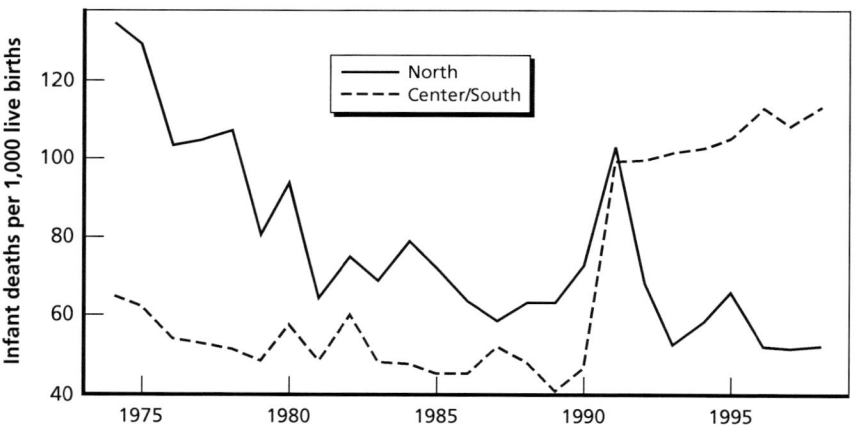

SOURCE: John Blacker, Gareth Jones, and Mohamed M. Ali, "Annual Mortality Rates and Excess Deaths of Children Under Five in Iraq, 1991–98," *Population Studies*, Vol. 57, No. 2, 2003, pp. 217–226.
RAND *MG321-8.2*

---

[5] United Nations Children's Fund, *The Situation of Children in Iraq.*

health care.[6] This two-tiered fee system enabled individual hospitals to generate revenue that would cover approximately 50 percent of their budget, including such items as staff salaries and infrastructure construction and maintenance.[7] Low-income groups paid about one-quarter of what middle- to higher-income groups paid. Those who could not afford to pay were seen for free, although the eligibility criterion for free health care was determined by each facility rather than standardized.[8]

Whatever effect these changes had on the provision of care, they were overshadowed by a drastic cut in public health expenditures. Despite a 10 percent to 15 percent increase in the total population, the Ministry of Health's overall annual budget decreased from $450 million before 1990 ($24.9 per capita) to approximately $22 million in 2002 ($1 per capita)—a 96 percent cut in spending per capita.[9] The decline in GDP in the 1990s partially explains the drop in public health expenditures. Figure 8.3 depicts health expenditures as a percentage of GDP for Iraq and its neighbors. In Iraq, this percentage dropped from 5.6 percent in 1990 to 3.7 percent in 2000. Assuming that health expenditures in 2000 were approximately the same as in 2002 ($22 million), they would have been only $33 million in 2000, even if they had remained at the 1990 percentage-of-GDP level.

However, the deterioration of Iraq's health system is not entirely attributable to the UN sanctions. Several other factors likely played a role:

- The 1991 Gulf War contributed to a large number of casualties. Estimates of military deaths range from 50,000 to 120,000, and

---

[6] United Nations Children's Fund, *The Situation of Children in Iraq.*

[7] International Study Team, *Our Common Responsibility: The Impact of a New War on Iraqi Children*, January 2003, www.warchild.ca/docs/final_report_report_january_29v1.1.pdf.

[8] International Study Team, *Our Common Responsibility*; Center for Economic and Social Rights, *The Human Costs of War in Iraq.*

[9] United Nations Children's Fund, *The Situation of Children in Iraq.*

Figure 8.3
Health Expenditures as a Percentage of Gross Domestic Product, Iraq and Other Countries in Region

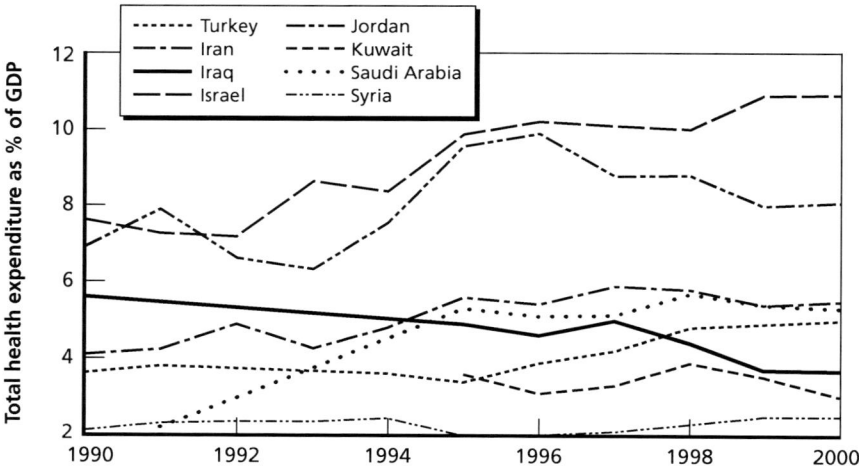

SOURCE: World Bank, *World Development Indicators 2003*.
RAND *MG321-8.3*

estimates of civilian deaths range from 3,500 to 15,000.[10] The number of deaths, however, underestimates the effect of these events on the population. At a minimum, one should consider the burden caused by injuries and by the mental health problems of the survivors. These have not been measured, but they may be large.

- Civil war erupted in March 1991, when the Kurds in the north and the Shia population in the south rose up against Saddam Hussein and were brutally crushed. Estimates of deaths caused

[10] Beth Osborne Daponte, "A Case Study in Estimating Casualties from War and Its Aftermath: The 1991 Persian Gulf War," *Physicians for Social Responsibility Quarterly*, Vol. 3, Nos. 57–66, 1993, www.ippnw.org/MGS/PSRQV3N2Daponte.html; E. Hooglund, "The Other Face of War," *Middle East Report*, July/August 1991; Medact, *Collateral Damage: The Health and Environmental Costs of War in Iraq*, November 2002, www.medact.org/tbx/docs/Medactpercent20Iraqpercent20report_final3.pdf; United Nations, *Ahtisaari Report*, Report to the secretary-general on humanitarian needs in Kuwait and Iraq in the immediate post-crisis environment by a mission under secretary general for administration and management, United Nations, March 1991.

by civil war and other post-war violence range from 20,000 to 35,000.[11]

- There was a massive exodus of refugees throughout the 1990s. The government's repression of the Kurdish and Shia populations spurred an estimated 1.8 million people to flee to Iran and Turkey. Refugee flows are usually associated with higher communicable disease rates and a lack of shelter, sanitation, food, and basic medical care. This wave of refugees alone is estimated to have led to the death of 15,000 to 30,000 people.[12]

- In 1991, the regime started draining the marshes in the south as an act of vengeance in response to the uprising of the local Shia population. Large numbers of people were displaced, and an area that had thrived with life became an ecological disaster of large proportions.[13, 14]

- The regime murdered many of its political opponents, as confirmed by the discovery of numerous mass graves. The precise number of killings and their timing are not known.

- Numerous chemical and biological plants and stores were destroyed during the Gulf War. In 1991, a UN mission found 650 out of 1,330 oil wells ablaze, and large oil spills were documented. The effects of the resulting contamination of air and water supplies are unknown but may be large.[15]

- The regime may have deliberately taken actions that worsened the effects of the UN sanctions in order to gain sympathy from abroad.

---

[11] United Nations, *Ahtisaari Report*, Daponte, "A Case Study in Estimating Casualties from War."

[12] United Nations, *Ahtisaari Report*.

[13] Eyal Benvenisti, "Water Conflicts During the Occupation of Iraq," *American Journal of International Law*, Vol. 97, No. 4, October 2003, pp. 860–872.

[14] Peter Clark, *The Iraqi Marshlands: A Pre-War Perspective*, March 7, 2003, www.crimesofwar.org/special/Iraq/news-marshArabs.html (as of December 10, 2005).

[15] Medact, *Collateral Damage*; E. Hoskins, "Public Health and the Persian Gulf War," in B. Levy and V. Sidel (eds.), *War and Public Health,* New York: Oxford University Press, 1997.

- Corruption is likely to have contributed to the deterioration of health conditions, as Oil-for-Food resources were improperly diverted to the regime.[16]

Health Challenges

This section examines the health of Iraq's population leading up to the 2003 U.S.-led invasion so that the challenges and difficulties of the reconstruction process can be better understood. As part of the examination, we present, whenever possible, the values of important health indicators immediately preceding the conflict, the historical values, and the possible reasons for the temporal pattern.

Public Health

We start with standard health indicators for Iraq over time. To put the numbers in perspective, we also show the corresponding time series for Iraq and other countries in the region. Figure 8.4 depicts infant mortality rates (number of infants per 1,000 live births that die before the age of one) and adult male mortality rates (defined as the probability that a 15-year-old male, if subject to the current age-specific mortality rates, will die before reaching age 60). The 1991 Gulf War is denoted by a vertical line in each of the figure's two panels.

As with many of the health indicators for Iraq, mortality rates steadily improved after 1960 and then sharply deteriorated in the early 1990s.[17] The mortality indicators can be interpreted in at least two ways. First, infant mortality in Iraq in 1990 was at 40 deaths per 1,000 live births, which was slightly higher than the rates of Iraq's neighbors Syria (34 deaths), Saudi Arabia (19), and Jordan (35), and much lower than Turkey (61) and Iran (54). By 1995, Iraq was at 98

---

[16] Independent Inquiry Committee into the United Nations Oil-for-Food Programme, *Report on Programme Manipulation*, www.iic-offp.org/story27oct05.htm.

[17] United Nations, www.un.org/Depts/oip/background/index.html.

Figure 8.4
Infant and Adult Male Mortality Rates, Iraq and Other Countries in Region

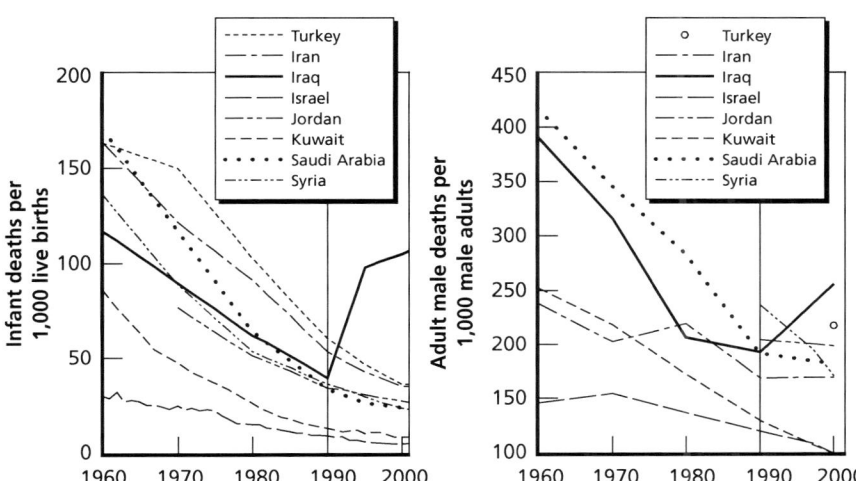

SOURCE: World Bank, *World Development Indicators 2003.*
RAND *MG321-8.4*

deaths per 1,000 births, equal to its 1967 level. In other words, the gains of 23 years were erased in the five years following the Gulf War. A similar computation for adult mortality shows that the gains of 10 and 13 years for females and males, respectively, were erased in the first seven years following the Gulf War.

A second way to interpret the health indicators is to look at the excess mortality rate for children under five years of age. Using the best available current data, it has been estimated that if the mortality rates observed for children under five in the period from 1986 to 1990 had remained constant between 1991 and 1998, Iraq would have experienced about 380,000 fewer deaths than it did experience in the under-five population.[18] Alternatively, if mortality rates had continued to decline at the pre-1990 rates in the 1991–1998 period,

---

[18] Blacker, Jones, and Ali "Annual Mortality Rates and Excess Deaths of Children Under Five in Iraq, 1991–98."

Iraq would have experienced about 480,000 fewer deaths in that population.[19]

To understand what mechanisms have been driving the dramatic changes in the health of Iraqi people in the last decade, it is helpful to examine morbidity patterns after the Gulf War. We do that next, focusing primarily on diseases that affect children under age 14, who constitute 40.7 percent of Iraq's population.

Communicable Diseases. After the 1991 Gulf War, Iraq experienced a sharp increase in the incidence of many infectious diseases. Part of the reason this happened is that the war destroyed a large number of facilities, ranging from water purification plants to sewage treatment networks. Iraq had the capabilities needed to rebuild the damaged facilities before the war, but the task became much harder in the post-war period because of the import restrictions linked to the UN sanctions imposed in 1991.

Figure 8.5 presents four panels showing different aspects of incidence and coverage of some communicable diseases in Iraq. The post-war lack of safe water and poor hygienic conditions led to an increase in the incidence of diseases such as cholera, typhoid, dysentery, hepatitis, giardiasis, and brucellosis, which had been almost under control before the war. The upper left panel in Figure 8.5 shows the incidence of some of these diseases. For one of these, cholera, the incidence is small relative to that of the other diseases; its case fatality rate, however, has been quite high, varying between 5 percent and 40 percent.[20] The UN reports that cholera was eradicated by 2003 in the northern governorates but was still lingering in the rest of the country.[21] Cases of diarrhea increased from an average of 3.8 episodes per child per year in 1990 to 15 episodes per child per year in 1996,[22] and the percentage of deaths from diarrhea increased from 20.7

---

[19] Blacker, Jones, and Ali, "Annual Mortality Rates and Excess Deaths."

[20] World Health Organization, *Communicable Disease Profile: Iraq*, WHO/CDS/2003.17, 2003, www.who.int/infectious-disease-news/IDdocs/whocds200317/1profile.pdf.

[21] United Nations, Office of the Iraq Programme, Oil for Food, www.un.org/Depts/oip/background/fact-sheet.html.

[22] United Nations Children's Fund, *The Situation of Children in Iraq*.

before 1991 to 38 after the Gulf War.[23] Although water safety and sanitation conditions improved after 1997, the levels of diarrheal diseases remained extremely high. Diarrheal diseases and acute respiratory infections accounted for 70 percent of childhood mortality; and the case fatality rates of diarrheal diseases and acute respiratory illness in children in 1999 stood at 2.4 percent and 1.4 percent, respectively, which is a tenfold increase over the rates of the previous decade.[24]

A striking feature of the top left panel in Figure 8.5 is the spike in malaria, a disease not endemic to Iraq before the 1991 Gulf War. This increase has been attributed to poor government policy interacting with the UN sanctions. After 1990, the government of Iraq unsuccessfully attempted to increase rice production. But without proper irrigation and pesticides—whose import was forbidden by the UN sanctions—stagnant water in the rice fields provided a breeding ground for malaria-carrying mosquitoes.[25] Recent data show that malaria is now roughly under control.

Figure 8.5's top right panel shows incidence rates for some diseases that can be prevented with vaccines. As is evident, these also witnessed sharp increases after the Gulf War. These increases cannot be attributed to a cold-chain failure, since the cold chain for vaccines was generally well maintained using kerosene refrigerators distributed by the government.[26] The most likely cause was a combination of disruptions in vaccination programs (such as the WHO expanded program on immunization) and massive refugee movements. The two lower panels in Figure 8.5 show reported coverage superimposed on reported incidence for both measles and pertussis, two vaccine-

---

[23] Richard Garfield and Ron Waldman, *Review of Potential Interventions to Reduce Child Mortality in Iraq*, November 2003, www.basics.org/publications/abs/abs_iraq_child_health. html.

[24] United Nations Children's Fund, *The Situation of Children in Iraq*.

[25] World Health Organization, *Communicable Disease Profile: Iraq*.

[26] Cold chain is the name of the system for vaccine transportation and storage; vaccine needs to be maintained between 2° C and 8° C (International Study Team, *Our Common Responsibility*).

Figure 8.5
Reported Incidence and Coverage of Various Diseases, Iraq

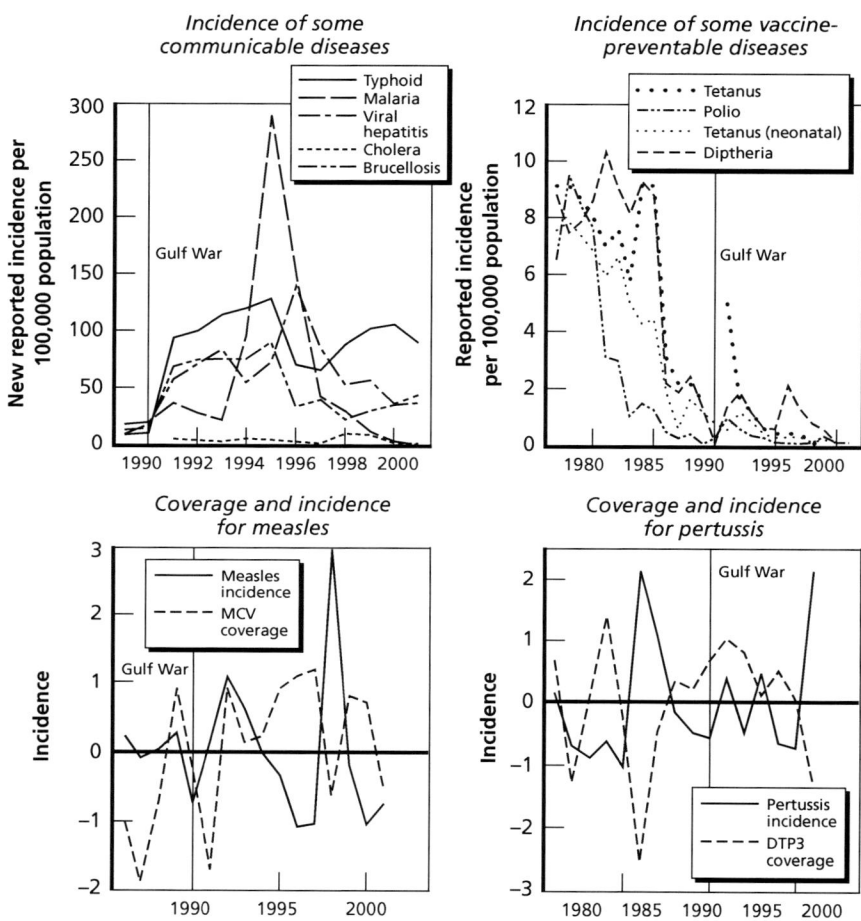

SOURCES: (Top left) Iraq Ministry of Health, *Communicable Diseases in Iraq, 1989–2001*, Baghdad: Iraq Ministry of Health, 2003. (Top right) World Health Organization, Disease Incidence Data Set, Geneva: WHO, 2005. (Bottom row) World Health Organization, Disease Incidence Data Set, 2005; World Health Organization, Immunization Coverage Data Set, Geneva: WHO, 2005.

RAND *MG321-8.5*

preventable diseases. Large variations in vaccination rates can be seen for both diseases, and drops in coverage are clearly associated with increases in incidence. Notice the higher-than-expected level of pertussis in 2001,[27] which could possibly be related to the increased risk of infection that accompanies poor nutrition. Fortunately, the UN reports that the incidence of measles and other communicable diseases was reduced in the central/south regions of Iraq in 2002 and 2003, and that polio appears to have been completely eradicated in 2000.

Water and Sanitation. Before the 1991 Gulf War, Iraq had a modern physical infrastructure of water treatment plants and effective distribution systems that provided safe and potable drinking water to its urban population. The Gulf War harmed the water and environmental sanitation sector in more than one way. Facilities could not be properly restored and maintained because of the sanctions—the needed replacement parts could not be imported. In addition, low and intermittent power generation levels did not allow the water and environmental sanitation sector to function properly. The United States had damaged 85 percent to 90 percent of the power grid during the Gulf War, and maintenance was difficult because of the lack of replacement parts.[28]

As a result, water treatment plants were operating at 30 percent to 70 percent of design capacity, and only 60 percent of the population had access to safe potable water. UNICEF and CARE reports indicate that of the 177 water and treatment plants in the central and southern parts of the country, 19 percent were classified as good, 55 percent as acceptable, and 26 percent as poor.[29] Similarly, 50 percent of the sewage treatment plants were inoperable, and those that

---

[27] World Health Organization, *Communicable Disease Profile: Iraq.*

[28] Coalition Provisional Authority, *Request to Rehabilitate and Reconstruct Iraq,* September 2003 (government publication; not releasable to the general public); United States Department of Energy, *Iraq: Country Analysis Brief,* Washington, D.C.: DoE, 2004, www.eia.doe.gov/emeu/cabs/iraq.html.

[29] United Nations and World Bank, *Joint Iraq Needs Assessment: Water,* October 2003.

were operable were operating at 33 percent to 48 percent capacity.[30] This implies that about 500,000 tons of raw sewage were being dumped in water bodies every day, contaminating the water supply.[31]

Nutrition. Before 1990, malnutrition in children was not considered a public health problem in Iraq. The government heavily subsidized the food market and controlled its prices to guarantee that all citizens had access to affordable and adequate food supplies. The Gulf War changed this picture dramatically. Although the UN sanctions allowed the importation of food and some medicines, Iraq's inability to sell oil, its main resource, left the Iraqi population with little money to spend. In 1991, the government established a rationing system, which probably averted a famine. But it was not sufficient to meet the needs of the population, and malnutrition became a serious problem, one that was particularly hard on children and pregnant women. Figure 8.6 reports the rates of acute and chronic malnutrition in children and of children underweight. Also shown is the amount of calories distributed per capita as a percentage of an estimated pre-war level of 3,315. Notice that after 1995, there was an inverse relationship between malnutrition and calorie intake.[32]

Health Care Delivery

Facilities, Providers, and Training. A substantial body of conflicting information attempts to describe the structure of Iraq's health system immediately before and after the 2003 conflict. The World Bank and UN joint assessment of Iraq's needs identifies 250 hospitals and at least 1,200 health clinics, of which only one-third are equipped to provide emergency obstetric care.[33] The joint assessment also reports that Iraq maintains an average of 17 health facility beds

---

[30] International Study Team, *Our Common Responsibility.*

[31] United Nations Children's Fund, "Iraq Watching Briefs: Water and Environmental Sanitation," July 2003.

[32] United Nations Children's Fund, "Iraq Watching Briefs: Water and Environmental Sanitation," October 2003; Garfield and Waldman, *Review of Potential Interventions.*

[33] United Nations and World Bank, *Joint Iraq Needs Assessment: Health.*

Figure 8.6
Malnutrition and Underweight Rates for Iraqi Children

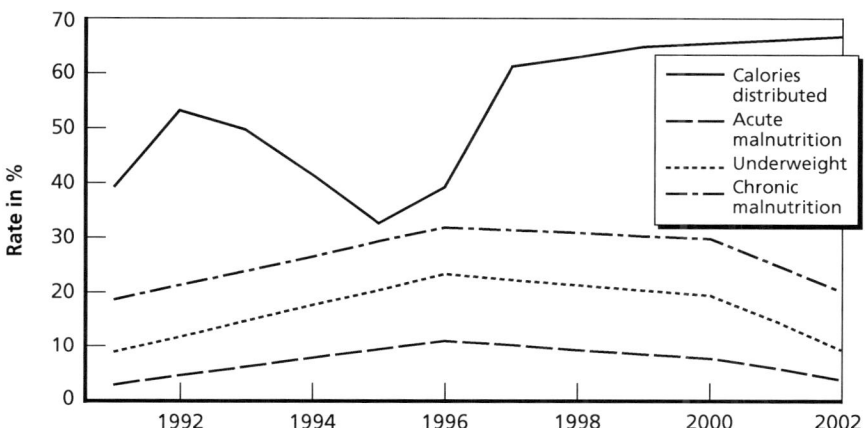

SOURCES: Richard Garfield and Ron Waldman, *Review of Potential Interventions to Reduce Child Mortality in Iraq*, November 2003; Food and Agriculture Organization of the United Nations, and World Food Programme, *FAO/WFP Crop, Food Supply and Nutrition Assessment Mission to Iraq*, September 23, 2003.
RAND *MG321-8.6*

per 10,000 people, which is slightly below the regional average and the averages of comparable-income countries. Hospital occupancy rates are low, and most of the health facility structures are old and poorly maintained. As a result, the assessment concludes that the health system is inefficient and access is inequitable.

Although the physician-to-population ratio has increased over time, it is still relatively low, at 4.7 per 10,000. The body of physicians is also unbalanced, with an excess of specialists and an insufficient number of physicians focusing on primary health care. The nurse-to-population ratio decreased with the exodus of foreign workers in 1990 and remains low, at 5.2 per 10,000 people. This implies that there is about one nursing staff per physician, compared to the three to six nursing staff per physician in most countries of the region. The nurse population is characterized by low training levels; less than one-third of nurses have received training in programs beyond high school.

Consumables, Equipment, and Utilization. Soon after economic sanctions went into effect, the government of Iraq began a rationing system for drugs. WHO estimates that between 1990 and 1997, Iraq contributed between $40 million and $50 million per annum for medicines, covering 10 to 15 percent of overall needs. Even after the Oil-for-Food Program, the health care system was still far from pre-embargo status. Medical equipment had greatly deteriorated, and drugs and other essential medicines were in short supply. According to the UN Health Coordination Group, only one-quarter of the medical equipment available in health care facilities was estimated to be operational in 1997.[34] Drugs and other medical supplies were rationed, and drugs were often administered at doses lower than would generally be accepted as standard treatment for specific health conditions. Laboratory investigations were hampered by lack of laboratory reagents, often resulting in poor diagnoses and over-prescription of antibiotics. Both the number of laboratory tests and the number of surgeries per capita dropped after 1990, as Figure 8.7 shows. Although these numbers started to rise again after 1997, they have remained at extremely low levels.

Mental Health. Although Iraq did offer mental health services, they were never fully integrated into the health system. Mental disorders were largely viewed as spiritual matters in need of traditional healing. By the mid-1970s, Iraq had established a formal psychiatric training program for physicians, but psychiatry never advanced as a field in Iraq, forcing many trained specialists to leave the country to pursue their careers. Psychiatric support was typically provided in clinics or by family members. The only institutional alternative, Al Rashad, was in Baghdad, with approximately 1,200 beds.[35]

---

[34] Center for Economic and Social Rights, *The Human Costs of War in Iraq.*

[35] Medact, *Working Paper No. 3: Mental Well-Being in Iraq—Six Months After the Start of Operation Iraqi Freedom*, 2003, www.medact.org/tbx/ACFC374.doc.

Figure 8.7
Surgeries and Laboratory Tests Per Capita, Iraq

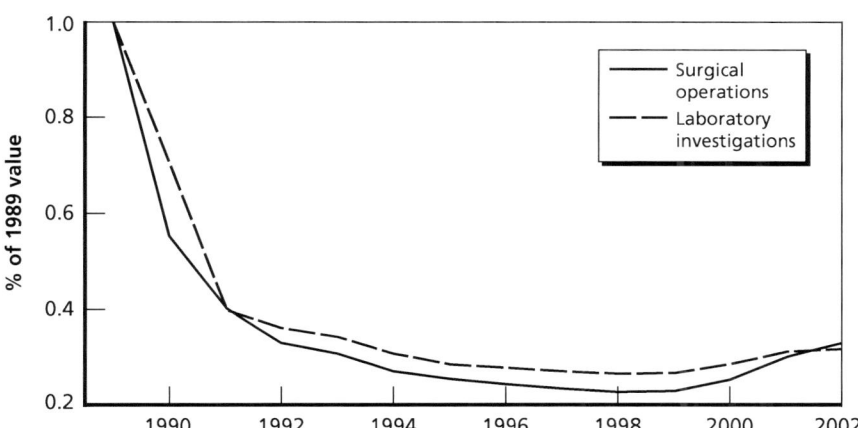

SOURCE: Center for Economic and Social Rights, "Health Data Tables," March 2003.

RAND *MG321-8.7*

Following the 1991 Gulf War, psychiatric services experienced the same constraints as other public services under sanctions. However, during 2001 and 2002, the International Committee of the Red Cross worked to refurbish Al Rashad and to develop a program for occupational therapy. Still, psychiatric services were limited in terms of access to mental health medications, physicians, and services for adolescents or young adults. According to Medact, fewer than 100 psychiatrists were available for a population of 25 million prior to the 2003 conflict. Furthermore, there are no available service-use data for broad mental health issues (such as domestic violence or substance abuse), and no available epidemiological data on mental health prevalence rates or suicide rates. In a society burdened by decades of systemic violence and oppression, this dearth of both services and existing data indicates an enormous unmet need within the health care system.[36]

---

[36] Medact, *Working Paper No. 3.*

Health Approach and Assessment

The reconstruction effort in Iraq is best characterized as a mix of short-term humanitarian assistance and longer-term reconstruction goals. Major challenges have included the unstable security environment and the poor state of Iraq's health infrastructure and population. The 1991 Gulf War triggered a decline in Iraq's health system and the health of the population. Numerous entities have contributed to the more recent immediate post-conflict and longer-term reconstruction efforts.[37] They can be roughly categorized as U.S. agencies, U.S. and coalition military forces, UN agencies and major international organizations, NGOs, commercial institutions, and contractors.

Key Participants and Donors

Between May 2003 and June 2004, the Coalition Provisional Authority (CPA)—which was headed by U.S. Ambassador L. Paul Bremer III—oversaw all reconstruction efforts in Iraq. On June 30, 2004, the CPA transferred sovereignty back to Iraq and ceased to exist. At the same time, two temporary offices were established: the Iraq Reconstruction and Management Office (IRMO) and the Project and Contracting Office (PCO). IRMO was a U.S. Department of State organization in charge of facilitating the transition of the reconstruction effort to Iraq. Its responsibilities included strategic planning and resource prioritization, allocation, and monitoring. The PCO was staffed, funded, and overseen by the U.S. Department of the Army; its responsibilities included contracting for and delivering services, supplies, and infrastructure funded by the U.S. Congress.[38]

Funding for the reconstruction effort came from several sources. The U.S. Congress appropriated $2.5 billion for relief and recon-

---

[37] T. Coipuram, *Iraq: United Nations and Humanitarian Aid Organizations*, Congressional Research Service, Washington, D.C.: U.S. Department of State, August 2003, fpc.state.gov/documents/organization/24059.pdf.

[38] Government Accountability Office, *Rebuilding Iraq: Status of Funding and Reconstruction Efforts*, GAO-05-876, July 2005.

struction efforts in April 2003, to carry through September 2003. It then appropriated, in November 2003, $18.4 billion for reconstruction efforts through September 2006 (this was called the Iraqi Relief and Reconstruction Fund, or IRRF). Another source of funding was the $13 billion in international grants and loans that was pledged by international donors, International Monetary Fund, and World Bank at the Madrid donors' conference in October 2003.[39] Donors agreed to channel their funds to Iraq either bilaterally or through a multi-donor trust fund facility managed by World Bank and the UN (called the International Reconstruction Fund Facility for Iraq, or IRFFI). Another considerable source of funding was Iraq itself: $2.7 billion from seized and frozen funds, and $18.1 billion from the Development Fund for Iraq, which consists mainly of proceeds from export sales of oil and gas and from uncommitted funds from the Oil-for-Food Program.[40]

U.S. Agencies. During the U.S.-led occupation, the CPA oversaw all reconstruction activities in Iraq, including essential services, economic development, security, governance, and strategic communications. Within the CPA, the Program Management Office, established in November 2003, was in charge of overseeing the reconstruction effort and administering the $18.4 billion appropriated in November under Public Law 108-106. The Program Management Office did not award contracts itself; instead it directed agencies such as USAID and the U.S. Army Corps of Engineers to award contracts.[41] The funds allocated directly to health constituted 4.2 percent of the total. However, a much larger share of the funds was allocated for reconstruction of the water and environmental sanitation sector,

---

[39] Congressional Budget Office, *Paying for Iraq's Reconstruction,* CBO Paper, January 2004. ftp.cbo.gov/49xx/doc4983/01-23-Iraq.pdf; Coalition Provisional Authority, *Quarterly Report to Congress,* Inspector General of the Coalition Provisional Authority, March 30, 2004, www.cpa-ig.org/reports_congress.html.

[40] Government Accountability Office, Rebuilding Iraq: Resource, Security, Governance, Essential Services, and Oversight Issues, GAO-04-902R, Washington, D.C.: GAO, June 2004.

[41] J. Spinner, "War Dangers Don't Deter U.S. Workers," *Washington Post,* May 17, 2004, p. A01.

which is directly related to health. The combined budgets of the two sectors amounted to 27 percent of the total in the original allocation of Public Law 108-106. The increased security challenges and the January 2005 election in Iraq led to a strategic review of the original allocation that resulted in funds being shifted from the electricity and water sector to the security, law enforcement, and public safety sectors. The original and the current funding allocations are shown in Table 8.1.[42]

UN Agencies. Numerous UN agencies have participated in the health reconstruction efforts in Iraq. Two of the most active are UNICEF and WHO. UNICEF, which had been in Iraq for many years before the 2003 conflict, received an $8 million grant to provide basic health services to the most vulnerable populations, with emphasis on the repair and rehabilitation of the water and environmental

Table 8.1
Allocation of $18.5 Billion Iraqi Relief and Reconstruction Fund and Its Strategic Revision

Sector	Public Law 108-106 Allocation	Increase	Decrease	Oct 5, 2005 Allocation
Security, law enforcement	3,235.00	1,809.6		5,044.60
Justice, public safety	1,484.00	460.5		1,944.50
Electricity	5,464.50		(1,074.55)	4,389.95
Oil infrastructure	1,701.00			1,701.00
Water and sanitation	4,246.50		(1,935.55)	2,310.95
Transport and telecommunications	499.50			499.50
Roads, bridges, construction	367.50			367.50
Health care	786.00			786.00
Private sector development	183.00	660		843.00
Education, refugees, human rights	259.00	80		339.00
Administrative expenses	213.00			213.00
Total	18,439.00		(3,010.10)	18,439.00

---

[42] Bureau of Resource Management, *Section 2207 Report on Iraq Relief and Reconstruction,* October 5, 2004, www.state.gov/s/d/rm/rls/2207/oct2004/html.

sanitation sector. UNICEF also received money from other sponsors; by June 2003, it had received $28.8 million in contributions for reconstruction of the water and environmental sanitation sector.

WHO worked with the Ministry of Health to identify and address the most immediate and short-term health needs of the population, while also strengthening health sector policy and systems such as health information. Specific activities supported under the grant include monitoring diseases and health status, responding to outbreaks of communicable diseases, rehabilitating health facilities and laboratories, training health staff, and assisting in the management and coordination of donor support and health partners working in Iraq. In addition, WHO has provided technical expertise to the Ministry of Health at the local and national levels. Its goal has been to strengthen the overall capacity of the Ministry of Health in several areas: health policy analysis and strategic planning, monitoring and evaluation, management of human resources, service delivery, and administration of health institutions.

The UN and its agencies—and their work in Iraq—have been directly affected by the unstable security environment. On August 19, 2003, Iraqi insurgents targeted the UN office in Baghdad with a truck bomb, killing 20 people and the UN special representative, Sergio Vieira de Mello. After the attack, nearly two-thirds of the UN's 600 non-Iraqi staff were evacuated.[43]

Non-Governmental Organizations. NGOs have assumed key roles in health, shelter, food distribution, water and sanitation, and other activities. Although NGOs operate in many different areas, the vast majority of them are involved in the health or health-related sectors, such as water and sanitation. By July 14, 2003, approximately 80 NGOs were registered in the UN Humanitarian Information Center database as carrying out 317 projects.[44] The NGO sector is highly fragmented. A large number of NGOs have been involved in

---

[43] *The Economist,* "We Won't Be Sacrificial Lambs," August 30, 2003.

[44] Humanitarian Information Center, *Who's Doing What, Where?* Map Reference 271, July 14, 2003, www.humanitarianinfo.org/iraq/maps/271-A1-WhoWhatWhere.pdf (as of February 9, 2005).

three or fewer projects, while two large NGOs (CARE and Premier Urgence) have been involved in more than 40 projects. The UN reported in March 2004 that "up to 85 aid agencies may currently be working in Iraq."[45] That number likely decreased in late 2004 and 2005, however, since the security situation induced some NGOs to leave.

Coordination has been a major challenge. Prior to the conflict, the International Medical Corps and several leading NGOs established the Joint NGO Emergency Preparedness Initiative to address coordination problems. The initiative was intended as a short-term project to respond to the needs of the international and local NGOs, UN agencies, and government authorities; it served to establish a clearinghouse for information, assessments, and experiences. For the longer term, the NGO Coordination Committee for Iraq (NCCI) was established as the legitimate coordinating body of NGOs. Its purposes were to coordinate and exchange information, monitor humanitarian issues, provide shared services to the NGO community, and support Iraqi NGO development.

There appeared to be little cooperation between NGOs and the CPA. For example, the NGO Coordination Committee for Iraq reported in January 2004 that the CPA was not fully aware of the Committee's role and involvement in Iraq and requested that the UN provide a letter of endorsement.[46] In addition, Order 45, which required all NGOs operating in Iraq to register with the CPA through the NGO Assistance Office of the Ministry of Planning and Development Cooperation, was divisive. Registration for tax status is the norm for NGOs operating in any country. But many NGOs complained that the decision was made without their input, that the

---

[45] United Nations Assistance Mission for Iraq (UNAMI), "Iraq: International NGOs Discuss Exit Strategies," Newsroom, News and Events, www.uniraq.org/newsroom/story.asp?ID=260.

[46] United Nations Assistance Mission for Iraq, "Minutes of the UNAMI Coordination Meeting, January 14, 2004, www.uniraq.org/coordination/minutes.asp.

amount of information requested was either too intrusive or too detailed, and that the process was too bureaucratic.[47]

A further deterioration in their relationship came during the intense fighting between coalition forces and insurgents in Fallujah and Najaf. On April 13, 2004, the NGO Coordination Committee for Iraq issued a statement condemning several practices of the coalition forces that had been witnessed: the closing of the main teaching hospital of Fallujah, shooting at ambulances, and using health facilities as bases for military operations.[48] The lack of security in Iraq has seriously limited the NGOs' operability by making it difficult for them to move around the country. It has also led to numerous inefficiencies, since repaired facilities are often redamaged by insurgents or criminals. Moreover, NGOs have spent large amounts of money on operations, such as water tankering, that would not have been necessary had facilities not been damaged. In many cases, inadequate security has driven NGOs out of the country or caused them to reduce their presence.

U.S. and Coalition Military Forces. The Iraqi and coalition military forces are responsible for ensuring a secure and stable environment so that reconstruction and nation-building can proceed. U.S. troops have made up the bulk of the coalition forces: In May 2003, they totaled 150,000, while the other coalition members' troops stood at 23,000.[49] The number of U.S. troops decreased—despite reports of increasing insecurity—until they reached a low of 115,000 in February 2004. U.S. troops were then rapidly increased after February 2004, as attacks on both military forces and civilians intensified. At the same time, the number of non-U.S. troops slightly decreased, as Spain and Honduras withdrew their troops in May 2004. The

---

[47] Global Policy Forum, "Iraq: NGO Registration Causes Controversy," Integrated Regional Information Network, January 13, 2004, www.globalpolicy.org/ngos/aid/2004/0113contro. htm.

[48] Relief Web, "International NGOs call for an end to hostilities in Iraq," April 13, 2004, www.reliefweb.int.

[49] Brookings Institution, *Iraq Index: Tracking Variables of Reconstruction and Security in Post-Saddam Iraq,* Washington, D.C.: The Brookings Institution, April 2004, www.brookings. edu/fp/saban/iraq/index.pdf.

number of troops and the number of fatalities are reported, respectively, in Figures 8.8 and 8.9.

Military forces occasionally participated in the health reconstruction efforts in Iraq. The U.S. Army Corps of Engineers took part in rebuilding water and sanitation plants, as well as hospital facilities. As lack of security caused NGOs, major international organizations, and contractors to lose much of their mobility, coalition forces were increasingly drawn into the reconstruction process.[50] The U.S. military also has the ability to bring in medical supplies where no other entity can, but it seems to do this only sporadically. Similarly, military doctors took good care of wounded Iraqis but did not seem to be otherwise involved in caring for the Iraqis. There may be some reason

Figure 8.8
Number of U.S. Troops in Iraq

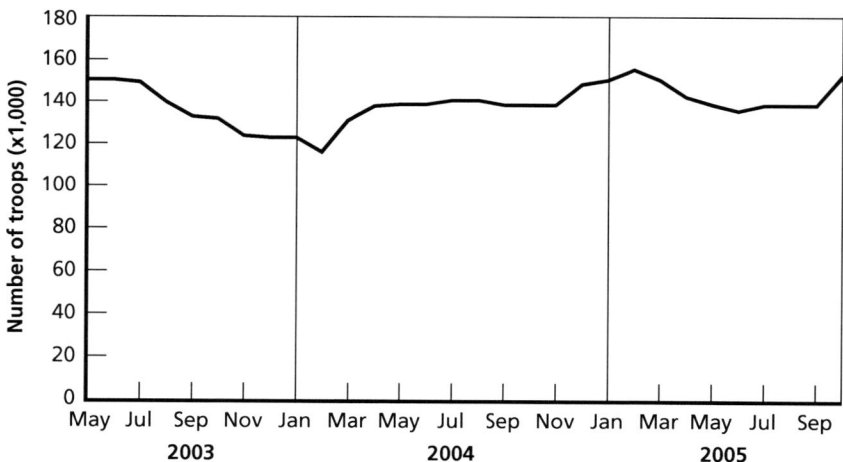

SOURCE: Brookings Institution, *Iraq Index*.
NOTE: Number of other coalition troops remained at about 23,000 during period.
RAND *MG321-8.8*

---

[50] F. Hiatt, "In Iraq, Focus and Idealism," *Washington Post*, June 28, 2004.

Figure 8.9
Number of U.S. Troop Fatalities in Iraq

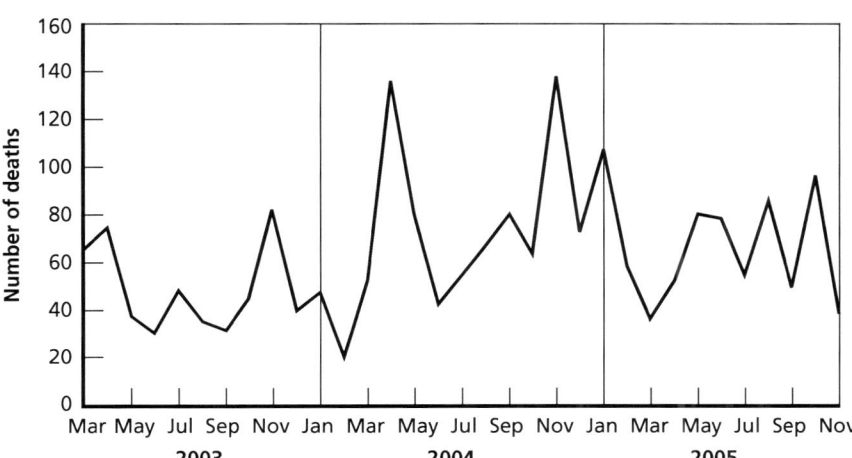

SOURCE: United States Department of Defense, *Military Casualty Information*, 2004.
NOTE: Numbers include fatalities from non-hostile causes, which on average
constitute 18.5% of all deaths.
RAND *MG321-8.9*

that it is infeasible or inadvisable for military doctors to play a significant role in rebuilding health, but the image of U.S. forces may suffer
as a consequence. This possibility should not be underestimated,
since small incidents sometimes produce large amounts of negative
press.

Private Sector. The private sector has carried out a large part of
the overall reconstruction effort in Iraq but has done relatively little
in the health sector. One notable exception is Abt Associates, a large
government and business consulting firm that has many years of experience in health care delivery and financing, as well as a widespread
international presence. Commercial enterprises will contribute significantly to the reconstruction of the water and sanitation sector. For
example, USAID awarded Bechtel two contracts, one for $1 billion
and one for $1.8 billion, for the repair and rehabilitation of Iraq's
infrastructure, including water and sanitation facilities. Bechtel will

do part of the work itself but will subcontract most of it, giving a large number of the contracts to Iraqi firms.

Public Health

In the post-conflict period, J. K. Haveman, former public health director for the state of Michigan, ran the Ministry of Health. In September 2003, he ceded the position to an Iraqi health minister, Khudair Fadhil Abbas. However, the Ministry of Health was not officially turned over to the Iraqis until March 28, 2004, when it became the first autonomous Iraqi ministry.

The Iraqi population has mixed views about the current status of the health care system. Results from the February 2004 National Survey of Iraq,[51] a nationally representative survey conducted by Oxford Research International, suggest that about one-half of the population at that time was unhappy with the availability of medical care. However, the same survey shows that about 45 percent of the population rated their current situation as an improvement over the pre-invasion period, and only 16 percent believed that things had worsened in terms of medical care availability. The unhappiness of a large portion of the population may stem at least partly from the fact that much of what the Ministry of Health has been actively doing is not visible. Activities such as redesigning the university medical training curriculum, identifying target regions, assessing the costs of providing primary care, and designing disease surveillance systems—all of these will bring benefits that are not immediately tangible or obvious but are nonetheless crucial to the health of much of the population.

To provide a clearer picture of how Iraq's health has changed since the recent conflict, the next sections analyze what happened in sectors that affect health.

Water and Sanitation. The water and sanitation sector is tightly linked to the health sector. According to a UNICEF assessment in May 2003, 40 percent of the water and sanitation network in Bagh-

---

[51] Oxford Research International, *National Survey of Iraq*, February 2004, news.bbc.co.uk/nol/shared/bsp/hi/pdfs/150304iraqsurvey.pdf.

dad was badly damaged. The pipes and other infrastructure were fragile because of improper maintenance and could not withstand the vibrations caused by bombing and tanks.[52] As a result, 50 percent of the water supply was lost due to ruptures in the system in the immediate post-conflict phase. Additionally, looting deprived water treatment plants of necessary equipment and directly damaged pipes. As Pat Carey, CARE's Senior Vice President for Programs, argued in July 2003: "The goal of restoring basic services in Baghdad to pre-war levels has clearly not been achieved. Indeed, the trend in the last month has been going in the wrong direction."[53]

Progress in restoring basic services has been slow and has proved to be a major source of frustration for the Iraqi people. To understand the situation, it is useful to understand the Iraqis' point of view on this matter. The water and environmental sanitation sector and the electricity sector were heavily damaged in the 1991 Gulf War, but they were then restored fairly quickly. Many Iraqis saw American reconstruction efforts as slow and had trouble understanding why the CPA could not make repairs as quickly as Saddam Hussein's regime did.[54] The argument that the security environment was the main cause was problematic, since the CPA was in charge of security as well. However, the current reconstruction effort began with a system that was falling apart because of years of under-maintenance, whereas the system before the 1991 Gulf War was in comparatively good shape.

---

[52] United Nations Children's Fund, *Crisis Appeal for Iraq's Children*, December 2003.

[53] Patrick Carey, "Humanitarian Assistance Following Military Operations: Overcoming Barriers—Part 2," Committee on Government Reform, Subcommittee on National Security, Emerging Threats and International Relations, July 18, 2003.

[54] C. Hanley, "Six Months After War's End, Most Iraqis Still Jobless; Lack of Work Leads Some to Claim They Were Better Off Before," *Pittsburgh Post-Gazette*, October 19, 2003; J. Spinner, "Lights Are Coming On, Slowly, in Iraq; Citizens Frustrated by Continuing Problems with Power Generation, Distribution, *Washington Post*, February 7, 2004; D. Baker, "Bechtel Under Siege, Iraqi's Seethe at Sabotage, Red Tape, Slow Repair Effort, *San Francisco Chronicle*, September 21, 2003; R. Chandrasekaran, "Troubles Temper Triumphs in Iraq; Problems Persist in Reconstruction Despite Gains," *Washington Post*, August 18, 2003.

During the summer of 2003, when Iraqis were anxious to get their public utilities restored, they saw American contractors coming in, surveying the facilities, and then leaving without doing any work, because their goal at that time was to perform a comprehensive assessment of what needed to be done.[55] Iraqis had no choice but to rely on a patchwork of emergency assistance and temporary measures, such as portable generators and trucked water. They grew angrier with every blackout.[56]

Formerly state-owned companies in Iraq were banned from reconstruction contracts as part of the de-Ba'athification process. And because of Iraq's high level of centralization prior to the conflict, numerous skilled Iraqi workers were ineligible to assist in the rebuilding.[57] Contractors such as Bechtel have put substantial effort into hiring Iraqis, but there are still complaints. For example, Iraqis commonly say that they get too small a share of the reconstruction funds or only get lower-level jobs; that they have neither been asked how they want their infrastructure system to be rebuilt nor given a say in how reconstruction funds are spent; and that they could perform repairs and maintenance much better, much quicker, and for less money than foreign contractors.[58]

---

[55] D. Baker, "Bechtel Under Siege, Iraqi's Seethe at Sabotage, Red Tape, Slow Repair Effort, *San Francisco Chronicle*, September 21, 2003; D. Struck, "Engines of Industry Sputtering in Iraq," *Washington Post*, July 10, 2004; A. Eunjung Cha, "Iraqi Experts Tossed with the Water: Workers Ineligible to Fix Polluted Systems," *Washington Post*, February 27 2004, p. A01.

[56] P. Constable, "Beyond Oil, Iraqi Industry Struggles Despite Freedom; Factories Working Far Below Capacity," *Washington Post*, August 28, 2003; A. Shadid, "In Basra, Worst May Be Ahead; As Southern Iraq Bakes, British Also Frustrated by Shortages," *Washington Post*, August 11, 2003.

[57] A. Eunjung Cha, "Iraqi Experts Tossed with the Water: Workers Ineligible to Fix Polluted Systems," *Washington Post*, February 27 2004, p. A01; S. Schifferes, "The Challenge of Rebuilding Iraq," *BBC News*, October 21, 2003, news.bbc.co.uk/1/hi/business/3176934.stm.

[58] *The Economist*, "Who'll Help Us? We Ourselves, Mostly," Special Report, September 13, 2003; J. Glanz, "Western Ways Force Iraq to Trim Water Projects," *New York Times*, July 26, 2004; A. Cha, "$1.9 Billion of Iraq's Money Goes to U.S. Contractors," *Washington Post*, August 4, 2004; M. Rubin, "Trust the Iraqis: Silent Majority," *New Republic*, June 7, 2004; J. Spinner and A. Cha, "U.S. Decisions on Iraq Spending Made in Private," *Washing-*

The only measure currently available for determining the progress being made in the water and environmental sanitation sector is number of hours per day of water service (regardless of quality). The U.S. Department of Defense made governorate-level data on this measure available in a January 2004 briefing[59]. Water service was reported for three time periods: before the conflict, after the conflict, and in January 2004. We do not know for sure what period of time is being indicated by "after the conflict," but we think it likely to be the summer of 2003. The exact timing does not change the general conclusions, however.

A measure of progress can be obtained by comparing the values on January 2004 with a baseline, which could be either the value before or the value after the conflict. If we choose the before-conflict value as the baseline, we obtain a measure of progress from the viewpoint of the Iraqis, because their starting point is what they had before the conflict, or what they were accustomed to. If we choose the after-conflict value, we obtain a measure of progress from the viewpoint of the people who have done the work, since their starting point would be what existed right after the conflict. Table 8.2 shows the water service in Iraq. The left-most set of three columns shows the Department of Defense data—i.e., the number of water service hours per day. Population for the governates is in the middle, and the right-most set of three columns shows the number of water service hours per day per million people served—i.e., the number of water service hours per day multiplied by the population with access to water service within the governorate, expressed in millions.

The last three rows in the table show the hours of service averaged over the governorates and the percent change compared to the baseline before-conflict measure and the baseline after-conflict measure. The percent-change numbers suggest that as of January 2004

ton Post, December 27, 2003; *The Economist*, "Cleaner, But Still Bare," October 4, 2003; J. Glanz, "In Race to Give Power to Iraqis, Electricity Lags," *New York Times*, June 14, 2004.

[59] United States Department of Defense, *Iraq Status,* Draft working papers, January 4, 2004, www.export.gov/iraq/pdf/dod_wklyrpt_012004.pdf.

Table 8.2
Water Service in Iraq

Governorate	Water (service hours/day)			Population with Access to Water	Water (service hours per million population served/day)		
	Before Conflict	After Conflict	Jan. 20, 2004		Before Conflict	After Conflict	Jan. 20, 2004
Baghdad	19	11	17	6,116,063	116.21	67.28	103.97
Nineveh	19	15	17	2,181,558	41.45	32.72	37.09
Arbil	24	24	24	1,177,655	28.26	28.26	28.26
Diyala	13	9	13	1,150,311	14.95	10.35	14.95
Basrah	19	15	17	1,126,432	21.40	16.90	19.15
Dhi-Qar	23	23	24	977,756	22.49	22.49	23.47
Anbar	17	12	13	964,758	16.40	11.58	12.54
Suliamaniyah	23	23	24	912,222	20.98	20.98	21.89
Babylon	15	16	23	832,623	12.49	13.32	19.15
Salah Al-Din	23	10	19	759,271	17.46	7.59	14.43
Dohuk	18	17	17	726,419	13.08	12.35	12.35
Najaf	15	11	23	687,866	10.32	7.57	15.82
Wassit	20	19	23	635,446	12.71	12.07	14.62
At-Ta'mim	14	16	16	621,123	8.70	9.94	9.94
Qadissiyah	12	8	19	540,555	6.49	4.32	10.27
Karbala	17	17	23	537,429	9.14	9.14	12.36
Maysan	14	16	16	526,912	7.38	8.43	8.43
Al-Muthanna	18	17	18	264,042	4.75	4.49	4.75
Average hours of service	17.9	15.5	19.2		21.4	16.7	21.3
Percent change over before-conflict measure		−0.14	0.07			−0.22	−0.003
Percent change over after-conflict measure			0.24				0.28

SOURCE: U.S. Department of Defense, *Iraq Status*, Draft working papers, December 15, 2003, www.export.gov/iraq/pdf/dod_wklyrpt_121503.pdf.

there was a 7 percent improvement with respect to the pre-conflict situation and a 28 percent improvement with respect to the post-conflict situation. However, because the Department of Defense simply averages over the governorates, the figures obtained are misleading in that they do not take into account the population differences among the governorates. What we care about is the welfare of the entire population, so to measure benefits we have to multiply the number of hours of access to water by the number of people who have access to that water (the served population).[60] The resulting measure, the number of million person hours of access to water, can then be easily aggregated to produce the total benefits to the population. When we measure benefits in this way, the improvement over the before-conflict baseline is only three in a thousand.

This result is driven by the fact that access to water is not equal throughout the country. Better conditions are usually found in the northern governorates, and some of the large improvements have occurred in relatively small governorates, such as Najaf, Qadissiyah, and Karbala. The large Baghdad governorate experienced a decline in conditions. In general, reconstruction progress is perceived differently by the Iraqi population, who use the before-conflict conditions as their baseline, than it is by the people involved in reconstruction activities, who use the after-conflict conditions as their baseline. The "Iraq Quality Survey Reports" of February 2005 show that only half of the population rated the level of water supply as good or very good.[61] Although progress was made, the overall progress of U.S efforts was difficult to estimate because of the lack of performance data, measures, and appropriate records.[62]

---

[60] Data on access to water are from United Nations Children's Fund, *Situation Analysis of Children and Women in Iraq*, April 1998, www.childinfo.org/Other/Iraq_sa.pdf.

[61] Government Accountability Office, *Rebuilding Iraq: U.S. Water and Sanitation Efforts Need Improved Measures for Assessing Impact and Sustained Resources for Maintaining Facilities*, GAI-05-872, September 2005; United Nations Development Programme, *Iraq Living Conditions Survey 2004, Volume II, Analytical Report*, www.iq.undp.org/ILCS/PDF/Analytical%20Report%20-%20English.pdf.

[62] Government Accountability Office, *Rebuilding Iraq: U.S. Water and Sanitation Efforts*.

The sewage sector experienced problems similar to the water sector. Iraq has 13 major sewage plants. As of March 2004, the three Baghdad plants, which make up 75 percent of the nation's sewage treatment capacity, were still reported to be inoperable.[63] According to UNICEF, the sewage plants were kept from operating by a breakdown in the fuel supply line, lack of maintenance, and looting.[64] Consequently, the waste of 3.8 million people was flowing untreated into the Tigris, putting the Iraqi population at high risk of communicable disease outbreaks. During May 2003, WHO observed a tenfold increase in the cases of cholera compared to the previous year, and WHO officials issued a warning that massive outbreaks were possible.

In May 2004, the Kerkh wastewater treatment plant began operating at full capacity for the first time in 12 years.[65] And GAO reported that six sewage treatment plants were repaired by Bechtel as of September 2005.[66] In general, however, most Iraqis have been unhappy with the quality of sanitation services. According to GAO, the "Iraq Quality of Life Survey" of February 2005 found that less than 20 percent of the population rated the quality of wastewater disposal as good to very good, and that rates of dissatisfaction were particularly high in southern Iraq.[67]

Infectious Diseases and Immunization. In the immediate aftermath of the conflict, the country experienced increased rates of infectious diseases. After WHO reported the first outbreak of cholera in Basra, on May 15, there was widespread reporting of pertussis and diphtheria, especially in the south. WHO also reported that diarrheal disease represented 22 percent of all medical consultations, a threefold increase over the previous year.[68] Three months after the conflict

---

[63] www.usaid.gov/press/factsheets/2004/fs040318.html.

[64] www.unicef.org/infobycountry/iraq.html.

[65] http://www.usaid.gov/iraq/accomplishments/watsan.html.

[66] Government Accountability Office, *Rebuilding Iraq: U.S. Water and Sanitation Efforts.*

[67] Government Accountability Office, *Rebuilding Iraq: U.S. Water and Sanitation Efforts.*

[68] Carey, "Humanitarian Assistance Following Military Operations."

began, an estimated 210,000 babies were born in Iraq, none of whom received the necessary immunization.

In addition, measles vaccination rates in the 1990s had been low, which meant that older children were now also at higher risk. No epidemic of measles was observed in the conflict's immediate aftermath, although the scenario had been greatly feared. The country's vaccine supply was stored in Baghdad at the Vaccine and Serum Institute, which was struck by a missile in early 2003 and lost electricity. Looting made emergency repair impossible. Consequently, the cold chain was disrupted and all vaccine stocks were lost. UNICEF eventually replaced the vaccine stock and resumed national routine immunization by mid-June 2003.[69] Additional vaccine shortages have been reported, but USAID has stated that three million (out of a total of 4.2 million) children under five years of age have been immunized. In addition, 700,000 pregnant women have been vaccinated for tetanus, and five million children between the ages of six and 12 have been immunized against measles, mumps, and rubella.[70]

Another critical aspect was the disease surveillance system, which allowed public health agencies to monitor disease incidence and plan responses. This system was, of course, disrupted by the conflict, but efforts to reestablish it began very quickly. At the beginning of May 2003, WHO developed and carried out an early warning surveillance protocol in Basra. By the end of 2004, WHO had developed a tool, the *Public Health Problem Identification and Verification List*, that public health professionals could use to help identify and monitor public health emergencies.[71]

Food and Nutrition. There have been no signs of starvation in Iraq, but there have been widespread signs of chronic malnutrition,

---

[69] United Nations Children's Fund, "Routine Immunization of Children Re-established Across Iraq," Press release, June 2003. www.unicef.org/media/media_9414.html.

[70] United States Agency for International Development, www.usaid.gov/iraq/accomplishments/health.html.

[71] World Health Organization, *Iraq Annual Report*, 2004, http://www.emro.who.int/iraq/pdf/annualreport04.pdf.

especially in children and mothers. Figure 8.10 charts the prevalence among children age five and under of chronic and acute malnutrition. Malnutrition rates sharply increased after the 1991 Gulf War, peaked in 1996, and then dropped, most likely because of the Oil-for-Food Program. The 2003 conflict appears to have reversed the downward trend: The percentage of children who were underweight or had acute malnutrition increased, while the proportion of children with chronic malnutrition seemed stable. Malnutrition was concentrated in the central and south regions, which is consistent with the general finding that the north had been in better shape than the rest of the country prior to the conflict and was less affected by the conflict. The high prevalence of chronic malnutrition, which manifests itself as low height-for-age ("stunting"), is particularly worrying, because it is

Figure 8.10
Malnutrition Rates in Children Age Five and Under, Iraq

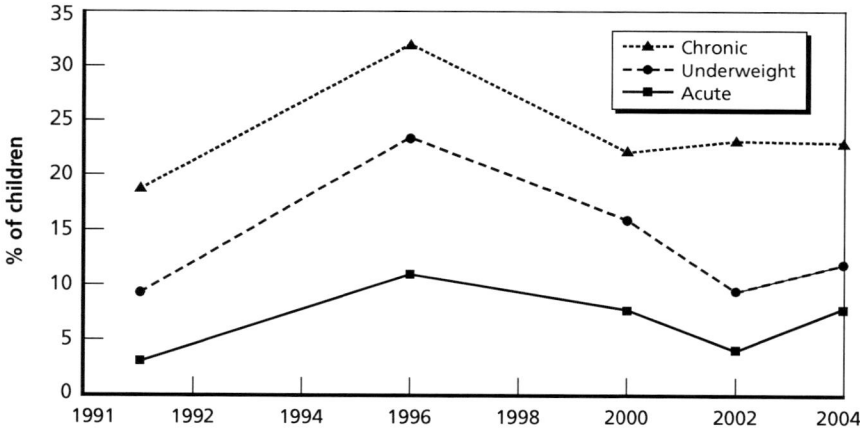

SOURCES: Food and Agriculture Organization of the United Nations, and World Food Programme, *FAO/WFP Crop, Food Supply and Nutrition Assessment Mission to Iraq*; United Nations Development Programme (UNDP), *Iraq Living Conditions Survey 2004*. Data for 1996 are from the International Study Team household survey; data for 1996 and 2000 are from the MICS household survey; data for 2002 are from the UNICEF-NRI household survey; data for 2004 are from the UNDP Iraq Living Condition Survey.
RAND *MG321-8.10*

widely believed that stunting at a young age can lead to cognitive deficits and a high burden of morbidity in adulthood.[72]

Despite good agricultural production in 2003 and the end of economic sanctions, 55 percent of Iraqis were poor, 44 percent had insufficient food, and 80 percent were in danger of having insufficient food if the public distribution system broke down.[73] The three leading causes of insufficient food were assessed as unemployment, chronic poverty, and death of the head of household. Food rationing, at first disrupted, started again in June 2003. By the second half of 2004, the Iraq Living Condition Survey[74] reported that 96 percent of Iraqis were receiving food rations and 25 percent of Iraqi families were highly dependent on them. There appears to be no correlation between the figures on food rations and the malnutrition rates. This can be partly justified by reports that the incidence of diarrhea in children was at high levels, and frequent bouts of diarrhea in children can lead to malnutrition because of malabsorption of nutrients. In addition, even when food rations supply adequate levels of calories, they may not supply needed micronutrients, such as iron, vitamin A, and iodine.[75]

Overall, several factors helped prevent starvation and a major epidemic. One important factor was that Iraq conducted its own planning before the conflict. For example, it distributed a three-month supply of consumables for the operation of water treatment plants before the conflict, and in August 2002, it started providing an additional advance monthly food ration.[76] In addition, the conflict

---

[72] D.S. Berkman et al., "Effects of Stunting, Diarrhoeal Disease, and Parasitic Infection During Infancy on Cognition in Late Childhood: A Follow-Up Study," *Lancet*, Vol. 359, 2002, pp. 564–571; F. Branca and M. Ferrari, "Impact of Micronutrient Deficiencies on Growth: The Stunting Syndrome," *Annals of Nutrition & Metabolism*, Vol. 46, Suppl. 1, 2002, pp. 8–17.

[73] Food and Agriculture Organization of the United Nations, and World Food Programme, *FAO/WFP Crop, Food Supply and Nutrition Assessment Mission to Iraq.*

[74] United Nations Development Programme, *Iraq Living Conditions Survey 2004.*

[75] United Nations Development Program, *Iraq Living Conditions Survey 2004.*

[76] International Study Team, *Our Common Responsibility.*

phase was relatively short, produced fewer casualties than expected, and did not lead to a large number of refugees or internally displaced persons. Had mass migration occurred, the food distribution system would likely have broken down. The ensuing refugee situation could then have greatly increased the spread of communicable diseases, bringing the country even closer to a full-scale epidemic.

Mortality Indicators. Estimates of such indicators as infant mortality are difficult to obtain for the immediate post-conflict phase. However, the U.S. Department of Defense stated that a goal for 2005 was "to reduce infant mortality rate by half to 50/1000," which implies that the 2004 infant mortality rate was considered to be around 100 per 1,000 live births.[77] This rate is plausible, since the infant mortality rates for 2000, 2001, and 2002 were 105, 107, and 102 per 1,000 live births, respectively.[78] The instability, looting, and destruction of medical records in 2003 made more-accurate estimates unlikely.

The problem for adult mortality is even more serious. Mortality statistics will be affected by the number of Iraqis who died during or in the aftermath of the conflict. However, it is U.S. policy not to produce estimates of civilian casualties. There are conflicting reports about whether the Iraq Ministry of Health compiled such statistics, but no official figure has been made available to date. Numerous organizations do their own estimates of civilian casualties from media reports and eyewitnesses, but these are not very accurate. The Iraq Index argues that the number of civilian casualties between March 2003 and October 2005 was between 15,800 and 27,800.[79]

---

[77] U.S. Department of Defense, *Iraq Status,* Draft working papers, December 15, 2003.

[78] We noticed that in the period around June 2004, the CIA's *World Factbook* updated its 2004 value of infant mortality to 52.71. It is extremely unlikely that this number is correct. If it were, it would represent a success of huge proportions, which would have certainly been publicized by agencies such as USAID, WHO, and UNICEF. Since the CIA *World Factbook* does not report data sources, it is impossible to tell the source of this estimate. Our attempts to contact the CIA *World Factbook* staff about this issue were unsuccessful.

[79] Brookings Institution, *Iraq Index: Tracking Variables of Reconstruction & Security in Post-Saddam Iraq*, Washington, D.C.: Brookings Institution, www.brookings.edu/iraqindex. The

By setting a target reduction in infant mortality rates, the Department of Defense provided an easy way to quantify delays in achievement of this goal. We can start by letting *dstart* and *dtarget* be, respectively, the current and target infant mortality rates per 1,000 live births, and letting T be the number of months during which the intervention to reduce infant mortality takes place. Let us assume for simplicity that mortality decreases linearly during the intervention and remains constant after the intervention.[80] If we denote the number of births occurring every year by b, then the number of children D who will die if the intervention achieves its target at time $T + \Delta T$ but would not have died otherwise is:

$$D = \Delta T \times b/12{,}000 \times (dstart - dtarget)/2 \,,$$

where *b/12,000* is the number of births per month per 1,000 population.

This formula shows that a one-month delay in the intervention translates into an additional number of infant deaths equal to *b/12,000 × (dstart − dtarget)/2*. We set *dstart* = 100 and *dtarget* = *dstart/2*, according to CPA figures.[81] For the number of births, we use the latest figure from the UNICEF Website, b = 867,000. As a result, a delay of one month in achieving the infant mortality target translates into D = 1,806 infant deaths (that is, deaths that would have been avoided in the absence of the delay). To put things in perspective, consider an infant mortality rate of 100 per 1,000 live births, which would put the number of deaths each month at 7,200.

Security and Personal Safety. Soon after the conflict ended, it was clear that security would be a major concern. Two weeks after the end of major combat operations, the WHO representative in Baghdad said that the three most urgent problems for health in Iraq were "security, security, security," and that the lack of security was posing a

---

Brookings Institution has compiled and continues to update an Iraq Index that includes a collection of indicators on Iraq.

[80] This will tend to underestimate the effect of delays.

[81] U.S. Department of Defense, *Iraq Status*, Draft working papers, December 15, 2003.

serious challenge to the health system.[82] Health care professionals and patients stayed away from health care facilities because they feared being attacked by looters. In addition, medical records were destroyed, equipment was looted, and the intact facilities were overburdened by the flow of patients from damaged facilities. The work of NGOs, international organizations, and contractors was either slowed or halted. And people's personal safety was being directly affected by the increased incidence of crime, mass casualties from car bombings, improvised explosive devices, shootings, and civilian casualties caused by coalition military operations.

The security situation quickly deteriorated after May 2003.[83] However, there are no good indicators of security available. One of the indicators on Iraq from the Iraq Index, the number of Iraqi civilians killed, is reported in Figure 8.11.

Another source of information about security is public opinion polls of Iraqis. In February 2004, Iraqis reported that lack of security was the most significant problem. Nearly two-thirds of the respondents cited regaining security in the country as the first priority for the next 12 months.[84] According to a nationwide poll conducted by CNN/USAToday/Gallup at the end of March 2004, 32 percent of 3,444 respondents were sometimes afraid to go outside of their home since the occupation began, whereas only 7 percent had been afraid to do so before the occupation. Furthermore, 94 percent of Baghdad residents believed that the city was more dangerous at the time of the polling than it had been before the invasion.[85]

---

[82] World Health Organization, "Health Briefing on Iraq," UN Humanitarian Briefing, May 14, 2003, www.who.int/features/2003/iraq/briefings/wednesday14/en/; O. Dyer, "Poor Security Is Biggest Impediment to Health Care in Iraq," *British Medical Journal*, Vol. 326, No. 7399, May 24, 2003, p. 1107.

[83] *The Economist*, "A Wider War, a Wider Worry," April 10, 2004, pp. 35–36; *The Economist*, "The Spectre of a Civil War," February 14, 2004; A.E. Cha and J. Spinner, "Some U.S. Workers Say the Risk Is Too Great," *Washington Post*, April 15, 2004; M.P. Flaherty and J. Spinner, "In Iraq, Contractors' Security Costs Rise," *Washington Post*, February 18, 2004.

[84] Oxford Research International, *National Survey of Iraq*.

[85] Brookings Institution, *Iraq Index*.

Figure 8.11
Number of Iraqi Civilians Killed

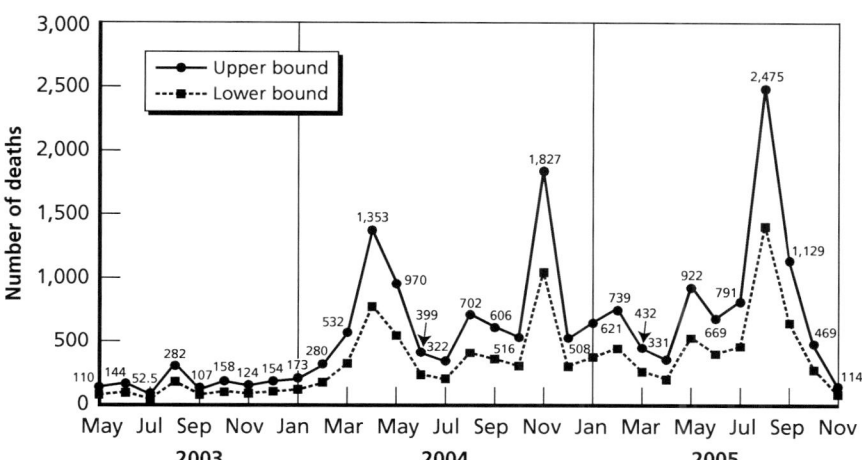

SOURCE: Brookings Institution, *Iraq Index*.
RAND *MG321-8.11*

The situation has been particularly difficult for Iraqi women and young girls, who have been placed at increased risk of sexual assault and abduction. In general, violent acts against women are largely unreported. According to Human Rights Watch, the perception on the ground following the war indicated a sharp increase in the cases of sexual violence. Interviews with Iraqi police officials substantiated these reports. As one police officer reported:

> There is no safety, and there is too much crime, too many cases, even to pursue. Some gangs specialize in kidnapping girls, then sell them to Gulf countries. This happened before the war too, but now it is worse, they can get them in and out without passports. We have so many cases, we have no authority to solve or investigate them.[86]

---

[86] Human Rights Watch, "Climate of Fear: Sexual Violence and Abduction of Women and Girls in Baghdad," Human Rights Watch, 7(E), July 2003.

Despite the significant effort invested in restoring security, the insurgency in Iraq intensified through 2004 and has remained strong, with frequent attacks against the United States, other coalition forces, and the civilian population.[87,88]

Health Care Delivery

Hospitals and Clinics. Iraqi health care facilities sustained considerable damage in the immediate aftermath of the conflict, severely limiting their capacity to respond to medical crises. While some damage was caused by aerial bombing and other military operations, a large portion was caused by looting. The best-known documented case of looting took place at Al Rashad, the only long-term psychiatric hospital in Iraq, which housed 1,400 patients. In April 2003, U.S. troops opened the gates of the compound and knocked down several walls. Patients with severe mental illnesses, including those with violent criminal histories, escaped from the hospital, and women were raped. Looters destroyed medical records and stripped the facility of air conditioners, heaters, beds, food supplies, and antipsychotic medication. Although security was eventually restored and some patients returned, Al Rashad remains in poor condition and in urgent need of repair.[89]

The reconstruction and repair of health facilities took approximately one year. In June 2004, the Ministry of Health reported that all 240 Iraqi hospitals and more than 1,200 primary health centers were operating, though many were still in poor condition. In addition, the Ministry was able to monitor facilities' service distribution,

---

[87] Seth G. Jones, Jeremy M. Wilson, Andrew Rathmell, and K. Jack Riley, *Establishing Law and Order After Conflict,* MG-374-RC, Santa Monica, California: The RAND Corporation, 2005.

[88] Government Accountability Office, *Rebuilding Iraq: Enhancing Security, Measuring Program Results, and Maintaining Infrastructure Are Necessary to Make Significant and Sustainable Progress,* GAO-06-179T, October 2005.

[89] Guy Raz, "Baghdad Mental Hospital on Life Support," Washington, D.C.: National Public Radio, May 1, 2003, www.npr.org/news/specials/iraq2003/raz_030501.html; M. Valentinas, "Iraq: Filth and Deprivation Rack Baghdad's Only Mental Hospital," 2003, www.globalsecurity.org/wmd/library/news/iraq/2003/05/iraq-030526-rfel-162816.htm.

cost information, and building condition through a database built with help from USAID and Abt Associates. In 2004, most of the population had some access to health centers and, to lesser degree, public hospitals, although there was less access in rural areas.[90] What is not known, however, is the quality of care received at these facilities. The U.S. Department of State tracked only the number of completed facilities as an indicator of increased access to care; it did not monitor staffing, training, and equipment levels.[91] Meaningful measures of the reconstruction program's success are thus difficult to produce.

Drugs and Consumables. Reports indicate that drug and supply distributions were slow to be reestablished and that many of the problems encountered stemmed from the power vacuum, lack of management, looting, attacks on convoys carrying supplies, and inoperable factories. Reports also indicate that facilities continued to experience shortages in essential medications and equipment through 2005. There have been shortages in, for example, antibiotics, diabetes medications, anticancer drugs, intravenous lines, tuberculosis test kits, oxygen, and equipment such as ventilators and incubators for premature babies. The Ministry of Health itself reported that as much as 65 percent of equipment in Iraq's hospitals was not functional or needed repair or replacement.[92] By May 2005, the delivery of 600 medical equipment kits was virtually complete. Lack of security and problems in the procurement process were the main causes of the delays.[93]

---

[90] United Nations Development Program, *Iraq Living Conditions Survey 2004.*

[91] Government Accountability Office, *Rebuilding Iraq: Enhancing Security, Measuring Program Results, and Maintaining Infrastructure.*

[92] A. Eunjung Cha, "Iraqi Hospitals on Life Support: Babies Dying Because of Shortages of Medicine and Supplies," *Washington Post*, March 5, 2004, p. A01; S. Faramarzi, "Iraqi Kids Suffer at Underfunded Hospital," *Associated Press,* June 4, 2004; S.N. Yacoub, "Iraqi Hospitals Prepare for Attacks," *Associated Press,* April 29, 2004; S. Chan, "Iraqis Take Control of Health Ministry," *Washington Post*, March 29, 2004, p. A15; K. Dilanian, "Iraqi Hospitals Remain Bleak Without U.S. Aid," *Knight Ridder/Tribune News Service*, March 5, 2004.

[93] Government Accountability Office, *Rebuiliding Iraq: Status of Funding and Reconstruction Efforts.*

Doctors, Nurses, and Medical Personnel. An additional problem concerns adequately trained nurses and physicians. The nurse population was low before the conflict began at about one nurse per physician. Nurses in Iraq are, on average, not very well trained, and only 300 nurses in the entire country currently have the equivalent of a bachelor's degree. Part of the reason for this inadequate nurse population is cultural: There is a stigma associated with nursing. Taboos prevent nurses from performing such tasks as bathing patients, which thus must be performed by physicians and residents or patients' relatives.[94] The inadequate security situation adds to the nurse shortage in that many nurses often are unable to get to work or are too afraid to leave the house.

The Ministry of Health has raised the salaries of health professionals in order to bring nurses back to work. This was possible because the budget for health increased, climbing from $16 million in 2002 to $950 million in 2004. One solution to the nurse shortage might be to import nurses from abroad, as was done prior to the Gulf War and as is commonly done in many countries in the Middle East. The security environment at this point rules this out as an option, however.

The Ministry of Health has also made training a top priority. By September 2003, more than 2,000 health care professionals had received training, with the assistance of USAID and Abt Associates. By March 2004, more than 1,000 health workers and volunteers had been trained to identify, treat, and monitor the growth of acutely malnourished children. Additional training and professional development have come through partnerships between American or British health organizations and selected Iraqi health care centers. Similar to a consortium of health care institutions in the United States, these partnerships provide professional and technical support and increase access to equipment, supplies, pharmaceuticals, and managerial expertise. The Iraq Minister of Health also requested assistance from

---

[94] D. Wood, "Nurses Help Rebuild Iraq's Health Care System," AMN Healthcare, Health Care News, 2003.

Bahrain in training health professionals by mutual exchanges of health teams.[95]

Lack of security has created significant problems for efforts aimed at improving health care delivery. During April and May 2004, more than 100 surgeons, specialists, and general physicians were abducted. In many cases, they were ordered to leave the country—a clear attempt to disrupt services in the country, along the lines of many other terrorist acts.[96] The abductions were largely concentrated in the Baghdad area. Based on a ratio of 4.7 physicians per 10,000 people, this means the abductions directly affected 213,000 patients. They also spread fear through Baghdad's hospitals and clinics.

Overall Assessment

This section analyzes and assesses some important aspects of the reconstruction effort. We start with security, since it has become very clear that lack of security profoundly affects the reconstruction effort. Even a large investment of effort and capital may lead to a poor outcome if the level of security is low.

Security. In its strategic plan, the CPA outlined a number of objectives and priorities for the achievement of a secure environment.[97] The list included such items as development of an accountable police system, creation of Iraqi security forces, and reform of the criminal/civil code and the penal system. Lack of security had several effects on reconstruction. First, it led to additional costs for the rebuilding efforts: security guards had to be hired, high insurance premiums had to be paid, and special transportation had to be arranged. In 2004 alone, an estimated 15,000 civilian security guards were op-

---

[95] "Iraq Keen to Learn from Bahrain Health Sector," *Bahrain Tribune*, May 25, 2004.

[96] E. Sanders, "Kidnappings Bleed Iraq of Doctors," *Los Angeles Times*, May 31, 2004; S. Peterson, "A Self-Rule Test at Iraq Ministry, *Christian Science Monitor*, May 19, 2004.

[97] Coalition Provisional Authority, *Strategic Plan,* Unpublished, 2003.

erating in Iraq (one for every 1,646 Iraqis), and a bodyguard could easily cost $1,000 per day.[98]

Second, lack of security took a toll on the size and effectiveness of the labor force. Although the flow of U.S. laborers willing to work in Iraq has not slowed significantly (for example, only one percent of Halliburton workers in the country have quit), some contractors and subcontractors (such as Creative Associates International and International Relief and Development Inc.) moved their workers out of Iraq.[99] General Electric and Siemens temporarily suspended most of their operations in late April 2004, delaying work on power plants by up to a month.[100] In central Iraq, a sewer repair project was suspended for four months in 2004 because of security concerns.[101]

When security is inadequate, many Iraqis are not willing to go to work. And even when workers do go to work, security checks may prevent them from working a full day. Overall, GAO found that security was responsible for more than 15 percent of the contract cost for eight of 15 reconstruction contracts it reviewed.[102] GAO also found that in the water and sanitation sector, low security increased project costs by 7 percent.[103]

For the health sector, the absence of security is associated with worse reconstruction outcomes. As a way to show this association, we built a measure of regional "success" using the data on person hours

---

[98] M.P. Flaherty and J. Spinner, "In Iraq, Contractors' Security Costs Rise."

[99] S. McNulty, "Come to Hell with Halliburton—the Pay's Good," *Financial Times*, June 14, 2004; A.E. Cha and J. Spinner, "Some U.S. Workers Say the Risk Is Too Great," *Washington Post*, April 2004; J. Spinner, "War Dangers Don't Deter U.S. Workers," *Washington Post*, May 17, 2004, p. A01.

[100] N. Pelham, "Baghdad Suicide Bomber Kills Five GE Contractors," *Financial Times*, June 15, 2004; J. Glanz, "Violence in Iraq Forces 2 Big Contractors to Curb Work," *New York Times*, April 22, 2004.

[101] Government Accountability Office, *Rebuilding Iraq: Enhancing Security, Measuring Program Results, and Maintaining Infrastructure.*

[102] Government Accountability Office, *Rebuilding Iraq: Enhancing Security, Measuring Program Results, and Maintaining Infrastructure.*

[103] GAO, *Rebuilding Iraq: U.S. Water and Sanitation Efforts Need Improved.*

of water service by governorate described earlier (see Table 8.2). We then attempted to correlate "success" with some regional security indicators, expecting to find a positive correlation between success and security. Finding security indicators by governorate was not an easy task. One possibility was to use the "Iraq Body Count," a dataset on civilian deaths that reports both time and place of death.[104] Another possibility was to use the data that *The New York Times* collected on number of insurgent attacks per 100,000 population within the month of September 2004.[105] We decided to use the number of attacks, since the number of civilian deaths may underestimate the magnitude of the security problem. The two measures correlate fairly well, though. When we excluded Baghdad, with its disproportionate number of casualties per attack, the correlation coefficient went from 0.5 to 0.8.

Our measure of success, then, is the percent change in the number of million person hours of access to water from the pre-conflict period to January 2004. Figure 8.12 plots our measure of success against the number of attacks per 100,000 population in September 2004 for the 18 Iraqi governorates. Although there is a large amount of noise, the data appear to support the notion that governorates with large numbers of deaths have made either little or negative progress with respect to the pre-conflict situation. To get a quantitative measure of security's effect on success, we divided the governorates into "higher" and "lower" security categories according to whether their number of attacks was below or above the median (three attacks per 100,000 population). Our calculations show that success was 4.8 times higher in the higher security governorates than in the lower security governorates.

---

[104] Available at www.iraqbodycount.org, this dataset, whose underlying collection methodology is well documented, uses news reports as data sources and thoroughly documents each event involving one or more deaths.

[105] J. Glanz and T. Shanker, "Iraq Study Sees Rebels' Attacks as Widespread," *New York Times*, September 29, 2004.

Figure 8.12
Success in Reconstructing Water Sector in Iraq as a Function of Insecurity

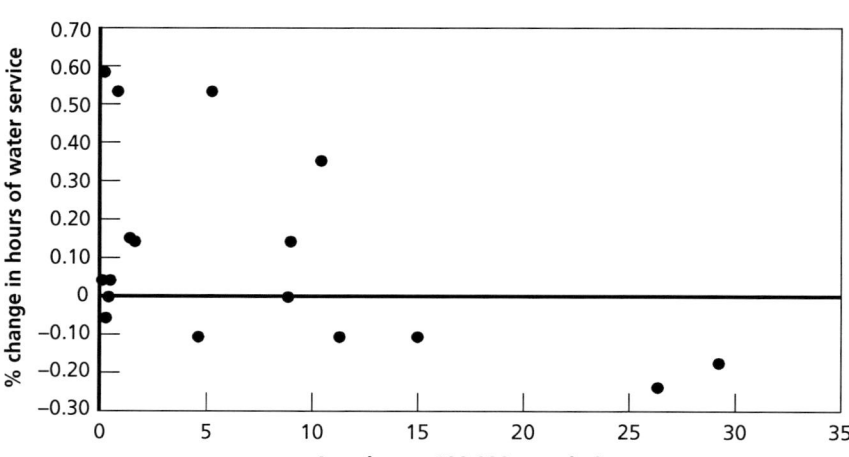

NOTE: Numbers do not include Iraqi civilians killed during major combat operations in March and April 2003.

RAND *MG321-8.12*

It should be noted that these results are preliminary, since the data were not reliable and we did not control for other, possibly confounding factors. However, the finding is in line with the expectation of a positive correlation between security and success.

Interaction Between Health and Other Sectors. Reconstruction of the health sector is tightly linked to progress in other sectors. For example, efforts to refurbish hospitals and clinics, train staff, and provide equipment will be nullified if electrical power is not always available. Hospitals and clinics in Iraq operated at partial capacity using power generators provided by different organizations.[106] This implies that many resources had to be diverted to this end rather than employed more directly in the health care sector. In addition, since the water and sanitation sectors also need electricity to function, power

---

[106] United Nations Children's Fund, *Routine Immunization of Children Re-established Across Iraq.*

generators had to be supplied to water and sanitation plants, and water had to be trucked to locations where it could not be pumped.

Consequently, protection of power generation and transmission systems from bombing and, even more important, looting, should be one of the highest priorities. And a large amount of resources should be invested in the electricity sector at the very beginning of the reconstruction effort—something that did not happen in Iraq. Part of the reason why this did not happen may be that few organizations other than Bechtel have the resources to do serious repair work in this sector. And Bechtel was slowed by the request to conduct full assessments and by security issues. A possible better strategy could have been to provide an initial, large amount of support to the efforts of NGOs and UN agencies to bring in portable generators, while at the same time making more use of Bechtel's expertise combined with Iraqi engineers' experience. This approach would have meant postponing the full assessments and probably would have led to some duplication of effort and similar inefficiencies. But it would have done much to alleviate the Iraqi people's frustration, which seems to have greatly fueled their anger and resentment and contributed to decreased levels of security.[107]

Procurement and Contracting. The Iraqi contracts awarded by the U.S. government—especially by the Department of Defense—constitute the largest single-country foreign aid package since the Marshall Plan, which implies that the related procurement activities constituted unprecedented challenges.[108] The speed in awarding the contracts did not have, unfortunately, a counterpart on the implementation side, at least for the water and sanitation sector. Part of the reason for this was the Defense Department's request that Bechtel perform a full assessment before starting the reconstruction work.

---

[107] E. Cody, "To Many, Mission Not Accomplished," *Washington Post*, June 3, 2004, p. A01; N. Riccardi, "For Iraqis, a Symbol of Unkept Promises," *Los Angeles Times*, June 1, 2004.

[108] J. Marburg-Goodman, "USAID's Iraq Procurement Contracts: Insider's View," *Procurement Lawyer*, Vol. 39, No. 1, Fall 2003.

Both the need for assessments and the need for a competitive bidding process are well grounded in arguments of efficiency, so it is unclear why, given the urgency of the situation, the U.S. government was willing to forgo some efficiency in the bidding process but not in the implementation process. This point is particularly relevant considering that the assessments took place in the summer, which is the time of year that Iraq usually experiences spikes in infectious diseases such as cholera, and that the delay in implementation thus could have been disastrous.

The issue of interest here is, given a fixed budget and time frame, what is the optimal spending pattern for infrastructure reconstruction? This issue is too complicated to address in full here, but we do want to stress an important aspect of it.

We begin by thinking of infrastructure as a form of capital, and thus as depreciating over time. The key observation is that the productivity of the reconstruction effort, measured by the improvement in infrastructure obtained by investing one unit of effort, depends on the level of infrastructure at the time the effort is invested. In addition, it is possible that productivity will remain low until the level of infrastructure exceeds a certain minimum threshold, at which point it will quickly increase as more infrastructure becomes available. This possibility is more likely when the infrastructure being rebuilt is basic, like electricity, so that some of it is needed to complete the reconstruction work.[109] When this is the case, it can be shown that it is more efficient to invest more effort at the beginning of reconstruction rather than later. In other words, if two spending patterns with the same total expenditures and time frame are available—one that increases spending over time and one that decreases it over time—the latter pattern will result in more reconstruction work being done by the end of the time frame. This pattern is also justified when security is taken into consideration. If we assume that slow progress in reconstruction leads to deteriorating security and that inadequate security hinders the reconstruction effort, then an initial high level of effort is

---

[109] For example, lack of electricity is likely to make the problem of rebuilding the electricity network more difficult.

necessary to keep security from deteriorating and thus hindering future work.

It seems implausible that the reason for the observed spending pattern in Iraq was lack of capital. UNICEF and WHO, both of which had the ability to move much quicker than Bechtel did and could have started their work right away, received initial awards of $8 and $10 million, respectively. These amounts were dwarfed by the size of the contracts that went to the private sector. And even if UNICEF and WHO had been awarded amounts five times larger than what they received, the total would have been only two percent of the appropriation for the water and environmental sanitation sector. In addition to UNICEF and WHO, other organizations could have been helpful in the early reconstruction phase. Several NGOs, such as CARE, were operating in Iraq before the conflict. By funding these organizations, the U.S. government could have leveraged their hands-on experience in the country.

One plausible reason for the U.S. government did not invest more at the beginning of the reconstruction phase was that it lacked sufficient staff to handle the larger number of contracts and grants. This hypothesis is consistent with a recent GAO finding that USAID lacks "surge capacity to respond to evolving foreign policy priorities and emerging crises."[110]

Planning and Pre-positioning. Before the 2003 conflict in Iraq, health experts had assessed the country to be much more vulnerable to the effects of a conflict than it had been in 1990. Although the 2003 conflict brought much suffering and disruption, the fact that there were no epidemics and no starvation can be considered a success. The conflict's tremendous impact on the water and sanitation system put the country at high risk for an epidemic of communicable diseases such as cholera and typhoid. In addition, the cold-chain disruption and low vaccination rates heightened the risk of an epidemic of diseases such as measles and polio. It seems unlikely that the reason no epidemics occurred was simply good luck.

---

[110] Government Accountability Office, *Strategic Workforce Planning Can Help USAID Address Current and Future Challenges,* Report to congressional requester, GAO-03-946, August 2003, www.gao.gov/new.items/d03946.pdf.

UN agencies and NGOs had several months to plan for humanitarian emergencies. A crucial part of planning is the acquisition of information. The UN had reasonable estimates of what was going to be available in Iraq if a conflict started. For example, the UN estimated that three to four months of certain types of medical supplies were available, that hospital power generators would not be able to work more than six hours on and off, that 70 percent of the standby generators in water projects were out of order, and that only half of the required number of ambulances were available.

In addition, UN agencies and NGOs pre-positioned supplies, equipment, and personnel in Iraq and neighboring countries. For instance, UNICEF and CARE pre-positioned water bladders, mobile water purification units, and fuel in Iraq. The International Committee of the Red Cross pre-positioned war-wounded kits and medical supplies in its warehouses. UNICEF pre-positioned high-protein biscuits in Iran and Jordan, and the World Food Programme pre-positioned food in neighboring countries. Another part of the preparation was to train local personnel to be prepared to respond to emergencies. For example, the UN trained people to monitor the food distribution system, and the World Food Programme trained its staff to be prepared for an emergency response. UNICEF immunized four million children against polio in February 2003 and launched a measles immunization campaign in March of the same year.

While there appears to have been no critical shortage of information essential for planning, the planning strategies were not as extensively implemented as they could have been. One reason for this was simply a lack of resources and funding. But it appears that another important factor was the reluctance of any government or UN agency to suggest that war was a foregone conclusion. This is particularly true in the case of the United States, where this reluctance was compounded by an internal coordination problem between the State and Defense departments, as accounted by F. M. Burkle, former deputy assistant administrator at USAID.[111]

---

[111] F.M. Burkle and E.K. Noji, "Health and Politics in the 2003 War with Iraq: Lessons Learned," *Lancet*, Vol. 364, October 9, 2004.

In January 2003, under presidential directive, the Pentagon created the Office of Reconstruction and Humanitarian Assistance to coordinate relief and reconstruction efforts both with U.S. and international entities. This was an unusual step, since this responsibility usually fell to the State Department. One consequence of this action was that most of the humanitarian planning was done in secrecy by military authorities, leaving the State Department agencies that typically would be involved in this kind of planning mostly in the dark.[112] Another consequence stemmed from the fact that the Office of Reconstruction and Humanitarian Assistance was under the control of the same military force that would eventually start the conflict. Many UN agencies and NGOs, worried about remaining independent and impartial, were not willing to coordinate and collaborate with the United States.

The issue was finally resolved by placing the disaster assistance response team under the Office of Reconstruction and Humanitarian Assistance's administrative control but allowing it to operate independently. While this move did allow collaboration with UN agencies and NGOs, it also resulted in a loss of trust on the part of relief organizations and projected an image of confused leadership.

Lessons Learned

It is difficult to make definitive conclusions about health efforts in Iraq because, as of the study's December 2005 end date, little time had passed since the end of major combat operations. Reliable data were difficult to gather, and often did not exist. Despite these challenges, we were able to make preliminary conclusions based on the anecdotal information available.

The basic lesson in Iraq is a familiar one: Little reconstruction takes place if the environment is not secure. In the health sector, the effects of inadequate security are pervasive. It hinders progress in re-

---

[112] Burkle and Noji, "Health and Politics in the 2003 War with Iraq."

building water plants and hospitals, it slows down immunization campaigns, it affects the labor force of providers by exposing them to intimidation and kidnapping, and it keeps patients from receiving care. An overall effect of this nature cannot be fixed by ad hoc measures, such as providing security guards to hospitals and by guarding water plants and pipes. The failure to provide adequate security is perhaps the single largest failure of the entire reconstruction effort in Iraq.

Lack of security is not, however, the only factor that affects progress in rebuilding the health sector. Health is tightly linked to the water, sanitation, and electricity sectors and progress in all of these sectors must occur in parallel. The value of a refurbished hospital is low if there is no reliable power and water supply. In more general terms, health outcomes are the result of a production process with many inputs, or production factors. Measuring the success of the reconstruction effort by one or several inputs (such as the number of facilities reopened) can be seriously misleading, because the values of those inputs depend on the values of all the other production factors.

Success is measured and perceived subjectively. Whereas Iraqis are likely to use pre-conflict conditions (perhaps augmented with a certain level of expectations) as benchmarks for success, agencies and agents involved in reconstruction are likely to use post-conflict conditions—which may be worse than pre-conflict conditions—as benchmarks. In addition, much of the reconstruction effort may go into activities whose benefits are not immediately apparent to Iraqis, such as constructing a surveillance system for epidemics or a database of hospitals and clinics. Failure to gauge success from the Iraqi point of view can cause reconstruction efforts to be misdirected and can generate much frustration in the population, further increasing the level of insecurity.

The most important success in the health sector—that there were no epidemics and no starvation—occurred in an area in which there were opportunities to plan. Agencies involved in this effort were international organizations, NGOs, and USAID, not private-sector entities. This underscores the fact that advanced planning and pre-positioning are not available as options to the private sector, which thus faces longer time-to-deployment and may be better suited for longer-term reconstruction efforts.

If the private sector is to play a crucial role in reconstruction, the amount of funding the government makes available to it must be matched with appropriate resources for the procurement, monitoring, and management side of the process. Both USAID and CPA have been assessed as being understaffed, which may have caused delays and contributed to funds not flowing smoothly. In other words, it can be relatively easy to appropriate large amounts of funds and yet quite difficult to spend them. In a country like Iraq, where the birth rates and infant mortality rates are high, delays in getting funds where they are needed can be especially costly.

CHAPTER NINE

Evaluating Health Reconstruction

How successful have past efforts to rebuild public health and health care delivery systems during nation-building operations been? What are the most important lessons for future missions? In this chapter, we answer these questions by bringing together data and lessons from the seven case studies presented in previous chapters. We define *success* as improvements in water and sanitation conditions, infectious disease rates, mortality and morbidity rates, and food and nutrition conditions over the course of reconstruction. More broadly, we consider how success in rebuilding health affects success in other areas of nation-building, such as security, economic stabilization, and infrastructure.

This chapter has two core arguments. First, nation-building efforts cannot be successful without adequate attention to health. Improvements in health are deeply interrelated with improvements in other areas of nation-building in two ways (see Figure 9.1): Health can have an independent impact on reconstruction and development, and others sectors can have an important impact on health. As Amartya Sen has argued, such areas as health, security, economic stabilization, and political development are deeply interrelated:

> Political freedoms (in the form of free speech and elections) help to promote economic security. Social opportunities (in the form of education and health facilities) facilitate economic participation. Economic facilities (in the form of opportunities for par-

ticipation in trade and production) can help to generate personal abundance as well as public resources for social facilities.[1]

Second, successful health reconstruction depends on two sets of factors: coordination and planning; and infrastructure and resources. The first factor includes the degree of coordination among the host government, non-governmental organizations (NGOs), international organizations, and donor states, as well as the establishment of a plan for health. The second includes the existence of functioning hospitals, other infrastructure (such as water and power systems), and donor support. External actors have significant control over some of these factors and little control over others, such as the condition of hospitals and clinics when reconstruction begins. Our case studies show that policymakers often fail to adequately plan and coordinate health reconstruction or to provide sufficient infrastructure and resources.

Figure 9.1
Health and Nation-Building

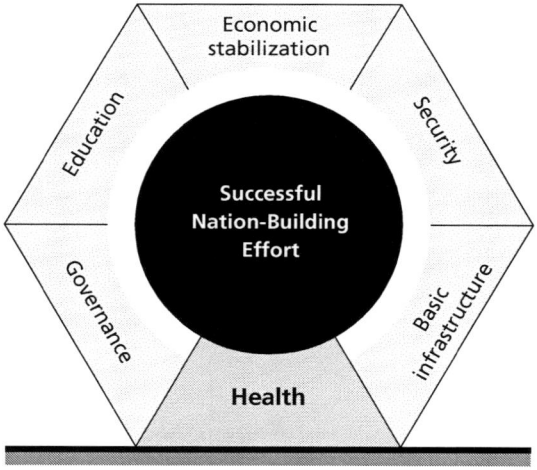

RAND *MG321-9.1*

---

[1] Amartya Sen, *Development as Freedom*, New York: Anchor Books, 2000, p. 11.

Several of the cases we reviewed suggest that health can have an important impact on security. In Iraq, there is evidence that poor health conditions—especially poor sanitation conditions—contributed to anti-Americanism and support for the insurgency.[2]

The rest of this chapter is divided into three sections. In the first of these, we use factor analysis to assess the outcome of health efforts in the seven cases. Of particular interest is finding those variables that contribute to success in rebuilding public health and health care delivery systems. In the second section, we compile and assess the major lessons learned across the cases. In the third, we briefly offer policy implications for future nation-building operations.

Comparative Analysis

This study faced a major obstacle: the challenge of compiling reliable data. Situations of conflict and societal upheaval are not conducive to the collection of good data, especially where a functioning central government does not exist. Therefore, we had to be creative in finding source materials that would allow for a degree of comparability. We examined qualitative accounts, conducted interviews, and collected quantitative data where available.

To compare data across cases, we wanted to conduct a rigorous quantitative analysis that assessed input and outcome data to find correlations. However, there were two main obstacles to this type of analysis. The first was the number of cases. With only seven countries, we did not have sufficient data to produce reliable statistical results. This problem was partially mitigated by the availability of some qualitative literature on health reconstruction. However, most of the literature focuses on domains other than health. The second obstacle was gathering reliable data. We found few variables that were avail-

---

[2] Major General Peter Chiarelli, Commander of the U.S. Army's First Cavalry Division, "Securing the Peace in Iraq," Briefing at RAND Corporation, Washington, D.C., March 10, 2005.

able across all countries. Data problems were particularly prevalent in Somalia, Haiti, Afghanistan, and Iraq. This was generally because there was no functioning central government that collected health statistics, or not enough time had elapsed to gather basic health indicators and measure change. While some data were available for individual countries, as discussed in each of the case study chapters, the same data did not exist across cases. The challenge, then, was to identify a way to compare findings across cases.

In response to these methodological challenges, we devised a strategy that is a hybrid of qualitative and quantitative analysis. We use our understanding of the cases to create simple numerical variables that are comparable across countries. We then perform a simple factor analysis of these variables to support our qualitative analysis. The specifics of our analysis are in Appendices A and B. The findings suggest that improvement in health depends on two sets of variables that we define as coordination and planning, and infrastructure and resources. The set of coordination and planning variables encompasses those factors that help determine the degree of coordination among different agencies involved in reconstruction. Coordination may be required between different agencies over space and time, but it may also be required within the same agency at different points in time. Therefore, variables that describe planning activities also belong to this category. The set of infrastructure and resource variables describe the level of effort devoted to improving health and the enabling conditions that allow progress to be made in building infrastructure.

Figure 9.2 plots the countries examined in this study. It includes coordination and planning on the x-axis, and infrastructure and resources on the y-axis. The countries are clustered into three quadrants. Japan and Germany are the most successful cases; Kosovo and Iraq are mixed cases; Haiti, Somalia, and Afghanistan are the least successful, and have low levels of all indicators.

Countries whose nation-building efforts lie in the lower left quadrant (low on infrastructure and resources, and low on coordination and planning) are those whose infrastructure either was poor

Figure 9.2
Outcome of Countries in Rebuilding Health

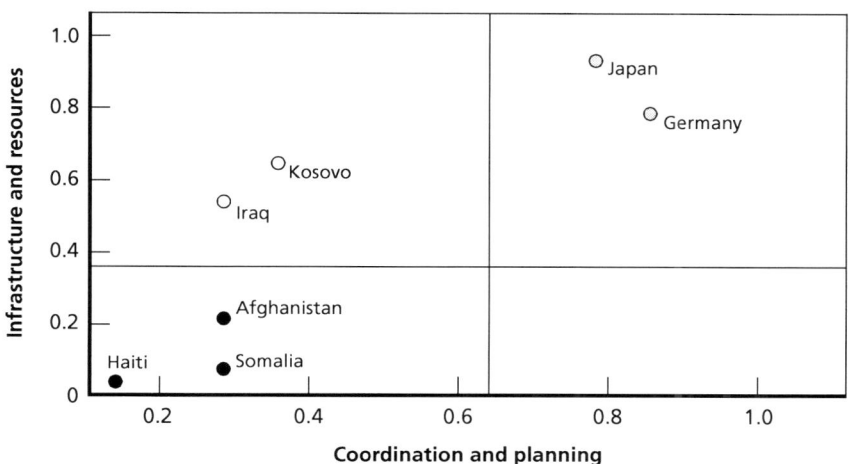

RAND *MG321-9.2*

before the conflict or was severely damaged by the conflict. In these countries, the overall coordination and planning efforts were also poor or inadequate, the health status of the population was poor, the health care system functioned poorly, and security was insufficient to support the nation-building effort. Afghanistan, Haiti, and Somalia's health care systems relied on NGOs and international aid even before their respective conflicts.[3]

Countries whose nation-building efforts fall in the upper left quadrant (high on infrastructure and resources but low on coordination and planning) are those that began reconstruction with a damaged but operational infrastructure and a system that did not rely on external support. Since these efforts were plagued by a lack of security, their infrastructure scores are not as high as those of Japan or

---

[3] These are often referred to as "rentier" states. See Charles Tilly, *The Formation of National States in Western Europe,* Princeton, New Jersey: Princeton University Press, 1975; Hazem Beblawi and Giacomo Luciani (eds.), *The Rentier State,* New York: Croom Helm, 1987.

Germany. These countries experienced multiple challenges within the coordination and planning dimension variables (see Table 9.2 later in this chapter). Kosovo and Iraq fall into this category.

The upper right quadrant holds the countries that were high in coordination and planning and in infrastructure and resources. They had a high level of security and a damaged yet still functional infrastructure. Japan and Germany fall into this category.

None of the seven case studies was in the lower right quadrant. Countries in this quadrant would have strong coordination and planning efforts but insufficient infrastructure and resources at the beginning of reconstruction. Several cases, such as the UN effort in East Timor that began in 1999, might fall into this category.

Lessons Learned

This section summarizes the major lessons learned from the case studies. It complements the quantitative analysis by presenting a series of qualitative findings. We believe that learning from and applying these lessons will not only improve the chances of success in rebuilding health, but also increase the likelihood of improving water and sanitation conditions, infectious disease rates, mortality and morbidity rates, and food and nutrition conditions. It will also increase the likelihood of achieving success in broader nation-building and development objectives. The lessons fall into the following categories:

- Health as an independent variable
- Impact of other sectors on health
- Coordination
- Sustainability and tipping points
- Exit strategies
- Performance metrics.

Health as an Independent Variable

Nation-building efforts cannot be successful if adequate attention is not paid to health. Indeed, health can have an important independent impact on nation-building and overall development. Several of the cases show that health can have a significant impact on security by helping to "win hearts and minds." This is an important objective in nation-building operations; cases such as Iraq and Somalia demonstrate that the inability to win hearts and minds contributes to insurgency, warlordism, and an unstable security environment. Counterinsurgency experts have long argued that winning hearts and minds is a key—if not *the* key—component in establishing peace.[4] And health can play a key role by, for instance, offering tangible health programs to the local population and meeting basic health needs, such as improving sanitation and nutrition conditions. These programs should be designed to gain support for the host country, rather than for the United States or other outside actors—the local government should be the entity winning the hearts and minds of the population. Following a review of U.S. health efforts during the Vietnam War, for example, Israeli General Moshe Dayan argued that "foreign troops never win the hearts of the people" and generally do not gain support for the host government.[5] In the early stages of nation-building operations, winning hearts and minds may be difficult if there is no local government. This was the case during the operations in Germany, Somalia, Kosovo, and Iraq. Over time, however, political authority invariably shifts to local control. When this happens, it is important

---

[4] Bruce Hoffman, *Insurgency and Counterinsurgency in Iraq*, Santa Monica, CA: RAND Corporation, 2004; U.S. Marine Corps, *Small Wars Manual*, Washington, D.C.: U.S. Government Printing Office, 1940; Julian Pagent, *Counter-Insurgency Campaigning*, London: Faber and Faber, 1967; Charles Simpson, *Inside the Green Berets: The First Thirty Years*, Novato, CA: Presidio Press, 1982; Robert J. Wilensky, *Military Medicine to Win Hearts and Minds: Aid to Civilians in the Vietnam War*, Lubbock, Texas: Texas Tech University Press, 2004.

[5] Quoted in Wilensky, *Military Medicine to Win Hearts and Minds*, p. 132. Also see General Moshe Dayan, National Archives, Record Group 319, Box 34 Folder: #32 History File, May 1–31, 1968, Folder 488.

to ensure that programs are designed to gain support for the local government.

Health can have an important impact on security—either a negative one or a positive one. In Iraq, for example, there is some evidence that poor health conditions—especially poor sanitation conditions—contributed to the levels of anti-Americanism and support for the insurgency.[6] Most early reconstruction efforts in Iraq's health sector went into activities that were not immediately visible to Iraqis, such as establishing a surveillance system and creating a statistical database of hospitals and clinics. In Japan, however, programs such as the introduction of powdered milk into schools, reversing the country's trend in childhood malnutrition, created a reservoir of good will that contributed to a benign security environment. Colonel Crawford F. Sams, Chief of the Public Health and Welfare Section, launched a nationwide effort to alter Japanese nutritional patterns after World War II. The centerpiece of this campaign was a school lunch program that included the delivery of adequate supplies of powdered milk. This simple program, which had a positive influence on millions of school children, created a reservoir of goodwill toward America and the Japanese government.

Maximizing the effectiveness of health as an independent variable means paying close attention to the sequence of health steps. Nation-building programs generally follow three broad, sequenced phases: immediate post-conflict, reconstruction, and consolidation. At least three types of emergency health situations should take priority during the immediate post-conflict phase. Failure to address them well and quickly can complicate reconstruction in other areas and lead to animosity among the local population. Success in addressing them well and quickly can help win hearts and minds.

The first of the three situations that should take priority is the clinical consequences arising after the use of weapons of mass destruction. In Japan, this situation was not addressed well or quickly. The treatment of survivors was left largely to the Japanese themselves, who

---

[6] Chiarelli, "Securing the Peace in Iraq."

initially treated the victims with vitamins, liver extract, and blood transfusions. Allied doctors eventually brought in penicillin and plasma, but the slow and inadequate treatment of victims contributed to high casualty rates. Many Japanese in Hiroshima and Nagasaki died of secondary diseases such as pneumonia and tuberculosis. The second situation is the outbreak—or potential outbreak—of communicable diseases, which needs to be addressed quickly to curtail spreading. The third situation is the provision of basic public health needs, such as food and sanitation. This also must be addressed as quickly as possible. Famine has been a particular concern. After Somali President Siad Barre was deposed in 1991, an estimated 300,000 people died of starvation over the next two years. The UN and United States provided immediate humanitarian assistance and saved an estimated additional 300,000 Somalis from famine.

Impact of Other Sectors on Health

Health conditions are deeply impacted by other sectors, including such key sectors as security, basic infrastructure (such as power and transportation), education, governance, and economic stabilization. Amartya Sen argues that the links among these sectors are empirical and causal:

> [T]here is strong evidence that economic and political freedoms help to reinforce one another. . . . Similarly, social opportunities of education and health care, which may require public action, complement individual opportunities of economic and political participation and also help to foster our own initiatives in overcoming our respective deprivations.[7]

Indeed, in successful reconstruction efforts, key indicators in health and other major sectors tend to be positive and improve over time. In failed efforts, however, key indicators across sectors tend to be negative.

---

[7] Sen, *Development as Freedom*, p. xii.

The health sector is particularly sensitive to security in at least two ways: through direct effects, such as the inability of patients to visit doctors; and through indirect effects, such as the inability of health care facilities to function properly. The absence of security can impede progress in the reconstruction of water plants and hospitals, slow immunization campaigns, restrict delivery of needed supplies to health care facilities, and affect the labor force by not protecting healthcare providers from being intimidated or threatened with kidnapping. Patients can also be deterred from seeking health care because of security concerns.

Several cases neatly illustrate how the absence of security impedes health efforts. In one case, in Iraq, fear of attack by looters prevented health care professionals and patients from going to health care facilities. Equipment was looted, medical records were destroyed, and intact facilities became overburdened by the flow of patients from damaged facilities. The work of NGOs, international organizations, and contractors was either slowed or halted. In addition, public safety was directly affected—by the increased incidence of crime and casualties from car bombings, improvised explosive devices, shootings, and U.S and coalition military operations. Such a pervasive lack of security could not be fixed by ad hoc measures, such as providing hospitals with security guards and guarding water plants and pipes.

In another case, this one in Afghanistan, NGOs frequently suspended, canceled, postponed, or significantly downsized health programs as a result of security issues. In 2004, the United States Agency for International Development (USAID) was scheduled to rebuild 121 health clinics and birth centers, but by March it had scaled back the plan to 72 facilities. Afghan women employed by international NGOs were the focus of particular threats by the Taliban and other insurgents. In 2004, Doctors Without Borders (Médecins sans Frontières) closed all medical programs in Afghanistan following a fatal attack on one of their vehicles in Badghis province.

In Somalia, security plagued the humanitarian relief operations. After the UN withdrew, the absence of security continued to make delivery of humanitarian assistance and the undertaking of any health sector reconstruction almost impossible. In Kosovo, instability in the region decreased the willingness of the private sector, international NGOs, and donor community to continue working in the area and commit resources.

At the same time, several cases demonstrate how the achievement of security can facilitate health efforts. In Germany, for example, the United States deployed a large number of forces to the U.S. sector and stabilized the country. U.S. forces suffered no casualties, despite initial concerns about German insurgent attacks. In May 1945, the United States had 61 divisions in Germany and a total of 1.6 million soldiers. These troops staffed border crossings, maintained checkpoints, and conducted patrols throughout the U.S. sector. Rapid demobilization then quickly reduced the force levels, but the security environment remained stable, facilitating health reconstruction by improving the freedom of movement and ensuring that water, sanitation, and other infrastructure were not damaged as they were built or refurbished.

In Japan, General MacArthur had 350,000 U.S. troops throughout the Japanese archipelago by the end of 1945. Much like Germany, the unconditional surrender and the devastation of defeat created a situation in which the population was unwilling or unable to resist. U.S. troops suffered no combat deaths during the occupation. The relative safety and stability of occupied Japan allowed the Pubic Health and Welfare authorities to focus on decreasing disease rates and rebuilding the health care infrastructure.

The success of the health sector is tightly linked with progress in other sectors, such as basic infrastructure. In Iraq, for instance, hospitals and clinics operated at partial capacity and had to use power generators provided by international organizations. In general, a lack of clean water, sanitation, or power increases the likelihood of epidemics and other acute disease outbreaks, and hampers efforts to build a functioning health system. International organizations may spend time and resources refurbishing hospitals and clinics, training staff, and providing equipment. But unreliable power nullifies much of this effort. The success of the health care system is also linked to the reconstruction of the financial, judicial, and education systems. For example, if financial systems are not working, it is difficult to acquire supplies and capital equipment, as well as to develop health financing mechanisms.

Coordination

The coordination of health efforts is a key challenge during reconstruction. Indeed, World Bank argues that past nation-building efforts have suffered from "a lack of an overarching nationally-driven plan to which all donors agree, resulting in fragmentation, gaps or duplication in aid-financed programs."[8] Poor coordination can have serious consequences. In particular, it can weaken fragile health systems by scattering assistance to an assortment of health projects and failing to sufficiently tackle key priorities.

In some ways, coordination and planning were simpler in the post–World War II cases of Germany and Japan because there were fewer actors involved. In Germany, for example, the U.S. Military Government only had to coordinate efforts with German authorities and a few NGOs, such as CARE, the International Committee of the Red Cross, and the United Nations Relief and Rehabilitation Administration. Communication and coordination in Japan were also less difficult. The U.S. Supreme Commander of the Allied Powers and the Japanese government implemented health reconstruction, with the international aid organizations, such as the Red Cross and CARE, playing only a minor role.

The number of actors involved in health reconstruction has exponentially increased since the end of the Cold War, and the greater the number of actors, the more difficult the coordination.[9] In Iraq, there were 80 NGOs registered with the United Nations Humanitarian Information Center database, and they carried out over 300

---

[8] United Nations Development Programme and World Bank, *An Operational Note on Transitional Results Matrices: Using Results-Based Frameworks in Fragile States*, New York: United Nations Development Programme and World Bank, January 2005, p. 2. Also see *Health Policy Formulation in Complex Political Emergencies and Post-Conflict Countries: A Literature Review*, London: London School of Hygiene and Tropical Medicine, November 2002.

[9] Mancur Olson, *The Logic of Collective Action: Public Goods and the Theory of Groups*, Cambridge, MA: Harvard University Press, 1971, p. 2.

projects. Two steps can help improve mission coordination: encourage and rationalize a lead state or lead organization system for health, and learn from and replicate successful on-the-ground organizational innovations.

First, there is a strong need to establish institutional arrangements that increase efficiency in rebuilding health in order to overcome coordination and collaboration problems. A variety of arrangement options are available: donor coordination units within a host state's Ministry of Health; a lead national actor; lead regional or local actors; regular collective Ministry of Health consultations with donors; and sector-wide approaches. A lead actor approach is usually the most effective strategy for coordinating planning and funding, especially when the host government is barely functional. In the health sector, experience suggests that the lead actor should be an international organization rather than a state. It can be difficult to agree on a lead actor, however, since donor states, international institutions, and NGOs generally have different priorities, interests, and strategies. Nonetheless, a lead actor is critical for ensuring efficiency and effectiveness. This actor's role can include coordinating and overseeing the undertaking of joint assessments, preparing shared strategies, coordinating political engagement, establishing joint offices, and introducing simplified arrangements (such as common reporting and financial requirements). In theory, the lead actor can be a donor state, international organization, or NGO. In practice, however, only states and international organizations have the resources and legitimacy necessary to be lead actors. Crucial to the task of establishing a lead actor is buy-in from the host government and support from key donors, international organizations, and NGOs.

Second, there is a strong need to consolidate lessons learned and best practices in coordinating mission activities. NGOs and other organizations have worked out effective ad hoc organizational arrangements at national and local levels to improve coordination. One important aspect of this step should be to coordinate with those international institutions and/or NGOs that were involved in health and health-related efforts before and during the conflict. Such experience provides an invaluable understanding of the health care system, the health status of the population, and the major health challenges within a nation. Since reliable statistical information on health conditions is often unavailable during the initial post-conflict phase, prior knowledge is crucial. Bilateral donors, international institutions, and NGOs should use actors with in-country experience to assist in coordination and planning. In Kosovo, WHO's prior knowledge of the health sector and the population's health care needs put it in a good position to help coordinate reconstruction efforts. In Haiti and Somalia, however, a key criticism of the planning process was its failure to involve actors with prior experience and knowledge.

Coordination in the case studies varied considerably. In Kosovo, for instance, there was no lead actor despite the establishment of a health action plan. UNMIK Health had insufficient capacity to take the lead role and to address the major policy, institutional, and budgetary problems in the health sector. WHO took the lead in developing policy guidance but was criticized by many NGOs for missing an important opportunity to direct the health effort and for not taking a stronger leadership role. WHO did not enforce the health policy framework or make NGOs abide by it. In Somalia, coordination was missing at many levels: among relief agencies and the military; among NGOs; and among the UN, United States, and other countries contributing troops. There were numerous impediments to coordination in Somalia:

- Failure to conduct adequate advanced planning and include all relevant players in the planning process.
- Frequent changes in UN personnel, humanitarian coordinators, and military and relief personnel.
- NGOs' desire to maintain an appearance of neutrality and their reluctance to cooperate with the U.S. and other militaries.
- Variations in the goals, missions, resources, and time in-theater of NGOs, all of which made it difficult for the military to determine which NGO's to support and how best to support their relief efforts.

In Afghanistan, there were numerous coordination problems. Several consultative and planning mechanisms attempted to coordinate donors and NGO activities and keep them aligned with the goals of the Afghan government. International organizations and NGOs did not successfully communicate or coordinate either among themselves or with the Afghan agencies that theoretically were in command. There were exceptions at both extremes. In several pockets of the country, such as Herat, there was little coordination, and NGOs implemented their own programs. In other places, such as Kandahar, NGOs and donor states established more-effective consultation mechanisms, in part because there were fewer agencies involved.

In Iraq, a small group of international organizations established the Joint NGO Emergency Preparedness Initiative to improve coordination. The initiative was a short-term project to provide a clearinghouse for information, assessments, and experiences for international and local NGOs, UN agencies, and government authorities. For the longer term, a group of NGOs in Baghdad established the NGO Coordination Committee in Iraq. Its activities included coordination and exchange of information, monitoring of humanitarian issues, and support for the development of Iraqi NGOs. While some cooperation may have occurred among NGOs, there was little between NGOs and the Coalition Provisional Authority (CPA). Significant tension arose over CPA Order 45, which required all NGOs operating in Iraq to register with the CPA. Many NGOs complained that the decision was made without their input, the amount of information requested was either too intrusive or too detailed, and the process was too bureaucratic. Their relationship deteriorated further during intense fighting between coalition forces and insurgents in cities such as Fallujah and Najaf. The Committee frequently accused coalition forces of closing the main teaching hospital in Fallujah, shooting at ambulances, and using health facilities as bases for military operations.

Sustainability and Tipping Points

Health sector reform must encourage long-term sustainability. Indeed, a key objective of health reconstruction should be to reach a tipping point—that is, the point at which the local government begins to assume substantial responsibility for managing the health sector and outcomes continue to improve. This point will be different in every nation-building case and will likely take longer to reach in less-developed states. As Figure 9.3 illustrates, the tipping point refers to the period at which the government and private sector are able to provide significant health care to most of the country without external assistance. This helps ensure that health conditions will continue to improve once external actors depart.[10]

Figure 9.3
The Health Tipping Point

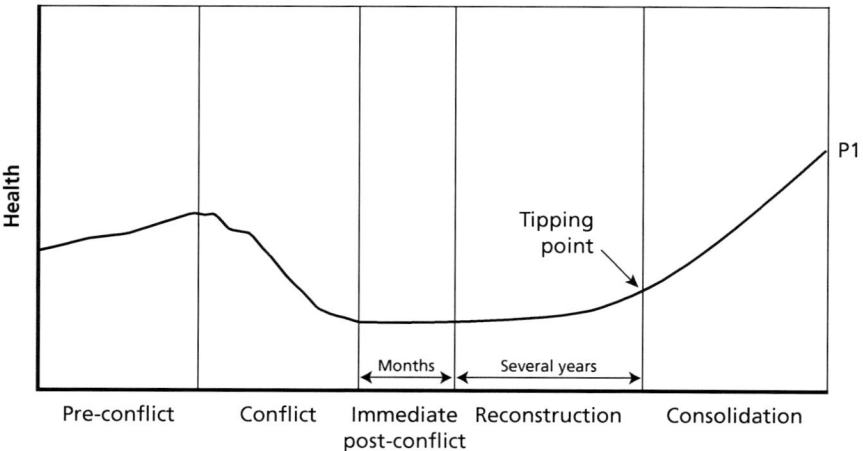

RAND *MG321-9.3*

---

[10] Tipping models have frequently been used to describe social and political developments, such as the shift from sporadic demonstrations to revolutions. Thomas Schelling, *Micromotives and Macrobehavior*, New York: Norton, 1978; David D. Laitin, *Identity in Formation: The Russian-Speaking Populations in the Near Abroad*, Ithaca, New York: Cornell University Press, 1998.

It took Germany approximately two and a half years to reach the tipping point. By January 1948, German and Laender health authorities took over full responsibility for health services from the U.S. Office of Military Government. But U.S. advisors continued to observe, inspect, advise, and report on health activities. In 1947, German health officials requested the assistance of American specialists in epidemiology, as well as materials such as respirators, in response to a poliomyelitis epidemic in Berlin. The specialists advised German authorities on measures to improve control and treatment of the disease and offered instruction to German doctors and nurses on the latest developments in therapy. They also offered instruction on the use of respirators, which German hospitals had not previously used.

Haiti never reached the tipping point. The United States largely withdrew after three years, and the Haitian government never developed the capacity to implement health programs and to administratively operate them. There was no functioning Ministry of Health or administrative personnel within the ministry who could receive donor support, oversee financial administration, and ensure effective implementation. Haiti lacked trained health care workers in the public sector. Since many Haitian professionals had left the country, the remaining personnel were often poorly trained and had little experience in administration or government. Aid organizations and donor states often funneled resources through the NGO community.

Training indigenous personnel is a critical aspect of sustainability. Otherwise, as Robert Wilensky argues, "the programs neither reflect favorably on the host government nor will they remain effective after withdrawal of outside forces."[11] Another key aspect is assessing the capacity of national and private health institutions to engage in needs assessment and implementation. Capacity has important implications for recovery and planning. From an operational perspective, it makes sense to distinguish between two types of post-conflict countries: those with strong national capacities and those with weak national capacities. These distinctions should not be regarded as abso-

---

[11] Wilensky, *Military Medicine to Win Hearts and Minds*, p. 132.

lute but as two ends of a continuum. Most countries are located between these extremes.

In countries with strong national health capacities, such as Germany after World War II, health progress may be more rapid. Since national contributions and ownership are likely to be high, planning can be oriented beyond the short-term (0 to 18 months) to include medium-term (18 to 36 months) recovery and development needs. In countries with weak health capacities, national and private health institutions usually do not have the capacity to make substantial contributions to the needs assessment and implementation. In Somalia, for example, warlords did not support relief efforts and attacked, looted, and extorted payments from relief convoys. Humanitarian assistance had the perverse effect of exacerbating tensions among rival groups within the country that were competing for the control of scarce resources. In Afghanistan, most of the country has historically been controlled by tribes and local warlords rather than by the central government. Without a viable central government, the country has long gone without health care leadership, competency, and capacity, making it difficult to create a self-sufficient and sustainable health system.

The variation in initial nation-building conditions places a premium on the ability to correctly determine the effectiveness of governance institutions and the nature of the conflict. Much like Afghanistan, states with a weak national capacity can face a series of challenges after major conflict:

- Severely deteriorating health conditions, especially if civilians and civilian structures have been targets of violence.
- Institutional collapse.
- Social cleavages among groups manipulated by the parties to the conflict.
- The absence of normal accountability mechanisms because there is no legitimate government.

The curves of decline and recovery for states with weak national capacity are likely to differ from those for states with strong national capacity, especially when there has been a long-term degradation of health. Challenges are more profound and progress toward the tipping point should be expected to be slower. The health infrastructure, administrative capacity, and physical infrastructure may have ceased to exist, or may never have existed at all. Such situations require a reconstruction effort strongly shaped by the goal of development. In Afghanistan, the international community geared up for a standard post-conflict reconstruction effort instead of acknowledging that what it largely faced was a development challenge. If development is the goal, an important question arises: Will health recovery plans perpetuate a tradition of national dependence on the external design, delivery, and financing of health care that will jeopardize sustainability? Unfortunately, the main health challenges in countries with weak national capacities are not amenable to quick fixes. The population must become stronger and healthier through improved nutrition and access to clean water and sanitation; a new generation of health care professionals has to be recruited, trained, and motivated to work in rural areas; and long-standing habits and attitudes (particularly related to marriage, family, and the status of women) must change. Moreover, the country needs years of stability and security for these changes to occur and take hold.

Finally, the cases we examined involved countries with widely different cultural and social backgrounds, which in some cases had a significant influence on health sector reform. International personnel must be aware of social and cultural norms and find ways to balance them with health concerns. In Afghanistan, for example, cultural and social factors influenced health in two ways. First, traditional beliefs about medicine, nutrition, and hygiene led to erroneous beliefs about what constituted safe health practices. For instance, many Afghans believed that any moving water was clean and that liquids should be withheld from children with diarrhea. Second, gender attitudes directly affected health. Examples in this case are the propensity to marry girls off at a young age, reluctance to spend money and resources on health care for daughters and wives, inequitable distribution of food within the family, frequent physical violence toward women and children, and reluctance to educate girls and women. In

Haiti and Somalia, the international community was strongly criticized for having an incomplete grasp of the socio-cultural realities and attempting to impose a strict Western health system. The majority of Haitians and Somalis, particularly in rural areas, were used to receiving their health care from traditional practitioners and healers, not from formal health care systems.

Exit Strategies

Short-term medical care is, of course, valuable; but to change a state's health care system requires time and sustained effort. In several cases we examined, such as Haiti and Somalia, outside powers wanted to withdraw as fast as possible. Our analysis suggests that the search for a fixed exit strategy is illusory, if this means a certain date in the near future when full control of health care facilities can be handed back to local authorities. Exit requires a functioning health care system that has at least reached the tipping point. This point will be different in every nation-building case, and will likely take longer to reach in less developed states.

Duration is a critical variable and cuts across all aspects of reconstruction. Based on the cases we examined, no effort to rebuild health after major combat has been successful in less than five years. In post-war Germany, efforts to rebuild health lasted from 1945 until at least 1950, though German federal and Laender health authorities took over most responsibilities by January 1948. In post-war Japan, health efforts also continued until at least 1950. In one sense, however, these cases *underestimate* the amount of time necessary to rebuild health, since Germany and Japan were both fairly developed countries in 1945. Nation-building efforts in developing countries, such as Somalia and Afghanistan in this study, would have to continue for much longer than five years to become successful. In cases such as these, which have little health infrastructure to begin with, the time needed for success has to include the time required to achieve local buy-in, build hospitals and clinics, conduct immunizations, train health personnel, and improve sanitation and nutrition conditions.

One important point to make here is that while staying for a long time does not always guarantee success, leaving early assures failure. U.S.-led efforts to rebuild Somalia and Haiti were short-lived. The bulk of health assistance lasted for only three years, and continuing political instability in Haiti led the international community to withhold all aid by 2000. Haiti and Somalia were also affected by political constraints in the United States. The Clinton administration defined its objectives rather narrowly and was influenced by domestic politics in making its decision to establish short exit strategies and departure deadlines. The cost of early departures is clear: it is difficult to ensure success in rebuilding health.

Performance Metrics

Health programs have often fallen into the trap of emphasizing outputs, rather than outcomes, as a measure of success. Success should not be measured by the number of hospitals constructed or the percentage of doctors and nurses trained. These are important steps, but they tell us little about the overall state of health.

Health assistance can be broken down into three categories: inputs, outputs, and outcomes. **Inputs** are the resources used in reconstructing health, such as the amount of financial assistance and the number of international personnel deployed. **Outputs** are the first-order results of the program. Examples include trained doctors and nurses, and functional hospitals. **Outcomes** are conditions that directly impact the public. They are not what governments and international institutions do but, rather, the consequences of what they do.[12] Many people mistakenly confuse outputs with outcomes, as U.S. policymakers did in Vietnam.

Table 9.1 is an example of a performance matrix that nation-building missions could create. It lists key health goals, inputs, outputs, and outcomes over time and should include information that has been gathered on baseline conditions and perhaps even relevant

[12] See Harry P. Hatry, *Performance Measurement: Getting Results*, Washington, D.C.: The Urban Institute Press, 1999; William T. Gormley and David L. Weimer, *Organizational Report Cards*, Cambridge, Massachusetts: Harvard University Press, 1999.

Table 9.1
Example of Performance Matrix

Key Health Goals	Baseline Conditions	Inputs	Outputs, First 6 Mos.	Outcomes	Broader Development Indicators
Address immediate health needs		Amount of financial assistance	Number and quality of doctors, nurses, and other personnel trained	Life expectancy rate	Level of security
Develop a cost-effective and sustainable health system	Quantitative and qualitative description of initial conditions	Number of international advisors		Birth rate	Quality of governance
		Amount and type of health equipment, drugs, and other consumables delivered	Number and quality of health facilities built or refurbished	Death rate	Economic conditions
Improve overall health conditions				Infant mortality rate	Education levels
			Institutional development and reform of Ministry of Health	Infectious disease rate	Provision of key services, such as power and water
				Malnutrition rate	

non-health indicators. Most important of all, however, is that it be used to track metrics over the course of reconstruction to monitor whether they are improving or getting worse.

If policymakers cannot measure performance, they have no objective method for judging success and failure in ongoing crises, which makes midcourse corrections more difficult. In Afghanistan, for example, the Government Accountability Office (formerly the General Accounting Office) found that USAID lacked "measurable goals, specific time frames, and resource levels," had not "identified external factors that could significantly affect the achievement of its goals," and did not "include a schedule for program evaluations" to assess progress against such goals. Key health outcome measures are life expectancy rate, birth rate, death rate, infant mortality rate, infectious disease rate, and malnutrition. Since these outcome measures may not always be readily available, more tactical and short-term measures may serve to give policymakers some indication of performance. Examples might include percentage of children under one year of age that have been immunized; percentage of births with skilled attendance; percentage of population with access to basic health services within two hours; and percentage of health facilities that report "stock outs" of essential drugs. Building such assessments into current and future assistance programs, and encouraging host nations to undertake such assessments, will make foreign actors better placed to optimize assistance programs.

We identified at least six criteria for compiling performance metrics for inputs, outputs, and outcomes.[13] First, inputs and outputs need to be tied to outcomes. Second, good indicators should be simple—that is, they must come in a clear format and be easy for all stakeholders to interpret. This is especially true in fragile states, where national capacities are thin, communication between stakeholders is usually limited, and the political dynamics may create fractures through which complex information could be lost or misused. Third, performance indicators should be selective. There must be a limited number of focused targets, and they must be prioritized to offer sequenced strategic direction. Fourth, they should be integrated. They need to link policy actions and donor interventions across all areas where lack of progress carries the risk of reversing the recovery process—from political and security issues to economic and health recovery. Fifth, effective indicators should be nationally owned. Ownership by national leadership is a necessary condition if reforms are to be promoted efficiently and sustained after the initial momentum of intense donor interaction fades. Sixth, indicators should get donor buy-in strong enough to translate promises into financial commitments, disbursements, and priority technical assistance. This type of buy-in may also help to avoid the fragmentation of donor dialogue and assistance and its associated high transaction costs.

Performance indicators should also vary somewhat according to a country's characteristics. For example, a more developed state may face a window of opportunity for fast structural reform, whereas a less

---

[13] See, for example, United Nations Development Programme and World Bank, *An Operational Note on Transitional Results Matrices*.

developed state could find rapid structural reform destabilizing and thus should instead see rebuilding familiar administrative and service delivery functions as its immediate priority. The timelines of performance measures should be adapted to country circumstances.

Moving Forward

What are the policy implications for international institutions, NGOs, and donor states in rebuilding health? Many of the recent cases, such as Afghanistan and Iraq, have reinforced well-worn lessons. Although the international community learned a great deal about health and nation-building during the 1990s, few of the lessons were applied in Afghanistan and Iraq.

The planning process is a particularly critical aspect of health reconstruction. Much can be lost or won during this early period, especially in connection with such issues as coordination, sustainability, and performance. Table 9.2 offers a sample planning matrix for designing a health mission, a matrix influenced by joint work conducted by the United Nations Development Programme, World Bank, and United Nations Development Group.[14] Reconstruction routinely takes place under extreme time constraints that offer little opportunity to think strategically about planning. This sample process aims to help make health reconstruction more effective by systematizing the analysis and suggesting more-efficient processes. It is meant to be illustrative rather than rigid, since order and timing can vary among cases. It includes 12 basic steps, beginning with a preparatory phase and concluding with a lessons learned phase. Key steps include reaching a political consensus on health objectives (step 2),

---

[14] United Nations Development Programme, World Bank, and United Nations Development Group, *Practical Guide to Multilateral Needs Assessments in Post-Conflict Situations*, New York: World Bank, August 2004.

Table 9.2
Sample Planning Process

Steps	Summary	Description	Products
1	Preparatory phase	Take a variety of steps, such as launching a donor conference, and do an initial needs assessment.	Memorandum of understanding Initial needs assessment report
2	Political consensus on health objectives and scope	Produce a health recovery strategy that is owned by national stakeholders and international community, making sure to involve key donors.	Memorandum of understanding
3	Coordination unit, including lead actor	Key donors, international institutions, and NGOs establish an institutional arrangement for coordinating assistance, including appointment of a lead actor, in order to support and manage the technical aspects of health reconstruction.	Coordinating body and lead actor
4	Long-term vision for health	Establish an overall vision for post-conflict health recovery by focusing on a small number of key objectives. This should be negotiated among the national authorities and the international community and should take local realties into account.	Briefing paper
5	Priority sectors and cross-cutting issues	Prioritize key health sectors in line with initial needs assessment. This should include identification of key multidimensional issues that cut across health and other areas (such as gender, environmental, and HIV/AIDS issues).	Briefing paper
6	Overall nation-building analysis	Conduct an analysis of security, political, economic, and other sectors that may impact health.	Briefing paper
7	Time requirements	Establish deadlines for completion of key health activities, taking into consideration that the time required may vary depending on the data, materials available, assessments already done, and initial conditions. This should include immediate recovery, medium-term, and long-term needs; and the resulting timeline should be revisited, modified, and updated as new information becomes available (step 11).	Timeline

Table 9.2 (continued)

Steps	Summary	Description	Products
8	Costing	Develop realistic and comprehensive cost estimates.	Sectoral cost estimates
9	Planning document	Establish a coherent planning document, detailing what should be achieved in each health sector and how this can be done. Such a planning framework is best derived by using an outcome-based approach and should provide a comprehensive definition of the principal objectives, vision, and scope of the health effort, as well as the priority sectors, timing, costs, and cross-cutting issues.	Plan for health
10	Team composition	Form primary group of experts who will collect data and analyze the actual health needs of the country, and who will be responsible for elaboration of sectoral analyses, planning frameworks, and technical reports.	Health team
11	Implementation and assessments	Implement plans and programs, monitor performance, and make necessary corrections.	Regular performance assessments tied to outcomes
12	Lessons learned	Compile major insights and lessons learned.	Lessons learned report

establishing a coordination unit that includes a lead actor (step 3), developing an outcome-based planning document that details what should be achieved in each health area and how this can be done (step 9), and compiling major insights and lessons learned (step 12). All of these steps should have specific outcome products and be tied to the overall vision and objectives for post-conflict health recovery.

Learning these lessons will not ipso facto guarantee success. But we believe it will vastly improve the chances of success, as measured by improvement in sanitation conditions, infectious disease rates, mortality and morbidity rates, and nutrition conditions. Our findings also support the use of these metrics as criteria for judging success. In anticipation of future nation-building missions, interdisciplinary experts may find it worthwhile to define prospectively the possible dimensions of "success." Even though nation-building missions will differ somewhat from each other in overall objectives and data availability, development of a framework for monitoring and measuring inputs and outcomes is nonetheless critical.

Methodology

The analysis discussed in Chapter Nine involved several steps. In the first of these, we created a set of input variables and one output variable. The input variables (covariates) described characteristics of the country being rebuilt as of the initial phase of reconstruction. The output variable summarized improvement in health and the tools a country can use to improve health, capturing both short-term gains and long-term potential gains.

The second step was to correlate the output variable with the input variables. Since we had about 20 covariates and only seven observations, we did not have sufficient information to run a meaningful regression analysis. Consequently, we performed a fairly radical dimensionality reduction step. Based on a highly simplified model of reconstruction, we took linear combinations of the 20 covariates to construct two new covariates, which we called "factors." These should be thought as new covariates that summarize characteristics of the case studies along two different dimensions: one relating to basic infrastructure and donor funding, and the other relating to the reconstruction effort's level of coordination and planning. Since these two factors are easily interpretable, they can be correlated with the output variable. The correlations we found provide a useful starting point for discussing the determinants of outcome.

Our third step arose from the fact that step 2, the dimensionality reduction step described above, was based on a simple model and some plausible arguments. To make our analysis stronger, we decided to use a standard statistical technique: factor analysis. It is blind to the meaning of the variables and allowed us to perform a similar dimensionality reduction. The factor analysis led us to define two factors that are fairly similar to the ones described above and are derived in a more intuitive manner. Since this is primarily a validation step—which supported our analysis without adding much new information and which contained mostly technical information—we present it separately, in Appendix B.

Definition of Input and Output Variables

This section defines the input and output variables and explains the methods we used in choosing them. We end up with a set of 20 covariates that represent specific characteristics of countries in the initial stages of reconstruction.

Input Variables

We constructed our input variables using a two-stage approach. We first had the authors of the chapters of this monograph and independent readers each make a list of relevant issues that might affect a reconstruction effort's success. We then produced a final list consolidating the individual lists.

Next, we asked the authors of each chapter to assign levels to items on the list, using a scale from 0 to 1. Some of the items, such as level of education, could have been quantified by a continuously valued variable. However, since we could not have made a detailed numerical analysis for all of them, we decided to convert all the values into three levels—low, medium, and high—which are represented by the numbers 0, 0.5, and 1, respectively. We could also have used a five-point scale, but we deemed this unlikely to add much to the analysis. Since the assignment of these numbers is somewhat subjective, we needed to rely on sensitivity analysis to make sure the findings were robust.

What issues did we put on the list? We started out by considering the different dimensions that may influence the success of a nation-building effort. That is, what did these countries' health sectors look like at the beginning of the nation-building effort? Or, to put it more specifically, what did the international community find at the end of the conflict, and what elements might influence the outcome of the reconstruction effort? The dimensions we considered included:

- Status of the health care system and health status of the population at the end of the conflict (i.e., at time 0, the start of the nation-building effort).
- Level of the international community's support for the nation-building effort.
- Status of key infrastructure and level of governance functioning.
- Expectations of the population and level of support for the nation-building effort.
- Coordination and planning activities, such as the level of coordination among key international players and NGOs and the comprehensiveness of the planning process.
- Complicating or enabling factors, such as level of security.

Table A.1 shows our final list of 20 items (covariates) and the three broad categories into which they fall. The first category is specific to the health sector; the dimensions in this category address the status of the health care system's infrastructure at time 0 and its level of functioning. For example, when the international community entered the country, was the health care delivery system functioning? How much damage had been sustained by the public health system's infrastructure and health care facilities? Was the public health information system intact? And what was the overall health status of the population? In addition, we identified enabling factors specific to the health sector, such as: To what degree had the health care system been dependent on international aid? What level of funding or aid was available to support health care reconstruction efforts? Was there a policy framework or plan to guide health sector rebuilding and reconstruction efforts?

Table A.1
List of Variables

Dimension	Germany	Japan	Somalia	Haiti	Afghani-stan	Kosovo	Iraq
Category 1: Status of Health Care System's Infrastructure and Level of Functioning							
1. Functioning health care system; is health care delivery occurring?	1	1	0	0	0	0.5	0.5
2. Trained health care professionals	1	1	0	0	0	0.5	0.5
3. Infrastructure of hospital and clinics (relative to pre-war: 1=no damage; 0.5=some damage; 0=complete damage)	0	0.5	0	0	0	0.5	0.5
4. Public health infrastructure, such as surveillance, prevention (damaged but in place)	1	1	0	0	0	0.5	0.5
6. Basic water, sanitation, and power infrastructure (damaged but in place)	1	1	0	0	0	1	1
8. Was there an overarching policy framework or plan for reconstructing health care system?	1	1	0	0	0	1	0
10. Level donor support/funding available for reconstruction (1=high); i.e., lack of funding not a major problem	1	1	0	0.5	0.5	1	1
12. Basic level of health status of population (1=good; 0.5=fair; 0=poor)	1	0.5	0	0	0	0.5	0
Category 2: Other Enabling Factors							
13. Level of security	1	1	0	0	0.5	0.5	0
14. Level of human capital	1	1	0	0	0	0.5	0.5
15. Level of transportation infrastructure	0	1	0	0	0	0.5	0.5
20. Functioning central government	0	1	0	0	0	0.5	0.5

Table A.1 (continued)

Dimension	Germany	Japan	Somalia	Haiti	Afghani-stan	Kosovo	Iraq
30. Population supportive of reconstruction effort	1	1	1	0	1	0.5	0
31. Government supportive of nation-building effort	1	1	0	0	1	1	1
Category 3: Coordination and planning							
5. Functioning public health information system to assess needs	1	0.5	0	0	0	0	0
22. International community appreciates full extent of problem in advance	1	1	0	0	0	0	0
24. Extent of reliance on NGOs (e.g., assumed role of nonfunctional government or ministry of health)	0	0	1	1	1	0	0
25. Level of coordination among international health agencies and NGOs	1	1	1	0	0.5	0	1
27. Level of coordination among NGOs, military, and international agencies	1	1	0	0	0.5	0	0

The second category contains dimensions for other enabling factors. Examples include the degree to which the local population and the government were supportive of the nation-building effort, the presence of a functioning central government, the status of the non-health infrastructure, and the level of security provided for the nation-building effort.[1]

Category 3 contains dimensions that address coordination and planning. These include the level of coordination among the key international agencies and non-governmental organizations (NGOs),

---

[1] The other dimensions with respect to infrastructure include the status of the transportation, communications, financing, education, and judicial sectors. These variables were highly correlated, so we retained the variable "level of transportation" to represent the infrastructure dimension in the shortened list of 20.

the degree to which the planning process reflected a full appreciation or assessment of the effort required, and the extent to which NGOs were relied on to fill other key roles.

Output Variable

The objective of health reconstruction efforts is to improve the population's health. Two ways in which this can be done are by direct health interventions run by the agencies involved in the reconstruction, and by providing the country with the tools to improve the health of its population. Therefore, it seems reasonable to use as an outcome variable one that summarizes progress made under these two dimensions. This variable is not necessarily a measure of success, however: one could argue that an operation was performed flawlessly, but the outcome was poor just because the problem was intrinsically hard to solve.

We used our qualitative assessments of the cases to score the different cases along these dimensions and produce a categorical outcome variable with three levels: high, medium, and low. The two countries that scored high on both dimensions are Germany and Japan. In these countries, we observed short-term health gains coupled with a long-term, sustained improvement. This recovery was facilitated by a significant effort to create or rehabilitate health institutions and improve capacity.

Haiti, Somalia, and Afghanistan scored low on both dimensions. There is little evidence of health gains in these countries and little indication that they are on a path of self-sustained improvement. There is a caveat for Afghanistan, since not enough time has passed and the reconstruction effort is ongoing. However, based on the current trends, it is hard to imagine that Afghanistan will follow a path similar to Japan.

This leaves us with Kosovo and Iraq, for which an assigned score of medium seems reasonable. The evidence of health gains in Kosovo is mixed, though the reconstruction effort has left Kosovo much better positioned than Somalia, Afghanistan, and Haiti for improvements in national health. Iraq is in the same situation as Afghanistan in that it is too early to provide a definitive conclusion. Short-term health gains have not materialized, and the country has been plagued by lack of clean water and proper sanitation. However, no major epidemics and no famine have taken place, and a large-scale immunization campaign was successfully and probably saved numerous lives. In addition, there are enough indications that, conditional on solving internal security issues, the country could put itself on a stable improvement path. For these reasons, we assigned an intermediate score to Iraq.

To summarize, we scored the seven cases along a summary measure that attempts to encapsulate both short-term health gains and long-term improvements in how the country is able to respond to health care needs in a sustained, independent fashion. We assigned a high score to Japan and Germany, an intermediate score to Kosovo and Iraq, and a low score to Haiti, Somalia, and Afghanistan.

Dimensionality Reduction

In the previous section, we compiled a set of 20 covariates that represent certain characteristics of the countries in the initial stages of reconstruction. These covariates are not independent of each other, and even a cursory inspection shows high correlation among them. For example, variables 1, 2, and 14 are perfectly collinear: they assume the same values. This suggests that we do not necessarily need 20 numbers to characterize each country, which is encouraging. Since we only have seven observations, we can afford to use only a small number of covariates. It is imperative that we find ways to reduce the number of covariates from 20 to only a few without losing much information (a process that, in accordance with standard nomenclature, we call "dimensionality reduction"). One way to reduce the problem's dimensionality is to drop some of the covariates, but we can also replace a number of them with a smaller number of their linear combinations. For example, when two variables describe similar concepts, they can both be dropped and replaced with the average of the two. The total number of covariates drops by one, but little information is lost.

Factor analysis is a standard statistical technique that can be used to figure out which covariates should be dropped and which linear combinations of the covariates should be retained. The problem with factor analysis is that even if its result can be interpreted in the end, the process leading to it is fairly technical and does not necessarily produce a "story" that is easy to tell. Therefore, we followed a different approach, proposing a "story" and a simple model that suggest a way to replace the 20 covariates with two interpretable covariates built as linear combinations of the original ones. We call these covariates "factors." Appendix B shows how we used factor analysis to perform a similar task; it also shows that the covariates suggested by factor analysis are quite similar to the ones obtained with our more intuitive story. Since we can show that factor analysis reduces the dimensionality of the problem while retaining most of the information contained in the original covariates, this result supports the notion that our two factors have a similar property. The following section describes a simple model and introduces our two factors.

A Simplified Model of Reconstruction

Let us consider a country in which people's health depend only on the availability of one good, which we will call "vitamin." A war disrupts vitamin's production and its distribution system enough that people's health deteriorates during the war. At the end of the war, an international organization enters the country to help reconstruct the vitamin production and distribution system. In an ideal situation, all operations go smoothly, and reconstruction proceeds smoothly in other areas, such as security, basic infrastructure, and economics. The improvement in the health of the population, measured after some reasonable time interval and denoted by Δ_H, depends only on F, the amount of funding available for the reconstruction: $\Delta\_H \propto F$. We are not concerned here about the functional form involved in this dependency.

Some complications may arise, though. For example, suppose the country has a poor transportation infrastructure system. Some vitamin will be spilled in truck accidents, so some of funds F may need to be spent to improve the transportation infrastructure, rather than to buy vitamin. As a result, only a fraction T (for transportation) of every dollar of funding really goes to improve health. The improvement in health is $\Delta\_H \propto FT$. We can think of T as an indicator between 0 and 1 that measures the efficiency of the transportation sector. What this formula says is that the same amount of effort spent in two countries having two different efficiency levels in the transportation sector will result in different improvements in health. Another way of stating the same concept is that transportation is an "enabler" for reconstruction of the health sector, where we use *enabler* to mean a feature that makes it easier for reconstruction to progress and appears multiplicatively in the formula for Δ_H.

Transportation clearly is not the only such enabler. Suppose that vitamin needs to be dissolved in water. If only a fraction W of the population has access to water, then the water sector is an enabler. The change in health will thus be $\Delta\_H \propto FTW$. In addition, it seems reasonable that H, the health status of the population itself will act as an enabler, since it may be easier to help a healthy set of people than a sick set of people. Moreover, H is a proxy for the efficiency of the health care itself. A larger value for H implies that the system was working well before and that the existing level of infrastructure was already high. Therefore, one can write $\Delta\_H \propto FTWH$. Finally, the level of security, S, is also an enabler, since it affects the efficiency of the overall reconstruction process. We thus write $\Delta\_H \propto FTWHS$.

Other variables, such as the extent to which there is a functioning government, may act as enablers. In general, we loosely refer to variables of this type as "infrastructure." The higher their values are, the more they are available to start building from—and the easier the reconstruction effort is. A characteristic of infrastructure variables is that they all appear multiplicatively in determining the improvement in health, and they are at least partially able to substitute for one another. However, another type of variables may play an important role in the reconstruction.

Consider the more complicated case in which vitamin is a compound of two substances (vitamin A and vitamin B) that have the same price but must be combined in a precise proportion. One unit of vitamin A must be combined with one unit of vitamin B to produce one unit of vitamin. This implies that if we have only one unit of vitamin A and multiple units of vitamin B, we can still only produce one unit of vitamin. In other words, the total amount of vitamin that can be produced depends on the minimum amount available of vitamin A or vitamin B. Suppose now that we have two international agencies working in the country, one investing F_A dollars to provide vitamin A and one investing F_B dollars to provide vitamin B. The total amount of vitamin that can be produced is then determined by the smallest of the numbers, F_A and F_B, which we denote by $\min(F_A, F_B)$. Taking into account the enablers previously defined, the improvement in health will then be given by the formula $\Delta\_H \propto TWH \min(F_A, F_B)$.

If this is the case, it is crucial that the two agencies coordinate their efforts so that the total amount of funding is equally split among them. In other words, giving more funding to only one of the agencies will not result in a larger improvement in health, and there is no substitution among the activities of the two agencies. Notice that the formula above can be rewritten as $\Delta\_H \propto [FTWH] \times \min(q_A, q_B)$, where q_A and q_B are the fraction of total funding F used by agencies A and B, respectively. This scenario can be easily generalized to more-complex cases. For example, we can introduce a time dimension. Vitamin A and vitamin B must be mixed not only in certain proportions, but also in a certain time frame; they might spoil if stored for too long. In this case, the final production of vitamin depends on both agencies performing their activities in a timely manner. Having one agency complete its task on time is fruitless if the other agency does not. Notice that a similar role can be played by variables that describe planning activities, which are often a prerequisite for coordination. All of these generalizations rely on the fact that to reach a given objective, certain things have to be done at certain times in a certain way; and certain activities are essential and cannot be substituted with others. This discussion suggests that a set of variables that may play an important role in reconstruction efforts may be the set that has to do with coordination and planning activities.

To summarize, the highly simplified model of reconstruction presented above suggests that improvement in health due to reconstruction efforts depends on two groups of variables:

- *Coordination and planning variables.* These help determine the level of coordination of the different agencies involved in reconstruction. Coordination may be required between different agencies over space and time, but also within the same agency at different points in time. Therefore, variables that describe planning activities also belong to this category.
- *Infrastructure variables.* These describe the level of effort devoted to improving health, or the efficiency with which the effort is transformed into health improvements. Numerous measures of public infrastructure belong to this category, as do the efficiency of government and the provision of security.

Definition of Factors

The discussion above suggests that two distinct groups of variables may influence the outcome of the reconstruction effort. This in turn suggests that one way to perform dimensionality reduction is to assign to each country two "indexes," or "factors," each built by averaging the values of the variables falling into that group. The variables included in the first factor, which we call "coordination and planning," are 25, 27, 22, 8, 13, and 5. The variables included in the second factor, which we call "infrastructure," are 4, 6, 3, 15, 24, 20, 31, 10, 30, 1, 12, and 13.

Notice that variable 13 appears in both definitions. Since it measures the level of security, it affects most aspects of the reconstruction effort. The numerical values of the factors are shown in Table A.2, and their definitions are discussed in more detail below.

Table A.2
Numerical Values of the Two Factors

	Coordination and Planning	Infrastructure
Germany	0.86	0.79
Japan	0.79	0.93
Kosovo	0.36	0.64
Iraq	0.29	0.54
Somalia	0.29	0.07
Afghanistan	0.29	0.21
Haiti	0.14	0.04

Defining Coordination and Planning

The first factor is the average of variables 25, 27, 22, 8, 13, and 5 taken from Table A.1. First is the level of coordination among the NGOs, military, and international communities (variables 25 and 27). Germany and Japan scored higher on these two coordination variables than did the other countries.

Second is whether (a) the international community fully appreciated the complexity and full extent of the needs and requirements of the nation-building effort, and (b) whether the international community was adequately prepared for the mission (variable 22). This variable represents the level and adequacy of the planning effort. Germany and Japan both scored high on this variable. For the other countries in the study, the overall level of preparedness by the international community was relatively low. For example, initial planning in Haiti was inadequate, and policymakers generally failed to fully appreciate the magnitude of the needs within the health sector.

Third is the extent to which there was a health policy framework or well-defined plan for rebuilding the health sector (variable 8). This variable captures whether there was an overarching health policy framework or plan developed to guide reconstruction of the health system. It also represents the degree to which key actors (such as donor states, international organizations, and NGOs) were supportive of the plan and adhered to its guidance. This was more the case in Germany, Japan, and Kosovo than it was in Somalia, Iraq, and Afghanistan.

Fourth is the level of security (variable 13). This variable indicates the average level of security during the reconstruction phase. Germany and Japan scored relatively high compared to Iraq, Haiti, Somalia, and Afghanistan.

Fifth is the extent to which the country has the ability to assess its public health needs (variable 5). This variable captures a country's ability to know what needs to be done, which is a critical element of planning. Germany scored high on this variable, followed by Japan, which had a semifunctional information exchange system.

In sum, Germany and Japan scored much higher on the "coordination and planning" factor than did the other countries, since the reconstruction efforts in those two countries were well planned and presented few coordination challenges. The absence of NGOs and international organizations made coordination and planning much easier. Iraq, Haiti, Somalia, and Afghanistan scored relatively low on this factor, their reconstruction efforts marred by coordination and planning problems. Kosovo scored in between the two extremes.

Defining Infrastructure

The second factor is the average of infrastructure indicators (what existed before the conflict, at time 0) and enabling factors, such as level of security and level of funding or support. The variables relevant in the second factor are 4, 6, 3, 15, 24, 20, 31, 10, 30, 1, 12, and 13 from Table A.1.

These are basic "infrastructure" variables. Variable 4 describes the presence of a public health infrastructure, such as prevention programs and disease surveillance systems, during the period prior to conflict. Variable 6 is similar to variable 4 but refers specifically to the status of the water and sanitation sectors. These variables attempt to capture the extent to which there is a public health system within a country, more than how well that public health system may have been functioning. These variables distinguish between countries such as Germany or Japan on the one hand, and Haiti or Somalia on the other. Variable 3 refers to the health system's level of physical infrastructure, such as hospitals and clinics, and whether that infrastructure was damaged during the conflict. Variable 3 is correlated with variable 4, but the scoring for the two is not always the same. Countries whose public health system was well developed but was substantially damaged during the conflict scored low on this variable (for example, Germany). Variable 15 incorporates the overall status of the country's infrastructure. For example, Somalia scored low on variable 15 because of the destruction of the Mogadishu ports and the lack of transportation infrastructure within the country to facilitate the movement of the relief convoys. In contrast, the transportation infrastructures of Kosovo and Iraq were relatively intact after the war, despite sustaining some damage.

Variable 24 incorporates the degree to which the health care sector was reliant on the NGO and international community. It describes the health sector's pre-conflict degree of dependence on NGOs and international aid agencies in delivering care and running the health care system. This is useful because it helps flag those countries that posed a challenge because they lacked local capacity or resources to build upon. For example, in Haiti, Somalia, and Afghanistan, the health sector was heavily reliant on international aid; NGOs and international agencies served almost as a de facto Ministry of Health. Even though this variable does not refer to physical infrastructure, we think of it as infrastructure, or an enabling variable.

Variables 20 and 31 include whether there was a functioning central government at the beginning of the reconstruction effort and whether the government was supportive of the nation-building effort. Variable 20 describes whether a functioning central government existed at the beginning of the reconstruction effort, which is important because it relates to the existence of a Ministry of Health. Variable 31 comprises the degree to which the central government or acting authority was supportive of the reconstruction effort. For example, Iraq did not have a central government at the beginning of the operations. But the Coalition Provisional Authority, which served as the acting authority, supported the effort. In Somalia, the warlords that ruled the country did not support the humanitarian relief or reconstruction efforts. These variables characterize the extent to which the international agencies involved in the reconstruction effort could rely on some sort of central, governing authority, and the infrastructure that goes with a functioning central government. We think of these as representing the "government infrastructure" variables.

Variable 10 quantifies the level of donor support by the international community and the flow of funding for the nation-building effort. This variable distinguishes, for example, Germany and Iraq from Somalia. Unlike most of the variables described above, which are of the "enabling" type, this variable describes the actual level of input into an operation. If we had to put a dollar amount for this variable, it would be the total aid received by a country, rather than the aid per capita. Since there are significant externalities, such as public goods and the fixed costs involved in the health care system, figures based on per capita might be misleading.

Variable 30 measures the degree to which the local population was supportive of reconstruction. This variable distinguishes cases such as Germany and Japan, where the local population was supportive of reconstruction, from cases such as Iraq or Somalia, where a notable segment of the population was either opposed to reconstruction or disengaged.

Variables 1 and 12 include, respectively, the extent to which health care delivery was occurring, and the health status of the population. These are our two "health care" variables. Germany and Japan had relatively high levels of health care delivery when the conflict ended. In comparison, Somalia, Haiti, and Afghanistan had health care systems that did not function as well. Variable 12 describes the general health status of the population and is only partially correlated with variable 1. For example, Japan, like Germany, had a functioning health care system, but the overall health status of the Japanese population at the end of the conflict was relatively poor. Finally, variable 13, security, is included here because of its strong enabling role.

In sum, the "infrastructure" factor aims to capture two important dimensions: the level of donor effort and support (an input), and enabling conditions that allow progress to be made using that input. These enabling conditions could be either standard infrastructure (variables 3, 4, 6, and 15) or the infrastructure related to the existence and support of a central government or authority (variables 20 and 31). Another enabling condition is measured by the degree of reliance on NGOs and the international community for health care delivery, which is an indicator of the degree to which a country has health care resources to build upon. Still another important enabling condition is security: a lack of security can seriously impede efforts to improve the functioning of the health care system. This explains why Somalia, Haiti, and Afghanistan all scored low on this factor. They are characterized by poor infrastructure, heavy reliance on NGOs and the international community, virtually no supportive central authority, and a low level of security.

Correlating Input and Output

Now that we have only two covariates for each country, we can examine the correlation between input and output. In principle, we could plot output as a function of input in three dimensions. However, since the output only assumes three levels, it is easy to plot where the countries stand in the two-dimensional plane defined by the factors. We can then label the countries with the value of the output variable: high, medium, or low.

As Figure A.1 shows, we split the plane, or "factor space," into four quadrants. The vertical line separates countries with relatively high scores from those with relatively low scores on the coordination and planning factor; the horizontal line does the same thing for the infrastructure and resources factor.

The upper left quadrant contains the countries whose infrastructure was damaged but still intact and whose health care system before the conflict was not heavily reliant on NGOs or the international community. However, the nation-building effort in these countries was characterized by poor coordination and planning, and by security that was inadequate relative to that of Japan and Germany. For Kosovo or Iraq to move closer to Japan and Germany, they would need a substantial increase in the level of security and improved coordination and planning.

Figure A.1
Distribution of Countries

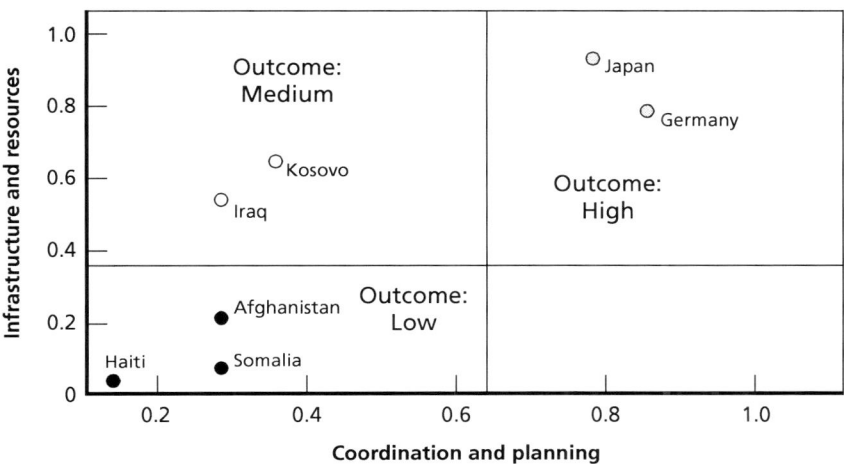

In the upper right quadrant are countries characterized by a high level of coordination and planning, a high level of security, and an infrastructure that was damaged but readily reparable. Germany and Japan are located here. Finally, the lower right quadrant is for countries with low levels of infrastructure but high levels of coordination and planning. None of our case studies fell within this quadrant, but we speculate that nation-building efforts such as the UN effort in East Timor might fall here.

In general, if the relative rankings of these nation-building efforts are considered in terms of success, they closely match the groupings shown in Figure A.1, which are based solely on the inputs. These findings suggest that the inputs identified in Figure A.1 help predict the overall success of a nation-building effort.

Security, Security, Security

It emerged from the comparative analysis that improvement in health (Δ_H) is a function of several determinants, some of which are outlined in the following formula:

$\Delta\_H \propto$ security

  $\times$ progress of reconstruction in the electricity sector

  $\times$ progress of reconstruction in the water and sanitation sector

  $\times$ progress of reconstruction in other basic public infrastructure

  $\times$ health status of population $\times$ level of healthy system development

  $\times$ prior level of dependence of the health sector on foreign aid

  $\times$ level of commitment by international community following the conflict

  $\times$ other factors (including coordination and planning) + exogenous shocks.

This formula helps underscore how changes in the level of security affect the success of reconstruction efforts.

The first term in the formula shows the direct effect of security on health improvement. Security also affects other sectors on which the health sector is strongly dependent, particularly the electricity and the water and sanitation sectors. Since progress in these sectors is also proportional to the level of security, the formula above contains the term *security_security_security*. In other words, the health sector gets hit by security issues at least three times: once for the direct effect, once for the indirect effect through the electricity sector, and once for the indirect effect through the water and sanitation sector.

However, since electricity and water/sanitation are not the only sectors on which progress in the health sector depends, the importance of security is being underestimated. For example, the transportation sector is also relevant. An important feature of the health sector is its close dependence on a large number of other sectors. This implies that ad hoc solutions to deal with the security problem, which might be available for less interdependent sectors, are unlikely to work for the health sector. For example, one can use troops and guards to maintain a higher level of security around important power hubs. Although expensive, this solution is feasible, because the electricity sector is less dependent on other sectors than is the health care sector. In sum, the success of rebuilding public health and health care delivery systems during nation-building missions is closely tied to the level of security.

Factor Analysis

As explained in Appendix A, we used factor analysis to strengthen our argument. To reduce the dimensionality of the problem, we used some standard tools that go under the names of principal component analysis (PCA) and factor analysis. Here we provide only an intuitive explanation of the dimensionality reduction, and refer the reader to standard references for the details.

The main idea is simple: It is possible that the only reason we need so many variables to describe the system of interest is that we have not chosen the "right" variables. In other words, it may be possible to define only a few variables, perhaps more complicated or abstract than the existing ones, that capture the same amount of information captured by the 17 rows of Table A.1. How can we find these more complicated but highly informative variables, which we call "factors"? If all our variables had only two levels (say, "yes" and "no"), one could think of forming complicated logical conjunctions of the variables. For example, a factor could be defined by the sentence "there are serious security problems, but the judiciary system is well functioning."

Since our variables are continuous, a similar approach is to form factors by taking linear combinations of the existing variables. For example, suppose we want to create a factor that captures the concept of "infrastructure" so that we can assign to each country a score representing the degree of infrastructure development. An easy way to do this is to form a linear combination of all the variables. We could assign 0 weight to any variables that have nothing to do with infrastructure, and a weight of 1 to all the infrastructure-related variables. This rule would assign the score 2 to Germany, 3 to Japan, and 0 to Haiti. To define a factor, we need to define a set of "weights," one for each variable. Once this is done, the score associated with the factor is simply computed as a weighted sum of the original variables.

The idea of factor analysis is that it may be possible to find a few factors that adequately summarize the information contained in the original variables. Obviously, if we start with 17 variables and summarize them with the scores of just three factors, some information is lost. This approach will work only if the original 17 variables are highly linearly correlated with each other. When this is the case, little information is lost in the dimensionality reduction process. The original table of 17 rows can be summarized in a table with a few rows. There is a rule (a linear map) that allows us to reconstruct the table with 17 rows from the table with three rows. Researchers do not know a priori when this process is possible, but they can verify it a posteriori. For any set of candidate factors, it is easy to check how well one can reconstruct the original variables from the factor scores. In more technical terms, one can compute how much of the variance in the original data is explained by the factor score, obtaining a natural measure of the reliability of a set of factors. This implies that one can find the optimal set of factors by simply maximizing this reliability of fit measure.

We applied these ideas to Table A.1 in Appendix A. Before processing the table, we first subtracted from each row the average score over the seven countries. This operation is harmless and creates a "centered" table, such that the average of each row is equal to 0. Then we looked for the two factors that could best explain the centered data. This means that we replaced the centered table of 17 rows with a table of only two rows. Every country is therefore uniquely associated to two numbers: the score of the first and second factors, respectively.

Because we are using only two factors, we cannot capture the entire variance in the data, and we leave about 13 percent of it unexplained. In other words, if we were to attempt to recover the original

17-row table using our two-row table, we would make a relative error of 13 percent. If we were to instead use three factors, the percentage of the variance left unexplained would drop to 6 percent, which is definitely reasonable. The reason we limit ourselves to two factors is that their interpretation is already difficult. We will come back to the third factor later in the discussion; now, we are ready to show where the countries are located in factor space.

Since each country is associated with two numbers, or factor scores, we can plot these numbers on a two-dimensional plane, as is done in Figure B.1. The horizontal and vertical axes show the score of each country on the first and the second factor, respectively. In terms of inputs, the countries are clustered the same way they were in Figure A.1. The question of interest is whether the interpretation of the factors is the same in both, so what we need is to understand the meaning of these factors. Remember that each factor is uniquely defined by a set of weights, one for each of the original variables (17 in our case). The score for each country is obtained by taking a linear combination of its variables using these weights. Therefore, each

Figure B.1
Distribution of Countries Using Factor Analysis

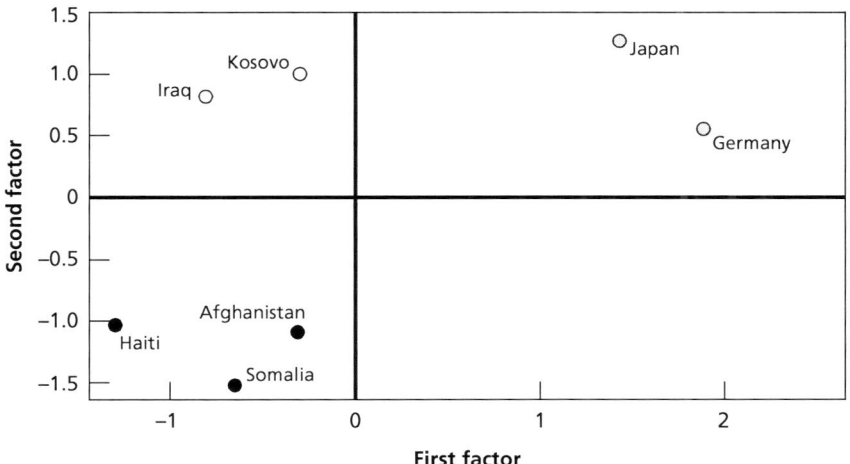

weight in a factor tells us "how much" of the corresponding variable is included in the factor.

If a weight is small, we can conclude that the corresponding variable is not important for defining the factor. Figure B.2 shows the values of these weights for both factors. For each factor, the horizontal axis runs through the variable names. For each variable, we plot the value of the corresponding weight as a vertical bar. For example, the first factor is mostly "made of" variables 27, 30, 22, 13, and 5.

To make things easier, we produced some "simplified" factors by setting to zero all factor weights smaller than 0.25. This threshold was chosen in such a way that the distribution of the countries remains qualitatively similar if the simplified factors are used instead of

Figure B.2
Weights for Each Factor

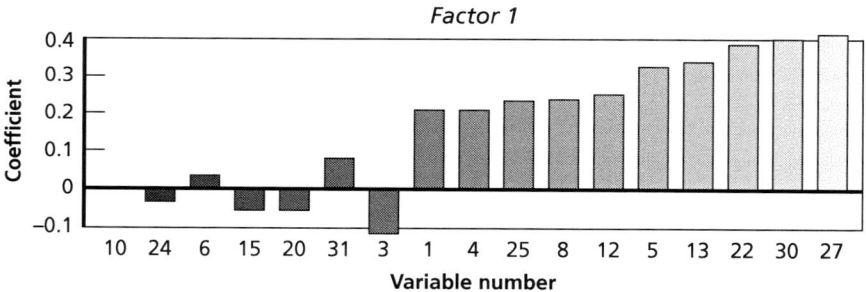

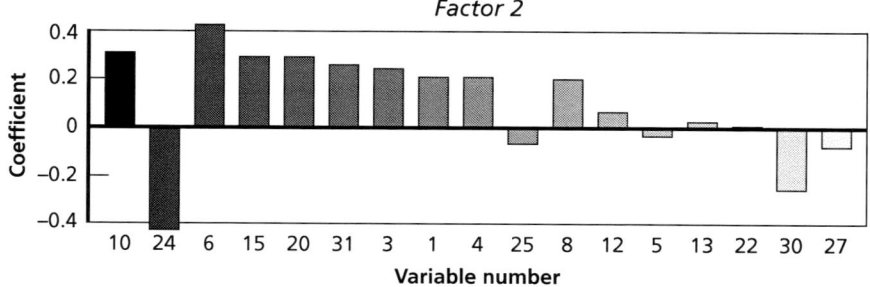

the original factors. The weights in the simplified factors, which are shown in Figure B.3, can be used as a starting point for analysis.

The First Factor

The variables that are relevant in the first factor are the following: 27, 30, 22, 13, 5, 12, 8, and 25. We can now come to an interpretation of the first factor and to why it distinguishes Germany and Japan from the rest. It seems that the first factor summarizes several dimensions: coordination and planning, security, health status, and population support. In a sense, this factor combines the smoothness of the flow of actions involved in reconstruction with the "starting point" in

Figure B.3
Simplified Weights for Each Factor

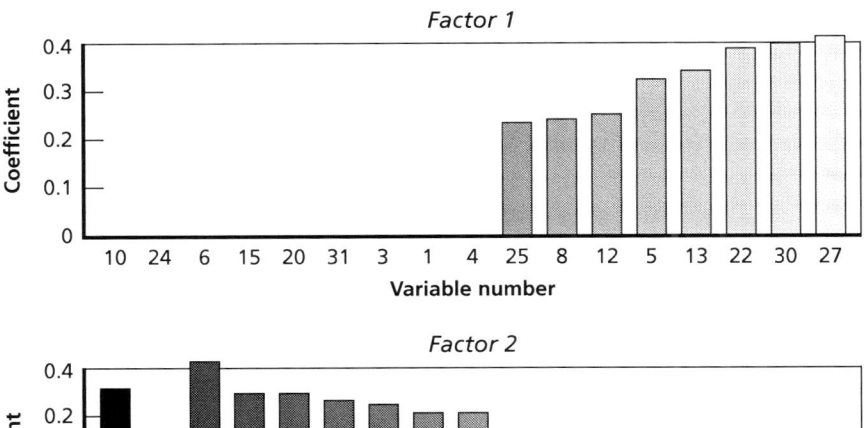

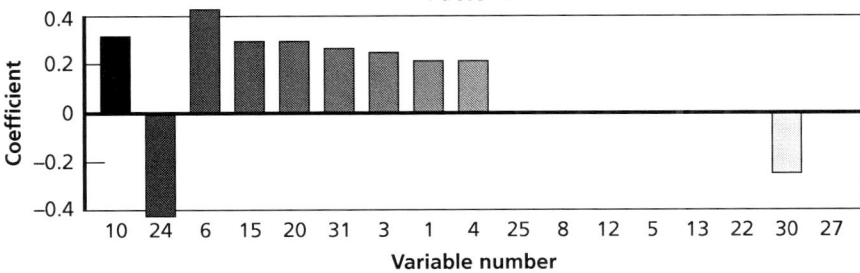

terms of health status. Consequently, it is not surprising that Germany and Japan score much higher on this factor than the other countries do. The reconstruction efforts in Germany and Japan were well planned, had few security problems, were highly supported by the population, and started from a relatively higher level in terms of health status and health care delivery. It is also not surprising to find that Iraq, Haiti, Somalia, and Afghanistan score low on this factor. Reconstruction efforts in these countries were marred by security, coordination, and planning problems. Kosovo is somewhere in between these two extremes.

This factor overlaps quite well with the coordination and planning factor described in Appendix A. The most important, and surprising, difference between the two is the presence of health status (variable 12) in the factor derived from factor analysis. In our more intuitive approach, health status is an enabler and appears with the infrastructure variables. The presence of population support (variable 30) in the first factor of Figure B.3 is not a concern, since we can easily think of it as playing an important role in the overall coordination of events. Despite this discrepancy, however, the meaning of these two factors is fairly similar. We must take into account the fact that factor analysis introduces constraints on how the factors are constructed: the two factors must be orthogonal. In addition, factors produced by factor analysis are not unique but are defined up to a multidimensional rotation. Criteria must be introduced in order to produce a unique choice. The criterion used in the analysis described in this appendix is that the weights in the factors must have the maximum number of zeros (or small numbers) to facilitate interpretation.

The Second Factor

The variables that are relevant in the second factor are 18, 24, 6, 15, 20, 31, 3, 1, and 4. When we look at the definitions of these variables, it seems that the second factor captures two important dimensions. One is the input, or the level of donor effort; the other is a set of enabling conditions, or those conditions that allow progress to be made using that input. The enabling conditions could be standard infrastructure (variables 3, 4, and 15) or the infrastructure related to the existence and support of a central governing authority (variables 20 and 31). Another enabling condition is the lack of reliance on NGOs for health care delivery (variable 24), which means that the country has some resources of its own. This explains why Somalia, Haiti, and Afghanistan all score low on this factor: they have poor infrastructure, complete reliance on NGOs, and lack a supportive central authority. This factor overlaps very well with the "infrastructure" factor derived in the previous section.

What Is Missing

Several things are missing from the analysis above, one of which is the proper location of Iraq. Iraq shares many features with Kosovo, since both had a somewhat functioning health care system, received significant attention from the international community, and certainly had potential for growth and success. But Iraq is a very special case, partly because not enough time has elapsed to measure success. This obviously does not show in the analysis if we only use two factors.

Preliminary analysis shows that using three factors allows us to separate Kosovo from Iraq. However, interpretation of the factors becomes more difficult, and it is not clear that an attempt to interpret three factors with only seven countries would be meaningful. Therefore, we decided not to pursue this avenue of research, which might be better explored with more case studies.

Bibliography

Ackerman, Seth, "Afghan Famine on and off the Screen," *Fair*, May/June 2002, www.fair.org/extra/0205/afghasn-famine.html.

Afghanistan Office of National Security Council, *National Threat Assessment*, Kabul, September 2005, pp. 4–5.

African Red Cross and Red Crescent Health Initiative 2010, "Landmines in Africa," www.ifrc.org/WHAT/health/archi/fact/fmines.htm (as of December 31, 2004).

Air Staff, "The Value of Incendiary Weapons in Attack on Area Targets," September 29, 1941, in Towns Panel of the British Bombing Survey Unit, *Effects of Strategic Air Attacks on German Towns*, London: Her Majesty's Stationery Office, 1947.

Allen, G.C., *A Short Economic History of Modern Japan, 1867–1970*, London: George Allen & Unwin Ltd., 1972.

Alley, Kate, John Richardson, and Jacques Berard, *Country Programme Evaluation 1992–mid-1996: Programme Choices in Political Crisis and Transition*, Haiti Evaluation Team, New York: UNICEF, December 1996.

———, *Programme Choices in Political Crisis and Transition*, UNICEF Latin America and the Caribbean Regional Monitoring and Evaluation Electronic Bulletin, No. 2, New York: UNICEF, September 1997.

Amnesty International, "Afghanistan, Justice Denied to Women," Amnesty International, 2003, www.web.amnesty.org/library/print/ENGASA1102 32003.

Anderson, Benedict, *Imagined Communities: Reflections on the Origin and Spread of Nationalism,* New York: Verso, 1991.

Asian Development Bank, "Improving Primary Health Care in Afghanistan Through NGOs," December 23, 2002, www.adb.org/Documents/News/2002/nr2002268.asp.

Bartsch, Jonathan, *Violent Conflict and Human Rights, A Study of Principled Decision Making in Afghanistan*, Peshawar: CARE, October 1998.

Beblawi, Hazem, and Giacomo Luciani (eds.), *The Rentier State*, New York: Croom Helm, 1987.

Benvenisti, Eyal, "Water Conflicts During the Occupation of Iraq," *American Journal of International Law*, Vol. 97, No. 4., October 2003, pp. 860–872.

Berkman, D.S., et al., "Effects of Stunting, Diarrhoeal Disease, and Parasitic Infection During Infancy on Cognition in Late Childhood: A Follow-Up Study," *Lancet*, Vol. 359, 2002, pp. 564–571.

Biddiscombe, Perry, *Werwolf! The History of the National Socialist Guerrilla Movement, 1944–1946*, Toronto: University of Toronto Press, 1998.

Bidinian, Larry J., *The Combined Allied Bombing Offensive Against the German Civilian, 1942–1945*, Lawrence, Kansas: Coronado Press, 1976.

Blacker, John, Gareth Jones, and Mohamed M. Ali, "Annual Mortality Rates and Excess Deaths of Children Under Five in Iraq, 1991–98," *Population Studies*, Vol. 57, No. 2, 2003, pp. 217–226.

Blanpain, Jan, Luc Delesie, and Herman Nys, *National Health Insurance and Health Resources: The European Experience*, Cambridge, Massachusetts: Harvard University Press, 1978.

Branca, F., and M. Ferrari, "Impact of Micronutrient Deficiencies on Growth: The Stunting Syndrome," *Annals of Nutrition & Metabolism*, Vol. 46, Suppl. 1, 2002, pp. 8–17.

Bornemisza, O., and E. Sondorp, *Health Policy Formulation in Complex Political Emergencies and Post-Conflict Countries: A Literature Review*, London School of Hygiene & Tropical Medicine, London: University of London, Department of Public Health and Policy, November 7, 2002.

Brookings Institution, *Iraq Index: Tracking Variables of Reconstruction and Security in Post-Saddam Iraq*, Washington, D.C.: Brookings Institution, April 2004, www.brookings.edu/fp/saban/iraq/index.pdf.

Brown, Macalister, and Joseph Zasloff, *Cambodia Confounds the Peacemakers, 1979–1998*, Ithaca, New York: Cornell University Press, 1998.

Buck, Alfred, et al., *Health and Disease in Rural Afghanistan*, Baltimore, Maryland: York Press, 1972.

Bureau of Resource Management, *Section 2207 Report on Iraq Relief and Reconstruction*, October 5, 2004, www.state.gov/s/d/rm/rls/2207/oct2004/html.

Burkle, F.M., and E.K. Noji, "Health and Politics in the 2003 War with Iraq: Lessons Learned," *Lancet*, Vol. 364, October 9, 2004.

Byman, Daniel, et al., *Strengthening the Partnership: Improving Military Co-ordination with Relief Agencies and Allies in Humanitarian Operations*, MR-1185-AF, Santa Monica, California: RAND Corporation, 2000.

Cardozo, Barbara Lopes, Alfredo Vergara, Ferid Agani, and Carol A. Gotway, "Mental Health, Social Functioning, and Attitudes of Kosovar Albanians Following the War in Kosovo," *Journal of American Medical Association*, Vol. 284, No. 5, August 2, 2000, pp. 569–577.

CARE International, *CARE International in Somalia*, Washington, D.C.: CARE International, 2004, www.careinternational.org.uk/cares_work/where/somalia/ (as of December 31, 2004).

Carey, Patrick, "Humanitarian Assistance Following Military Operations: Overcoming Barriers—Part 2," Committee on Government Reform, Subcommittee on National Security, Emerging Threats and International Relations, July 18, 2003.

Center for Economic and Social Rights, "Health Data Tables," Humanitarian Information Center for Iraq, Brooklyn, New York, March 2003, www.agoodplacetostart.org/download/unohci/Iraq.

———, *The Human Costs of War in Iraq*, Brooklyn, New York: CESR, 2003, www.cesr.org/iraq/.

———, *Who's Doing What, Where?* Map Reference 271, Humanitarian Information Center for Iraq, July 14, 2003, www.humanitarianinfo.org/iraq/maps/271-A1-WhoWhatWhere.pdf (as of February 9, 2005).

Central Intelligence Agency, *World Factbook*, Washington, D.C.: CIA, various years, www.cia.gov/cia/publications/factbook/geos/iz.html#Intro.

Chesterman, Simon, *You, The People: The United Nations Transitional Administration, and State-Building*, New York: Oxford University Press, 2004.

Chiarelli, (Major General) Peter, "Securing the Peace in Iraq," Briefing at RAND Corporation, Washington, D.C., March 10, 2005.

Clark, Peter, *The Iraqi Marshlands: A Pre-War Perspective*, March 7, 2003, www.crimesofwar.org/special/Iraq/news-marshArabs.html (as of December 10, 2005).

Clarke, Walter, and Jeffrey Herbst (eds.), *Learning from Somalia*, Boulder, Colorado: Westview Press, 1997.

Clay, Lucius D., "From General Lucius Clay Personal for Echols," May 18, 1946, CC 5314, in Jean E. Smith (ed.), *The Papers of General Lucius D. Clay: Germany 1945–1947* (2 vols.), Bloomington, Indiana: Indiana University Press, 1974, pp. 206–208.

Coalition Provisional Authority, *Quarterly Report to Congress*, Inspector General of the Coalition Provisional Authority, March 30, 2004, www.cpa-ig.org/reports_congress.html.

———, *Request to Rehabilitate and Reconstruct Iraq*, September 2003. Government publication; not releasable to the general public.

———, *Strategic Plan*, unpublished, 2003.

Coipuram, T., *Iraq: United Nations and Humanitarian Aid Organizations*, Congressional Research Service, Washington, D.C.: U.S. Department of State, August 2003, fpc.state.gov/documents/organization/24059.pdf.

Congressional Budget Office, *Paying for Iraq's Reconstruction*, CBO Paper, January 2004, ftp.cbo.gov/49xx/doc4983/01-23-Iraq.pdf.

Daalder, Ivo H., and Michael E. O'Hanlon, *Winning Ugly: NATO's War to Save Kosovo*, Washington, D.C.: Brookings Institution, 2001.

Daponte, Beth Osborn, "A Case Study in Estimating Casualties from War and Its Aftermath: The 1991 Persian Gulf War," *Physicians for Social Responsibility Quarterly*, Vol. 3, Nos. 57–66, 1993, www.ippnw.org/MGS/PSRQV3N2Daponte.html (as of December 10, 2005).

Davidson, Anders, and Peter Hjukstroem (eds.), *Afghanistan, Aid and the Taliban*, Stockholm: The Swedish Committee for Afghanistan, 1999.

Davis, L.M., S.D. Hosek, M.G. Tate, M. Perry, G. Hepler, and P. Steinberg, *Army Medical Support for Peace Operations and Humanitarian Assistance*, MR-773-A, Santa Monica, California: RAND Corporation, 1996.

Dayan, Moshe, National Archives, Record Group 319, Box 34 Folder: #32 History File, 1–31 May 1968, Folder 488.

Department for International Development, *Kosovo: Strategy Paper 2001–2004*, Section on organization of the health care system, August 2001.

de Ville de Goyet, C., and E. Sondorp, *Internal Evaluation of WHO Response in Kosovo*, June–December 1999, WHO/EHA, May 2001, p. 23.

Diefendorf, Jeffry M., "America and the Rebuilding of Urban Germany," in Jeffry M. Diefendorf, Axel Frohn, and Hermann-Josef Rupieper, *American Policy and the Reconstruction of West Germany, 1945–1955*, New York: Cambridge University Press, 1993.

Dobbins, James, et al., *America's Role in Nation-Building: From Germany to Iraq*, MG-1753-RC, Santa Monica, California: RAND Corporation, 2004.

———, *The UN's Role in Nation-Building: From the Congo to Iraq*, MG-304-RC, Santa Monica, California: RAND Corporation, 2005.

Doctors of the World, *Our Projects: Kosovo; WHO, Tuberculosis Action Plan: Kosovo, 2000*, Tuberculosis Technical Commission, WHO, January 2, 2004.

Doctors of the World/USA, *Doctors of the World/USA Maternal and Infant Health Project 1998–2002*, Final Report, New York: Doctors of the World/USA, 2002.

Dower, John W., *Embracing Defeat: Japan in the Wake of World War II*, New York: W.W. Norton & Company, 1999.

Doyle, Michael W., Ian Johnstone, and Robert C. Orr (eds.), *Keeping the Peace: Multidimensional UN Operations in Cambodia and El Salvador*, New York: Cambridge University Press, 1997.

———, *UN Peacekeeping in Cambodia: UNTAC's Civil Mandate*, Boulder, Colorado: Lynne Rienner, 1995.

Dyer, O., "Poor Security Is Biggest Impediment to Health Care in Iraq," *British Medical Journal*, Vol. 326, No. 7399, May 24, 2003, p. 1107.

East, James, "Afghanistan: Child Marriage Rate Still High," IRIN, July 13, 2004.

The Economist, "A Wider War, a Wider Worry," April 10, 2004.

————, "Cleaner, But Still Bare," October 4, 2003.

————, "The Spectre of a Civil War," February 14, 2004.

————, "We Won't Be Sacrificial Lambs," August 30, 2003.

————, "Who'll Help Us? We Ourselves, Mostly," Special report, September 13, 2003.

Fagan, Patricia Weiss, "Conflict Reconstruction and Reintegration: The Long-Term Challenges," in Edward Newman and Joanne Van Selm (eds.), *Refugees and Human Displacement in Contemporary International Relations*, New York: United Nations University Press, 2003.

Fearon, James D., and David D. Laitin, "Neotrusteeship and the Problem of Weak States," *International Security*, Vol. 28, No. 4, Spring 2004.

Food and Agriculture Organization of the United Nations, and World Food Programme, *FAO/WFP Crop, Food Supply and Nutrition Assessment Mission to Iraq*, September 23, 2003, ftp.fao.org/docrep/fao/005/J0465e/ J0465e00.pdf.

Frederiksen, Oliver J., *The American Military Occupation of Germany, 1945–1953*, Darmstadt, Germany: Historical Division, Headquarters, United States Army, Europe, 1953.

Fukuyama, Francis, *State-Building: Governance and World Order in the 21st Century*, Ithaca, New York: Cornell University Press, 2004.

Garfield, Richard, and Ron Waldman, *Review of Potential Interventions to Reduce Child Mortality in Iraq*, November 2003, www.basics.org/ publications/abs/abs_iraq_child_health.html.

Gellner, Ernest, *Nations and Nationalism*, Ithaca, New York: Columbia University Press, 1983.

General Headquarters, Supreme Commander for the Allied Powers, Public Welfare and Health Section, *Public Health and Welfare in Japan*, Annual Summary, 1948, 1949, and 1950.

George, Alexander L., "Case Studies and Theory Development: The Method of Structured, Focused Comparison," in Paul Gordon Lauren (ed.), *Diplomacy: New Approaches in History, Theory, and Policy*, New York: Free Press, 1979, pp. 43–68.

Global Policy Forum, "Iraq: NGO Registration Causes Controversy," Integrated Regional Information Network, January 13, 2004, www.globalpolicy.org/ngos/aid/2004/0113contro.htm.

Goodhand, J., and D. Hulme, "From Wars to Complex Political Emergencies: Understanding Conflict and Peace-Building in the New World Disorder," *Third World Quarterly*, Vol. 20, 1999, pp. 13–26.

Gormley, William T., and David L. Weimer, *Organizational Report Cards*, Cambridge, Massachusetts: Harvard University Press, 1999.

Gottesman, Evan, *Cambodia After the Khmer Rouge: Inside the Politics of Nation Building*, New Haven, Connecticut: Yale University Press, 2003.

Government Accountability Office [formerly General Accounting Office], *Afghanistan Reconstruction: Despite Some Progress, Deteriorating Security and Other Obstacles Continue to Threaten Achievement of U.S. Goals*, Washington, D.C.: GAO, July 2005.

———, *Afghanistan Reconstruction: Deteriorating Security and Limited Resources Have Impeded Progress—Improvements in U.S. Strategy Needed*, Washington, D.C.: GAO, June 2004.

———, *Rebuilding Iraq: Enhancing Security, Measuring Program Results, and Maintaining Infrastructure Are Necessary to Make Significant and Sustainable Progress*, GAO-06-179T, October 2005.

———, *Rebuilding Iraq: Resource, Security, Governance, Essential Services, and Oversight Issues*, Report GAO-04-902R, Washington, D.C.: GAO, June 2004.

———, *Rebuilding Iraq: Status of Funding and Reconstruction Efforts*, GAO-05-876, July 2005.

———, *Rebuilding Iraq: U.S. Water and Sanitation Efforts Need Improved Measures for Assessing Impact and Sustained Resources for Maintaining Facilities*, GAI-05-872, September 2005.

———, *Strategic Workforce Planning Can Help USAID Address Current and Future Challenges*, Report to Congressional Requester, GAO-03-946, August 2003, www.gao.gov/new.items/d03946.pdf.

Graig, Laurene A., *Health of Nations: An International Perspective on U.S. Health Care Reform*, 3rd ed., Washington, D.C.: Congressional Quarterly, 1999.

Hamerow, T.S. (ed.), *The Age of Bismarck*, New York: Harper and Row, 1973.

Hanouet, Stephanie, *Nutritional, Vaccination Coverage and Mortality Survey*, Kabul Province: Action Contre La Faim, February 1999.

Hatry, Harry P., *Performance Measurement: Getting Results*, Washington, D.C.: The Urban Institute Press, 1999.

Hazem, Adam Ghobarah, Paul Huth, and Bruce Russett, "Civil Wars Kill and Maim People—Long After the Shooting Stops," *American Political Science Review,* Vol. 97, No. 2, May 2003.

Health Policy Formulation in Complex Political Emergencies and Post-Conflict Countries: A Literature Review, London: London School of Hygiene and Tropical Medicine, November 2002.

Helander, B., "Getting the Most Out of It: Nomadic Health Care Seeking and the State in Southern Somalia," *Nomadic Peoples*, No. 25/27, pp. 122–132.

Henke, K.D., "The Federal Republic of Germany," in Richard Scheffler and L.F. Rossiter (eds.), *Advances in Health Economics and Health Services Research*, Greenwich, Connecticut: JAI Press, 1990, pp. 145–168.

Hjelm-Wallén, L., *Mother and Child Health Care in Desperate Need of Funds*, Kabul: Swedish Committee for Afghanistan, 2003.

Hoffman, Bruce, *Insurgency and Counterinsurgency in Iraq*, Santa Monica, CA: RAND Corporation, 2004.

Hooglund, E., "The Other Face of War," *Middle East Report*, July/August 1991.

Hoskins, E., "Public Health and the Persian Gulf War," in B. Levy and V. Sidel (eds.), *War and Public Health*, New York: Oxford University Press, 1997.

Human Rights Watch, "Climate of Fear: Sexual Violence and Abduction of Women and Girls in Baghdad," *Human Rights Watch*, Vol. 7(E), July 2003.

———, "Killing You Is a Very Easy Thing for Us: Human Rights Abuses in Southeast Afghanistan," HRW Index No. C1505, July 29, 2003.

———, "'We Want to Live as Humans': Repression of Women and Girls in Western Afghanistan," HRW Index No. C1411, December 17, 2002.

Humanitarian Information Center, *Who's Doing What, Where?* Map Reference 271, July 14, 2003, www.humanitarianinfo.org/iraq/maps/271-A1-WhoWhatWhere.pdf (as of February 9, 2005).

Humanitarian Information Centre for Iraq, *Health in Iraq: Facts and Figures*, Health Coordination Group, 2004, www.agoodplacetostart.org/download/health/HealthFacts.doc.

Independent Inquiry Committee into the United Nations Oil-for-Food Programme, *Report on Programme Manipulation*, www.iic-offp.org/story27oct05.htm.

International Development Project, "Survey of Maslakh Camp Shows Alarming Levels of Mortality," Global IDP Database, www.db.idpproject.org/Sites/idpSurvey.nsf/wViewCountries, July 2002.

International Federation of Red Cross and Red Crescent Societies (IFRC/RCS), *Health, Relief and Rehabilitation*, Somalia: IFRC/RCS, 1998.

———, "Humanitarian Action," in *International Federation of Red Cross and Crescent Societies Annual Report 1999*, Geneva: International Federation of Red Cross and Red Crescent Societies, 2000, www.ifrc.org/PUBLICAT/ar/ar1999/arch1.asp.

International Monetary Fund, *Haiti: Selected Issues*, IMF Staff Country Report No. 01/04, January 2001, www.imf/org/external/pubs/ft/scr/2001/cr0104.pdf (as of April 11, 2004).

International Peace Academy, *Lessons Learned: Peacebuilding in Haiti*, IPA Seminar Report 7, Permanent Mission of Canada to the United Nations, New York: International Peace Academy, 2002.

International Study Team, *Our Common Responsibility: The Impact of a New War on Iraqi Children*, January 2003.

Iraq Ministry of Health, *Communicable Diseases in Iraq, 1989–2001*, Baghdad: Iraq Ministry of Health, 2003.

Japanese Ministry of Health, Labor and Welfare, *Vital Statistics*, Japanese Statistics and Information Department, Minister's Secretariat, www.mhlw.go.jp/english/database/db-hw/populate/index.html.

———, *White Paper: Annual Report on Health and Welfare 1998–1999*, 1999.

JCS 1067, "Directive to Commander in Chief of United States Forces of Occupation Regarding the Military Government of Germany," in *Occupation of Germany: Policy and Progress, 1945–1946*, Washington, D.C.: Department of State, Government Printing Office, August 1947.

Jones, Seth G., Jeremy M. Wilson, Andrew Rathmell, and K. Jack Riley, *Establishing Law and Order After Conflict*, MG-374-RC, Santa Monica, California: RAND Corporation, 2005.

King's College London, *A Review of Peace Operations: A Case for Change*, London: King's College, 2003.

Kirkman-Liff, Bradford, "Physician Payment and Cost-Containment Strategies in West Germany: Suggestions for Medicare Reform," *Journal of Health Politics, Policy and Law*, 1990, pp. 69–99.

Kumar, Chetan, and Elizabeth M. Cousens, *Policy Briefing: Peacebuilding in Haiti*, New York: International Peace Academy, 1996.

Kunder, James (USAID Deputy Assistant Administrator for Asia and the Near East), "Reconstruction Situation in Afghanistan," Testimony before the House Committee on International Relations, Washington, D.C.: U.S. Department of State, October 16, 2003, www.state.gov/p/sa/rls/rm/25427.htm.

Laitin, David D., *Identity in Formation: The Russian-Speaking Populations in the Near Abroad*, Ithaca, New York: Cornell University Press, 1998.

Large, Frantz, *The Health of Children in Haiti: Facing Socio-Economic Realities*, Washington, D.C.: The Panos Institute, 2001.

Le Duc, Carol, and Homa Sabri, *Room to Manoeuvre*, Kabul, Islamabad: United Nations Development Programme, July 1996.

Leffler, Melvyn P., *A Preponderance of Power: National Security, the Truman Administration, and the Cold War*, Stanford, California: Stanford University Press, 1992.

Licklider, Roy, "The American Way of State Building: Germany, Japan, Somalia, and Panama," *Small Wars and Insurgencies*, Vol. 10, No. 3, Winter 1999.

Light, Donald W., "Values and Structure in the German Health Care Systems," *Milbank Quarterly*, Vol. 63, No. 4, 1985.

Light, Donald W., and Alexander Schuller (eds.), *Political Values and Health Care: The German Experience,* Cambridge, Massachusetts: MIT Press, 1986.

Marburg-Goodman, J., "USAID's Iraq Procurement Contracts: Insider's View," *Procurement Lawyer,* Vol. 39, No. 1, Fall 2003.

Martin, L.M., "Somalia: Humanitarian Success and Political/Military Failure," Washington, D.C.: Global Security Organization, 1995, www.globalsecurity.org/military/library/report/1995/MLM.htm (as of December 31, 2004).

Mason, P., "Kosovo After the Conflict: Rebuilding Pharmaceutical Services," *Pharmaceutical Journal,* Vol. 264, No. 7079, January 15, 2000, pp. 98–100.

Mearsheimer, John J., *The Tragedy of Great Power Politics,* New York: W.W. Norton, 2001.

Medact, *Collateral Damage: The Health and Environmental Costs of War in Iraq,* November 2002, www.medact.org/tbx/docs/ Medactpercent20Iraqpercent20report final3.pdf.

———, *Working Paper No. 3: Mental Well-Being in Iraq—Six Months After the Start of Operation Iraqi Freedom,* 2003, www.medact.org/tbx/ACFC374.doc.

Medecins Sans Frontieres (Doctors Without Borders), *Somalia: Enduring Needs in a War-Ravaged Country,* 2001, www.msf.org/content/page.cfm?articleid=45699808-3D87-4FD5-8C2BA1F84FE072CE (as of December 31, 2004).

Menkhaus, K., *Somalia: A Situation Analysis,* United Nations High Commissioner for Refugees, Centre for Documentation and Research, 2000.

Menkhaus, K., and R. Marchal, *Somalia 1999 Human Development,* 1999, http://meltingpot.fortunecity.com/lebanon/254/undp.htm (as of December 31, 2004).

Miller, Laurel, and Robert Perito, *Establishing the Rule of Law in Afghanistan,* Special Report 117, Washington, D.C.: United States Institute of Peace, 2004.

Milward, Alan S., *War, Economy, and Society, 1939–1945,* Berkeley, California: University of California Press, 1979.

Mitchell, B.R., *International Historical Statistics: Africa, Asia & Oceania, 1750–1993*, 3rd ed., New York: Grove's Dictionaries, Inc., 1998.

Montgomery, John D., and Dennis A. Rondinelli (eds.), *Beyond Reconstruction in Afghanistan: Lessons from Development Experience*, New York: Palgrave Macmillan, 2004.

Morkiawa, M.J., "Primary Care Training in Kosovo," *International Family Medicine*, Vol. 35, No. 6, June 2003, pp. 440–444.

Nash, D., "Pentagon Backgrounder," PMO Website, May 24, 2004.

National Academies Press, *Initial Steps in Rebuilding the Health Sector in East Timor*, Washington, D.C.: National Academies Press, 2003.

Natsios, A. S., and J. Kreczko, *Special Press Briefing on Humanitarian Assistance to Afghanistan*, Washington, D.C.: Department of State, 2002.

Nishimura, Sey, "Censorship of the Atomic Bomb Casualty Report in Occupied Japan," *Journal of American Medical Association*, Vol. 274, No. 7, August 16, 1995.

———, "The U.S. Medical Occupation of Japan and History of the Japanese-Language Edition of JAMA," *Journal of American Medical Association*, Vol. 274, No. 5, August 2, 1995.

Oakley, Robert B., Michael J. Dziedzic, and Eliot M. Goldberg (ed.), *Policing the New World Disorder: Peace Operations and Public Security*, Washington, D.C.: National Defense University Press, 1998.

Office of Management and Budget, "Section 2207 Report," Quarterly Reports on Iraq, April 5, 2004.

Office of Military Government for Germany, United States, *Public Welfare*, No. 9, April 20, 1946.

———, Report of the Military Governor, *Public Health and Medical Affairs*, various numbers (9–31), Washington, D.C.: Office of Military Government for Germany, United States, 1946–1949.

———, *Statistical Annex*, various numbers, 1946–1949.

Olson, Mancur, *The Logic of Collective Action: Public Goods and the Theory of Groups*, Cambridge, Massachusetts: Harvard University Press, 1971.

Oxford Research International, *National Survey of Iraq*, February 2004, news.bbc.co.uk/nol/shared/bsp/hi/pdfs/150304iraqsurvey.pdf.

Pagent, Julian, *Counter-Insurgency Campaigning*, London: Faber and Faber, 1967.

Pan-American Health Organization, *Core Health Data Selected Indicators*, 2002.

————, *Haiti Country Health Data*, Washington, D.C.: Pan-American Health Organization, 1998.

————, *Health Situation Analysis and Trends Summary*, Haiti Country Profile, Washington, D.C.: Pan-American Health Organization, 1998, www.paho.org/English/DD/AIS/cp_332.htm.

————, *Humanitarian Crisis in Haiti: Support to the Health Sector*, Washington, D.C.: Pan-American Health Organization, February 2004.

Pan-American Health Organization and World Health Organization, *Haiti's Country Health Profile, Basic Country Health Profiles,* Summary 1999, www.paho.org/English/DD/AIS/cp_332.htm.

————, *Health in the Americas,* 1998, http://165.158.1.110/english/sha/prflhai.html.

Pape, Robert A., *Bombing to Win: Air Power and Coercion in War*, Ithaca, New York: Cornell University Press, 1996.

Perito, Robert M., *The American Experience with Police in Peace Operations,* Clementsport, Canada: The Canadian Peacekeeping Press, 2002.

————, *Where Is the Lone Ranger When We Need Him? America's Search for a Postconflict Stability Force,* Washington, D.C.: United States Institute of Peace, 2004.

Physicians for Human Rights, *War Crimes in Kosovo: A Population-Based Assessment of Human Rights Violations of Kosovar Albanians by Serb Forces,* June 15, 1999.

"Progress Toward Poliomyelitis Eradication, Afghanistan, 1994–1999," *Morbidity and Mortality Weekly Report*, Vol. 48, No. 37, September 24, 1999, p. 2.

Public Nutrition Policy and Strategy 2003–2006, final draft for comment, Ministry of Health, October 30, 2003.

Rashid, Ahmed, *Taliban: Militant Islam, Oil and Fundamentalism in Central Asia,* New Haven, Connecticut: Yale University Press, 2000.

Raz, Guy, "Baghdad Mental Hospital on Life Support," Washington, D.C.: National Public Radio, May 1, 2003, www.npr.org/news/specials/iraq2003/raz_030501.html.

ReliefWeb, "Afghanistan: WFP Team Investigating Famine Reports," March 19, 2001, www.reliefweb.int.

―――, "International NGOs Call for an End to Hostilities in Iraq," April 13, 2004, www.reliefweb.int.

Rieff, David, *A Bed for the Night, Humanitarianism in Crisis*, New York: Simon and Schuster, 2002.

Rubin, M., "Trust the Iraqis: Silent Majority," *The New Republic,* June 7, 2004.

Salama, P., P. Spiegel, M. Van Dyke, L. Phelps, and C. Wilkinson, "Mental Health and Nutritional Status Among the Adult Serbian Minority in Kosovo," *Journal of American Medical Association*, Vol. 284, No. 5, August 2, 2000.

Sams, Crawford F., *Medic, The Mission of an American Military Doctor in Occupied Japan and Wartorn Korea*, Zabelle Zakarian (ed.), New York: M.E. Sharpe, 1998.

Schaller, Michael, *The American Occupation of Japan,* New York: Oxford University Press, 1985.

Schelling, Thomas, *Micromotives and Macrobehavior*, New York: Norton, 1978.

Schwartz, Thomas Alan, *America's Germany: John J. McCloy and the Federal Republic of Germany,* Cambridge, Massachusetts: Harvard University Press, 1991.

Securing Afghanistan's Future: Accomplishments and the Strategic Path Forward, Health and Nutrition Technical Annex, Prepared at the request of the Transitional Islamic Government of Afghanistan, January 2004, www.af/resources/mof/recosting/draft%20papers/Pillar%201/Health%20and%20Nutrition%20-%20Annex.pdf.

Sen, Amartya, *Development as Freedom*, New York: Anchor Books, 2000.

Simpson, Charles, *Inside the Green Berets: The First Thirty Years*, Novato, CA: Presidio Press, 1982.

Somalia Aid Coordination Body, *SACB Health Strategy Framework*, 2000, www.sacb.info/commitees/MainHealth.htm (as of December 31, 2004).

Spiegel, P., and P. Salama, *Kosovar Albanian Health Survey, September 1999*, International Emergencies and Refugee Health Branch, Centers for Disease Control and Prevention, 1999.

Starr, Joseph R., *Denazification, Occupation, and Control of Germany, March–July 1945*, Salisbury, North Carolina: Documentary Publications, 1977.

Stone, Deborah, "Professionalism and Accountability: Controlling Health Services in the United States and West Germany," *Journal of Health Politics, Policy and Law*, Vol. 2, No. 1, Spring 1977, pp. 32–47.

Suny, Ronald Grigor, *The Revenge of the Past: Nationalism, Revolution, and the Collapse of the Soviet Union*, Stanford, California: Stanford University Press, 1993.

Taft-Morales, Maureen, *Haiti: Issues for Congress*, Washington, D.C.: Congressional Research Service, 2001.

Tardif, Francine, *Building a Bridge for Peace or Servicing Complex Political Emergencies? A Study of the Case of the Health Humanitarian Programs in Haiti*, Port-au-Prince: World Health Organization, 1998.

Tarnoff, Curt, "Kosovo: Reconstruction and Development Assistance," *CRS Report for Congress*, Updated June 7, 2001, Order Code RL30453.

Tilly, Charles, *The Formation of National States in Western Europe*, Princeton, New Jersey: Princeton University Press, 1975.

Trachtenberg, Marc, *A Constructed Peace: The Making of the European Settlement, 1945–1963,* Princeton, New Jersey: Princeton University Press, 1999.

UNAIDS, *Epidemiological Fact Sheets*, who.int/globalatlas/pdffactory/hif/efs_pdfs/efs2004_ht.pdf/.

UNAIDS and WHO, *Haiti Epidemiological Fact Sheet on HIV/AIDS and Sexually Transmitted Infections*, Geneva: UNAIDS and WHO, 2004.

United Nations, *Ahtisaari Report,* Report to the secretary-general on humanitarian needs in Kuwait and Iraq in the immediate post-crisis environment by a mission under secretary general for administration and management, United Nations, March 1991.

————, *Assistance to Refugees in Somalia*, New York: United Nations General Assembly, 1989.

————, *The Comprehensive Report on Lessons Learned from United Nations Operation in Somalia (UNOSOM)*, April 1992–March 1995, 1995.

————, "Emergency Economic Recovery Program," United Nations' *International Report*, Vol. 1, No. A1, April 3, 1995.

————, "Recent Violence in Kosovo Shook UN Mission 'To Its Core,'" Security Council Told," News Centre, United Nations, May 11, 2004.

————, Supplement to *An Agenda for Peace: Preventive Diplomacy, Peacemaking, and Peacekeeping*, New York: United Nations, 1992.

United Nations and World Bank, *Joint Iraq Needs Assessment: Water*, October 2003.

United Nations Assistance Mission for Iraq, "Iraq: International NGOs Discuss Exit Strategies," Newsroom, News and Events, www.uniraq.org/newsroom/story.asp?ID=260.

————, "Minutes of the UNAMI Coordination Meeting," January 14, 2004, www.uniraq.org/coordination/minutes.asp.

United Nations Children's Fund, *Crisis Appeal for Iraq's Children*, December 2003.

————, "Iraq Watching Briefs: Water and Environmental Sanitation," July and October 2003.

————, "Routine Immunization of Children Re-established Across Iraq," Press release, June 2003, www.unicef.org/media/media_9414.html.

————, *Situation Analysis of Children and Women in Iraq*, April 1998, www.childinfo.org/Other/Iraq_sa.pdf.

————, "The Situation of Children in Iraq," UNICEF, 2003, www.unicef.org/publications/index_4439.html.

————, *Somalia: Programme Evaluation Final Report*, Nairobi: UNICEF, 2002.

————, "UNICEF Expresses Concern over Reports of Child Abduction and Trafficking in Afghanistan," Kabul: UNICEF, September 25, 2003, www.unicef.org/media/media_14783.html.

————, "World Health Day, Plight of Afghanistan's Children Cause for Concern," April 6, 2003, www.unicef.org/media/media_7203.html.

United Nations Development Programme, *Human Development Report, 2004: Cultural Liberty in Today's Diverse World*, New York: UNDP, 2004.

——, *Iraq Living Conditions Survey 2004, Volume II, Analytical Report*, www.iq.undp.org/ILCS/PDF/Analytical%20Report%20-%20English.pdf.

United Nations Development Programme and World Bank, *An Operational Note on Transitional Results Matrices: Using Results-Based Frameworks in Fragile States*, New York: United Nations Development Programme and World Bank, January 2005.

United Nations Development Programme, World Bank, and United Nations Development Group, *Practical Guide to Multilateral Needs Assessments in Post-Conflict Situations*, New York: World Bank, August 2004.

United Nations High Commissioner for Refugees, *Concept Paper on a Proposed Framework for Return of Refugees and Internally Displaced Persons to Kosovo*, Section 3, Planning Figures and Assumptions, UNHCR News, May 12, 1999.

United Nations Security Council Resolution 1546, on Iraq, June 8, 2004.

United States Agency for International Development, *Accomplishments: Water and Sanitation*, Washington, D.C.: USAID, March 2004, www.usaid.gov/iraq/accomplishments/watsan.html.

——, *CP FY 2000: Federal Republic of Yugoslavia*, Washington, D.C.: USAID, 2000.

——, *FY 1998 Congressional Presentation on Haiti*.

——, *Haiti Activity Data Sheet*, Washington, D.C.: USAID, 2002.

——, *Haiti Country Profile: HIV/AIDS*, 2003 and 2004.

——, *Haiti: Situation Overview*, Washington, D.C.: USAID, 2004.

——, *Kosovo CP FY 2001*, Washington, D.C.: USAID, 2001.

——, *Kosovo: Activity Data Sheet*, FY 2003 Program, Washington, D.C.: USAID, 2003.

——, *Kosovo. Health Issues: Reproductive Health Partnership*, Washington, D.C.: USAID, www.usaid.gov/missions/kosovo/Activities/Health_initiatives.htm (as of August 30, 2005).

————, *Kosovo: The Development Challenge*, Text taken from the FY 2003 Congressional Budget Justification, Washington, D.C.: USAID, wysiwyg://31/http://www.usaid.gov/pubs/cbj2003/ee/kosovo/ (as of January 19, 2004).

————, *Shelter in Kosovo: Challenges and Solutions*, Fact Sheet, Washington, D.C.: USAID, November 10, 1999.

————, *Somalia Strategic Plan 1997*, Washington, D.C.: USAID, 1997.

————, *USAID Congressional Presentation FY 1997: Somalia*, www.usaid.gov/pubs/cp97/countries/so.htm.

————, *USAID Fact Sheet on Special Initiatives: Kosovo*, Tuberculosis Control Partnership Program, Washington, D.C.: USAID, July 17, 2004, www.globalcorps.com/orgs/ngo/dotw/kosovo.html.

————, *USAID Mission in Kosovo: Data Sheet, FY 2004 Program*, Washington, D.C.: USAID, www.usaid.gov/policy/budget/cbj2005/ee/pdf/167-0410.pdf (as of August 30, 2005).

————, *USAID's Key Achievements: Meeting TB Challenges in Kosovo*, Washington, D.C.: USAID, www.usaid.gov/our_work/global_health/id/tuberculosis/achievements.html#kosovo (as of July 24, 2004).

————, *USAID's Strategy in Somalia*, Washington, D.C.: USAID, 2004, www.usaid.gov/locations/sub-saharan_africa/countries/somalia/ (as of December 31, 2004).

United States Department of Defense, *Iraq Status*, Draft working papers, December 15, 2003, www.export.gov/iraq/pdf/dod_wklyrpt_121503.pdf.

————, *Iraq Status*, Draft working papers, January 4, 2004, www.export.gov/iraq/pdf/dod_wklyrpt_012004.pdf.

————, *Iraq Status*, Working papers, June 15, 2004, www.export.gov/iraq/pdf/dod_wklyrpt_061504.pdf.

————, *Military Casualty Information*, Directorate for Information Operations and Reports, 2004, web1.whs.osd.mil/mmid/casualty/castop.htm.

United States Department of Energy, *Iraq: Country Analysis Brief*, Washington, D.C.: DoE, 2004, www.eia.doe.gov/emeu/cabs/iraq.html.

United States Department of State, *Ethnic Cleansing in Kosovo: An Accounting*, Washington, D.C.: DoS, December 1999.

———, *Kosovo Humanitarian Situation Report 1*, Bureau of Population, Refugees, and Migration, Washington, D.C.: DoS, March 31, 1999.

———, *Occupation of Germany: Police and Progress, 1945–1946,* Washington, D.C.: U.S. Government Printing Office, 1947.

United States Mission to Afghanistan, *Afghanistan Development Update*, Kabul: United States Mission to Afghanistan, 2004.

United States Strategic Bombing Survey, *The Effect of Bombing on Health and Medical Care in Germany*, Washington, D.C.: War Department, October 30, 1945.

———, *The Effects of Atomic Bombs*, Chairman's Office, June 30, 1946.

———, *The Effects of Atomic Bombs on Health and Medical Services in Hiroshima and Nagasaki*, Medical Division, Washington, D.C.: War Department, March 1947.

———, *The Effects of Bombing on Health and Medical Services in Japan*, Medical Division, Dates of Survey: 24 October–31 November 1945, Washington, D.C.: War Department, June 1947.

———, *Physical Damage Division Report (ETO)*, Physical Damage Division, Washington, D.C.: United States War Department, April 1947.

United States War Department, Office of the Adjutant General, Machine Records Branch, *Strength of the Army*, Washington, D.C.: United States War Department, December 1, 1945.

Valentinas, M., "Iraq: Filth and Deprivation Rack Baghdad's Only Mental Hospital," 2003, www.globalsecurity.org/wmd/library/news/iraq/2003/05/iraq-030526-rfel-162816.htm.

VanRooyen, M.J., and J.B. VanRooyen, "Somalia: Medicine and the Military," *Journal of American Medical Association*, Vol. 271, No. 12, March 23–30, 1994, pp. 904–905.

VanRooyen, M.J., S.B. VanRooyen, E.P. Sloan, and E. Ward, "Mobile Medical Relief and Military Assistance in Somalia," *Prehospital Disaster Medicine*, Vol. 10, No. 2, Apr–Jun 1995, pp. 118–120.

Vemuri, S., and M. Kellerman, *Somalia: A Cultural Profile—Looking at Healthcare*, Toronto: University of Toronto, 2002.

Waldman, Ronald, and Homaira Hanif, *The Public Health System in Afghanistan*, Afghanistan: AREU Afghan Research and Evaluation Unit, May–June 2002.

Westermeyer, J., "Health of Albanians and Serbians Following the War in Kosovo, Studying the Survivors on Both Sides of Armed Conflict," Editorial, *Journal of American Medical Association*, Vol. 284, 2000, pp. 615–616.

Wilensky, Robert J., *Military Medicine to Win Hearts and Minds: Aid to Civilians in the Vietnam War*, Lubbock, Texas: Texas Tech University Press, 2004.

Wood, D., "Nurses Help Rebuild Iraq's Health Care System," AMN Healthcare, Health Care News, 2003.

World Bank, *Afghanistan: World Bank Approach Paper, November 2001*, Washington, D.C.: The World Bank Group, November 29, 2001, www.reliefweb.org.

———, "World Bank Helps Afghanistan Meet Urgent Health Needs," News Release 2003/388/SAR, web.worldbank.org/WBSITE/EXTERNAL/NEWS/0.

———, *World Development Indicators 2003*, Washington, D.C.: World Bank, 2003, www.worldbank.org/data/wdi2003/index.htm (as of December 31, 2004).

World Food Programme, *Afghanistan Weekly Situation Report*, January 15, 2004, www.reliefweb.org.

World Health Organization, *Case Study of the WHO/DfID Peace Through Health Programme in Bosnia and Herzegovina*, Sarajevo: WHO, 1998.

———, *Communicable Disease Profile: Iraq*, WHO/CDS/2003.17, 2003, www.who.int/infectious-disease-news/IDdocs/whocds200317/1profile.pdf.

———, Core Health Data Selected Indicators, 2002.

———, Disease Incidence Data Set, Geneva: WHO, 2005.

———, "Health Briefing on Iraq," UN Humanitarian Briefing, May 14, 2003, www.who.int/features/2003/iraq/briefings/wednesday14/en/.

———, Immunization Coverage Data Set, Geneva: WHO, 2005.

————, *Iraq Annual Report*, 2004, www.emro.who.int/iraq/pdf/annualreport04.pdf.

————, *Kosovo Activities Update*, May 2000.

————, *Kosovo Health Sector Situation Report*, January 2000.

————, *Operations in Kosovo, Action Plan 2000*.

————, *Somalia: A Health System in Crisis*, 2000, www.hartford-hwp.com/archives/33/128.html (as of December 31, 2004).

————, *Somalia Country Profile*, 2001, www.emro.who.int/mnh/whd/CountryProfile-SOM.htm (as of December 31, 2004).

————, *The Transition from Relief to Development in the Context of Complex Humanitarian Emergencies and Natural Disasters*, ECOSOC 2002 Humanitarian Segment, WHO technical contribution to the panel, New York: WHO, July 16, 2002.

————, *WHO Annual Report*, 2000, Geneva: WHO, 2000.

————, *WHO Disaster Preparedness and Response Operation in Kosovo: Evaluation of Kosovo Programme, 1999–2000*, Pristina: WHO, 2002.

————, *WHO Somalia Fact Sheet 2002*, www.who.int/disasters/repo/8074.doc (as of December 31, 2004).

Ziemke, Earl F., *The U.S. Army in the Occupation of Germany, 1944–1946*, Washington, D.C.: U.S. Government Printing Office, 1990.

Zwi, A., *Post-Conflict: Health System Development in Kosovo*, London School of Hygiene & Tropical Medicine, London: University of London, www.lshtm.ac.uk/hpu/post_conflict_kosovo_project.htm (as of January 21, 2004).